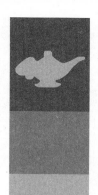

STUDY GUIDE FOR BLACK & HAWKS

Medical-Surgical Nursing
Clinical Management for Positive Outcomes

Eighth Edition

Cynthia M. Sublett, DNSc, RN
Adjunct Faculty
Xavier University
Cincinnati, Ohio

Meg Blair, RN, MSN, CEN
Associate Professor
Nebraska Methodist College of Nursing and Allied Health
Omaha, Nebraska

SAUNDERS

ELSEVIER

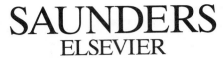

11830 Westline Industrial Drive
St. Louis, Missouri 63146

Study Guide for Medical-Surgical Nursing:
Clinical Management for Positive Outcomes, Eighth Edition

ISBN: 978-1-4160-5190-9

Notice

Knowledge and best practice in this field are constantly changing. As new research and experience broaden our knowledge, changes in practice, treatment and drug therapy may become necessary or appropriate. Readers are advised to check the most current information provided (i) on procedures featured or (ii) by the manufacturer of each product to be administered, to verify the recommended dose or formula, the method and duration of administration, and contraindications. It is the respon-sibility of the practitioner, relying on their own experience and knowledge of the patient, to make diagnoses, to determine dosages and the best treatment for each individual patient, and to take all appropriate safety precautions. To the fullest extent of the law, neither the Publisher nor the Authors assumes any liability for any injury and/or damage to persons or property arising out of or related to any use of the material contained in this book.

The Publisher

Previous editions copyrighted 2005, 2001, 1997, 1993

ISBN: 978-1-4160-5190-9

Managing Editor: Maureen Iannuzzi
Senior Developmental Editor: Jennifer Ehlers
Publishing Services Manager: Debbie Vogel
Cover Designer: Louis Forgione

Printed in United States of America

Last digit is the print number: 9 8 7 6 5 4 3 2 1

Working together to grow
libraries in developing countries

www.elsevier.com | www.bookaid.org | www.sabre.org

ELSEVIER   BOOK AID International   Sabre Foundation

Contents

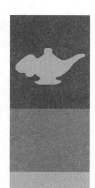

CHAPTER I

Health Promotion and Disease Prevention

CHAPTER OBJECTIVES

1.1 Compare and contrast various definitions of health.

1.2 Describe the nurse's focus of client care toward wellness during an acute care stay.

1.3 Define the term *illness* using each of the four models of health—clinical, role performance, adaptive, and eudaimonistic—including the response of the client in each definition.

1.4 Discuss the use of the "self-management support strategies" by the nurse to help clients adopt healthy lifestyles, including the core skills necessary for self-management.

1.5 Identify six strategies to assist a client to take action toward a health goal.

1.6 Discuss health promotion activities including nutrition, exercise, and stress management.

1.7 Discuss disease and injury prevention activities related to motor vehicle accidents, alcohol and drug abuse, smoking, safety for elders, elder abuse and neglect, domestic abuse, infectious diseases, and sexual activity.

1.8 Describe screening recommendations for cardiovascular disease; breast, prostate, and colorectal cancer; and depression.

UNDERSTANDING TERMINOLOGY

Relationships Among Health, Wellness, Illness, Disease, Client Perceptions

Match the following concepts with definitions below.

_____ 1. Dunn's concept of wellness

_____ 2. 1947 WHO definition of health

_____ 3. Disease

_____ 4. Illness

_____ 5. Travis concept of wellness

_____ 6. High-level wellness

_____ 7. Leininger's transcultural model

_____ 8. Model of health

_____ 9. Biomedical model

_____ 10. Relationship of health and disease

a. An integrated method of functioning oriented toward maximizing the potential of the individual within the environment where he or she is functioning

b. Equilibrium/disequilibrium

c. Self-actualization and maximizing potential

d. Failure of a person's adaptive mechanisms to adequately counteract stimuli and stresses, resulting in functional or structural disturbances

e. State of complete well-being, not just the absence of disease

f. Mismatch in needs and resources

g. Role performance

h. Disease and clinical manifestations

i. Wellness does not happen automatically

j. Culturally known beliefs and values used to maintain well-being

THEORIES AND TRENDS

Self-Management Skills

11. Identify three categories of self-management skills that promote health and give an example of each.

    a.

    b.

    c.

12. Define *health literacy*. State the implication this has for health.

Health Promotion

13. Match levels of health promotion with the appropriate health activity.

    _____ a. Primary prevention

    _____ b. Secondary prevention

    _____ c. Tertiary prevention

    1. Yearly mammogram
    2. Cardiac rehabilitation
    3. Wear a seatbelt

14. Name six strategies that help clients take action.

    a.

    b.

    c.

    d.

    e.

    f.

15. Match the Stages of Change from Prochaska and DiClimente's Transtheoretical Model to the appropriate description.

    Stages of Change

    _____ a. Precontemplation

    _____ b. Contemplation

    _____ c. Preparation

    _____ d. Action

    _____ e. Maintenance

    Description

    1. Taking steps to avoid relapse
    2. Thinking about making a change in the near future
    3. Making overt change
    4. Planning actively and starting a behavior change
    5. Thinking seriously about making a change

HEALTHY PEOPLE 2010: HEALTHY EATING, HEALTHY ACTIVITY, AND EFFECTIVE COPING WITH STRESS

16. According to the Institute of Medicine report on a healthy diet, the nurse would recommend total level of calories based on which of the following? (Select all that apply.)

    1. Age
    2. Gender
    3. Height
    4. Weight
    5. Body mass index (BMI)
    6. Body fat percentage
    7. Activity level

17. Obesity poses serious health risks. List the diseases that may occur as a result of obesity.

18. Explain why a 3-day dietary log is most helpful in recognizing problematic eating behaviors.

19. Which of the following principles is/are used to guide the development of a realistic plan for addressing problem eating patterns/behaviors? (Select all that apply.)
    1. Decreasing the amount of certain types of foods
    2. Substituting certain foods
    3. Totally eliminating certain foods
    4. Increasing certain foods

20. Current activity recommendations for adults state that they should accumulate _____ hour(s) of moderate activity every day.

21. Why is physical activity an effective intervention for stress management?

22. The goal of cognitive reappraisal is to change _____ or _____ of events as stressors.

REVIEWING YOUR KNOWLEDGE

23. Explain why it is important to have a broad definition of health.

24. Within the nurse-client relationship, which of the following reflect the nurse's role with regard to the client's health? (Select all that apply.)
    1. Display respect for the client's health choices and decisions.
    2. Assist the client to change his or her view of health.
    3. Support the client's participation in actualizing his or her health.
    4. Assist the client in understanding the priority of his or her values and perceptions.

25. High-level wellness requires what three actions?
    a.

    b.

    c.

26. What is the primary document that guides the United States' efforts to prevent disease and promote health?

27. True or False
    _____ Based on the epidemiology of how diseases originate and spread, interventions can be taken to reduce risk.
    _____ The ACS recommends increasing plant sources of foods to decrease health risks.
    _____ A client's definition of health remains static throughout his or her lifetime.
    _____ Wellness is the absence of clinical manifestations.
    _____ A person can have a disease without feeling ill.
    _____ Health requires mental, physical, and spiritual well-being.
    _____ Social support is believed to buffer individuals from the negative effects of stress.
    _____ Identifying a problem and developing a possible solution for the problem facilitates coping with stress.

28. Foods thought to reduce the risk of cancer are _____, _____, and _____.

29. Which of the following are true statements about healthy activity? (Select all that apply.)
    1. Sixty percent of adults get no leisure time physical activity.
    2. Women are more inactive than men.
    3. Physical activity improves mood.
    4. Physical activity decreases the mortality for heart disease.

30. List the four components of an exercise prescription:
    a.

    b.

    c.

    d.

31. True or False

    _____ To implement a successful healthy eating and physical activity prescription, a plan is needed to recognize and overcome probable barriers.

    _____ Tobacco is the single greatest cause of premature death in the United States.

    _____ Healthy eating is an effective intervention to resist stress.

32. The first step in helping a client manage stress is _____.

33. The nurse recognizes the goal of stress resistance is to _____ the body's response to stress.

34. Explain how each of the following interventions is helpful for cognitive reappraisal.
    a. Thought stopping

    b. Refuting irrational ideas

    c. Guided imagery

35. Young adults die prematurely for a number of reasons. Select the greatest causes of premature death in young adults. (Select all that apply.)
    1. Diabetes
    2. Motor-vehicle accidents
    3. Suicide
    4. Heart disease
    5. Stroke
    6. Homicide

36. CAGE is a mnemonic that guides assessment of problem drinking. Which of the following assessment questions would the nurse use to assess the "A" component?
    1. Have you ever been told to avoid drinking?
    2. How much alcohol do you consume per day?
    3. What activities are associated with your drinking?
    4. Have people annoyed you by criticizing your drinking?

37. True or False

    _____ Drug abuse is more common among men.

    _____ Drug abusers have decreased risk for communicable diseases.

    _____ Drug abuse assessment should be a part of a routine lifestyle assessment.

38. Which of the following statements applies to polypharmacy? (Select all that apply.)
    1. It has many consequences including adverse drug reactions.
    2. It is defined as the use of too many or unnecessary medications.
    3. It is a principal drug safety problem in the U.S.
    4. It is a major problem with older people.

39. A set of guidelines for intervening to help someone stop smoking is the _____ _____ _____.

40. Which of the following is a characteristic of women at risk for violence?
    1. High self-esteem
    2. Experience hopefulness
    3. Married at age 25 or older
    4. Living in households with high stress

41. Which of the following characteristics of a woman's partner increase her risk for abuse?
    1. Abused as a child
    2. Social drinker
    3. Shares relationship decision-making
    4. Verbally supportive

APPLYING YOUR KNOWLEDGE

42. Identify the four nursing actions that can be implemented to assist in meeting *Healthy People 2010* goals for young and middle-aged adults.
    a.

    b.

    c.

    d.

43. Which of the following clients would be classified as obese?
    1. BMI of 15
    2. BMI of 21
    3. BMI of 27
    4. BMI of 32

44. The nurse is conducting a nutrition class about decreasing cancer risk through healthy eating. Which of the following clients' diets would the nurse recognize as potentially decreasing cancer risk?
    1. Red meats, refined/processed grains, dairy products, and fruits
    2. Fish and poultry, complex and concentrated carbohydrates, and vegetables
    3. Fish, whole grains, fruits, and vegetables
    4. Fish, poultry, and red meats, refined/processed grains, fruits, and vegetables

45. A nurse is counseling a client experiencing stress. The goal is to help the client: (Select all that apply.)
    1. recognize stressors.
    2. cope effectively with stress.
    3. learn decision-making skills.
    4. learn positive thinking skills.
    5. recognize irrational thinking.

46. A nurse assesses a client for behavioral manifestation of stress. A positive finding would be:
    1. sore neck and shoulder muscles.
    2. increased blood pressure.
    3. anger.
    4. increased alcohol use.

47. When the nurse is planning a personalized eating and exercise prescription with the client, it is most important to consider:
    1. history.
    2. alternatives to exercise.
    3. perceived and actual barriers.
    4. penalties for noncompliance.

48. Key factors when assessing a client for stress are: (Select all that apply.)
    1. taking a history of manifestations.
    2. determining stressful situations.
    3. examining current coping behaviors.
    4. developing ineffective coping.
    5. developing a plan for coping.

49. When evaluating effectiveness of a stress management intervention, the nurse would know the intervention was effective when the client:
    1. overeats.
    2. has disrupted sleep.
    3. complains of a sore neck.
    4. practices relaxation techniques.

50. A nurse uses the Alcohol Use Disorders Identification Test (AUDIT) to assess a client for problem drinking. A client who scores _____ is considered a problem drinker.
    1. 2 or more
    2. 4 or more
    3. 6 or more
    4. 8 or more

51. A client is experiencing health consequences due to exposure to environmental tobacco smoke. Which of the following is the best example of a nurse acting in an advocacy role?
    1. Telling family members of the client to stop smoking
    2. Supporting social efforts to limit smoking in public places
    3. Advising the client to switch jobs
    4. Advising the client to wear a mask when exposed to environmental smoke

52. The highest priority nursing intervention for a client currently in a violent relationship is _____ _____.

53. The nurse assessing an older adult client finds the client has pressure ulcers and a fecal impaction. What is her next action?
    1. Call adult protective services
    2. Talk with the client about any abuse
    3. Assess for potential danger to the client and establish a safety plan
    4. Talk with the caregiver of the client about his or her stress

BEST PRACTICES

54. Which of the following is the best example of primary intervention?
    1. Screening for diabetes
    2. Referral to rehabilitation after injury
    3. Performing self-breast examination
    4. Immunization against hepatitis A

55. Which of the following is the best example of secondary intervention?
    1. Assessing a client's home for risk of falls
    2. Teaching a client to apply sunscreen before sun exposure
    3. Monitoring a client's blood pressure after starting antihypertensive medication
    4. Immunizing a client with the flu vaccine

56. Which of the following is the best example of tertiary intervention?
    1. Dental hygiene
    2. Physical therapy after a back injury
    3. Immunizing a client with the pneumonia vaccine
    4. Wearing seatbelts

57. A nurse is assisting a client to make a behavior change related to diet. Which of the following nursing actions is most likely to increase the client's self-efficacy?
    1. Providing the client with a handout on the Food Pyramid
    2. Giving the client several opportunities to select healthy foods from a food menu
    3. Admonishing the client when she makes an unhealthy food choice
    4. Telling the client she will never succeed unless she is willing to give up all sweets

58. A client comes to the clinic and presents with hypertension and diabetes. A health history reveals a 10-year, 2-pack-per-day smoking history. Using the stepped process for intervention, outline the five nursing actions to take with this client.
    a.

    b.

    c.

    d.

    e.

59. State the rationale for screening every female client for a history of or current abuse.

60. The two activities that are essential to protecting young adults from infectious diseases are:
    a.

    b.

61. When a woman reaches age 50, what preventive screening measures are completed on an annual basis?

62. Immunizations important for all adults regardless of age or health risk include:
    1. flu.
    2. hepatitis B.
    3. HPV.
    4. meningococcal meningitis.
    5. tetanus booster every 10 years.

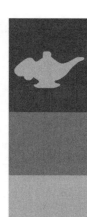

CHAPTER **2**

Health Assessment

CHAPTER OBJECTIVES

2.1 Compare and contrast the types of data collected during the health history and the physical examination.

2.2 Identify factors that can affect the accuracy of data collected during a health history.

2.3 Discuss how a history can be complete, yet brief if needed.

2.4 Describe an example of data collected from each portion of the health history.

2.5 Identify how symptom analysis expands the description of a current illness or problem.

2.6 Describe an example of data collected from each portion of a psychosocial history.

2.7 Identify how the stages of growth and development are used in health assessment.

2.8 Discuss how data collection from a social history can assist with planning discharge of a client.

2.9 Describe how various aspects of sexuality can be affected by illness.

2.10 Describe the process of determining the client's learning preference.

2.11 Identify the type of information gained from a review of systems.

2.12 Describe a section of a physical examination that is assessed using inspection, palpation, percussion, and auscultation.

2.13 Identify the body areas that normally produce each of the percussion sounds.

2.14 Describe the aspects of sounds heard during auscultation.

2.15 Explain the process of analyzing data collected during a health history and physical examination.

2.16 Discuss how the risk of pressure ulcers and falls can be identified during an initial health assessment.

2.17 Identify the importance of ongoing health assessment and how abnormal findings should be managed.

UNDERSTANDING TERMINOLOGY

1. The _____ is the client's subjective statement of the reason he or she is seeking health care.

2. Match each term related to symptom analysis to a description of that symptom's associated factor to explore during a symptom analysis (manifestation) with the appropriate description.

Associated Factor

_____ a. Onset

_____ b. Location

_____ c. Duration

_____ d. Characteristics

_____ e. Associated manifestations

_____ f. Radiation

_____ g. Treatment

Description

1. Determines how to proceed with the manifestation; e.g., orders for medication, phoning physician, etc.

2. Identifies where the manifestation occurs in the body and whether it is stationary or moves. May not be assessed if the answer is apparent.

3. Determines if anything else has occurred in conjunction with the manifestation.

4. Determines when the manifestation first occurred and what might have caused it.

5. Determines length of time the manifestation has been present, peak occurrences, etc.

6. Determines the progress of the manifestation in regard to how it occurs in 24-hour period, what self-treatment has been done, etc.

7. Asks the client to describe the manifestation in terms of qualities such as sharpness, dullness, etc.

3. Match each term associated with the mental status assessment with the appropriate definition.

Term

_____ a. Affect

_____ b. Mood

_____ c. Flat affect

_____ d. Blunted affect

Definition

1. Lack of any facial expression or emotional response accompanied by a monotonous voice

2. Reduced in intensity but still appropriate to the situation

3. Subjective description of a personal emotion that is pervasive and sustained

4. Observable, outward demeanor that depicts the current emotional state

4. Match terms related to the use of percussion in a physical examination.

Term

_____ a. Flatness

_____ b. Dullness

_____ c. Resonance

_____ d. Hyperresonance

_____ e. Tympany

Definition

1. Very loud, low-pitched sound; booming quality

2. Soft high-pitched, short sound from muscle tissue

3. A loud, high-pitched, moderately long sound that is drum-like

4. Moderate to loud sound of low pitch and long duration from air-filled lung tissue; hollow sound

5. Soft to moderately loud sound, moderate pitch and duration from fluid-filled tissue; thud quality

THEORIES AND TRENDS

5. Describe the advantages of using a computerized health history assessment.

6. List methods for organizing health history data.

7. From the website, add specific important aspects to components of the health history listed in the chapter.

8. Describe components of a cultural assessment as a part of the health history.

REVIEWING YOUR KNOWLEDGE

9. Which of the following describes nursing skills necessary to perform a health assessment? (Select all that apply.)
   1. It identifies physical and psychosocial needs.
   2. Advanced assessment techniques are required.
   3. It requires observation and decision-making skills.
   4. Proficiency requires practice.
   5. It requires ability to discriminate.
   6. It is comprised of several parts.

10. True or False

   _____ The health assessment begins with the physical examination.

   _____ If clients are unable to provide information during the health history, a family member or interpreter may provide the information.

   _____ Health history formats are standardized across health care settings.

   _____ The nurse must ask or validate the reason the client is in the hospital as the first question to ask the client.

   _____ The health history must be completed at the time of admission for all clients.

   _____ Past health history is unimportant to current reason for admission.

   _____ Asking about seatbelt use is relevant to the health history.

   _____ The purpose of the physical examination is to differentiate normal from abnormal physical findings.

   _____ The physical examination provides an excellent opportunity for the nurse to provide health teaching.

   _____ Assessing pressure ulcer risk and fall risk are not part of the normal health assessment.

   _____ Safety is a primary issue when identifying domestic abuse in a client.

   _____ General appearance can give a nurse much information about a client's mental status.

   _____ Stating "the client is depressed" is appropriate documentation on the client's chart.

   _____ Knowing if a client needs pictures to aid understanding of new information or if he/she prefers to read the information is important to the health assessment.

   _____ During the health assessment, the client can be used as his/her own "control" by comparing sides of the body with each other.

11. Compare and contrast the long versus the short health history format.

Long Format	Short Format

12. Identify the five essential components of a health history.
    a.

    b.

    c.

    d.

    e.

13. When gathering data about past health history, the nurse would *not* gather information about:
    1. usual childhood illnesses.
    2. family members' causes of death.
    3. hospitalizations.
    4. obstetric visits.
    5. allergies.

14. Which of the following variables affect a client's ability to respond to specific questions during a mental status exam? (Select all that apply.)
    1. Level of education
    2. Cultural background
    3. Degree of exposure to knowledge and information
    4. Familiarity with the language and vocabulary
    5. Perceived acceptance by the doctor

15. The cultural assessment is very broad in nature because it seeks information about:
    1. individual values.
    2. what the larger group's tenets mean to the individual.
    3. individual beliefs.
    4. individual behaviors.

16. Which of the following information is important to the social history? (Select all that apply.)
    1. Developmental level
    2. Personal habits
    3. Financial well-being
    4. Friends
    5. Sexual identity

17. Match each type of risk factor with the appropriate description.

Type of Risk Factor	Descriptor
_____ a. Genetic/biologic	1. Living in an area subject to floods
_____ b. Behavioral	2. Family history
_____ c. Environmental	3. High-fat diet

18. A foundation of _____ and _____ is key to developing skills in physical assessment.

19. List and describe each of the four primary techniques used in physical assessment.

    a.

    b.

    c.

    d.

20. The physical examination begins with_____
    _____.

21. True or False

    _____ a. Using the bell of the stethoscope, the nurse will hear low-pitched sounds such as murmurs.

    _____ b. Place the diaphragm of the stethoscope over bone to hear higher-pitched heart and lung sounds.

APPLYING YOUR KNOWLEDGE

22. It is important for the nurse to observe the client closely:
    1. throughout the health history.
    2. at the beginning of the interview.
    3. during psychological assessment.
    4. when assessing risk factors.

23. To ensure an accurate health history, the nurse should:
    1. obtain information from a secondary source.
    2. assume meaning if the client is reluctant to be forthcoming.
    3. be cognizant that the nurse's perceptions are always accurate.
    4. continually validate information gathered with the client.

24. During the family health history, the nurse assesses:
    1. immunization status.
    2. problems related to heart disease.
    3. quality, quantity, and duration of symptoms.
    4. frequency of social interactions.

25. During the general appearance component of the psychosocial assessment, the nurse assesses:
    1. grimacing.
    2. crying.
    3. orientation to time.
    4. manner of dress.

26. A client's motivation is influenced by:
    1. external resources.
    2. spiritual beliefs.
    3. personal needs and desires.
    4. genetic predisposition.

27. A client's socioeconomic status is influenced by:
    1. employment status.
    2. health habits.
    3. sleep patterns.
    4. leisure activities.

28. A nurse is assessing a client about the date a specific screening procedure was performed. Which question by the nurse is the best way to elicit this data?
    1. "You should have had a mammogram last month. Did you?"
    2. "Why haven't you been to the dentist in over 2 years?"
    3. "When was your last eye examination and what were the results?"
    4. "With your history, you do go for a Pap smear every year, don't you?"

29. Which of the following are true statements regarding the processing of physical assessment data? (Select all that apply.)
    1. Compare findings from one side of the body to the other.
    2. The human body is exactly symmetrical, which makes detection of abnormalities easier.
    3. Normal parameters are the benchmark for comparing findings.
    4. Examine suspected problem areas revealed during the health history carefully.

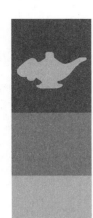

CHAPTER 3

Critical Thinking

CHAPTER OBJECTIVES

3.1 Define *critical thinking* and related terms.
3.2 Identify the cognitive processes needed to support clinical decision-making.
3.3 Describe the use of Universal Intellectual Standards by nurses.
3.4 Differentiate clinical decision-making of novice and expert nurses.
3.5 Relate the use of evidence-based practice to clinical decision-making in nursing.
3.6 Apply clinical preparation to specific client situations.
3.7 Identify important information to be presented in the pre-care conference.
3.8 Set priorities in client care.

UNDERSTANDING TERMINOLOGY

1. Define the terms *thinking* and *critical thinking*.

THEORIES AND TRENDS

2. List characteristics of a person who uses critical thinking skills.

3. True or False

    _____ Cognitive skills needed for critical thinking are learned early in a person's education.

    _____ Scientific process skills are essential for critical thinking.

    _____ Problem-solving skills and decision-making skills are similar.

    _____ The scientific process and the nursing process are very linear cognitive processes.

4. Universal Intellectual Standards, developed by Elder and Paul, describe critical thinking. List two questions that, if asked by the nurse, would represent these standards.

5. Based on the novice to expert work of Patricia Benner, the expert nurse will differ from the novice nurse in his or her ability to recognize changes in client conditions. Briefly explain this phenomenon.

REVIEWING YOUR KNOWLEDGE

6. Critical thinking in nursing practice affects client _____.

7. Critical thinking and decision-making in nursing practice include _____, _____, and _____.

8. Part of the decision-making process in client care requires the nurse to be _____ _____.

9. Evidence-based practice includes not only review of current research but also _____ and _____.

10. Steps necessary to solve clinical problems include:

    a.

    b.

    c.

    d.

    e.

APPLYING YOUR KNOWLEDGE

11. Student preparation for a clinical experience involves gathering all information about the client prior to the actual experience. Which of the following information will help you (the student) prepare adequately for the clinical experience? (Select all that apply.)

    a. The student asks about physician orders to determine relevance.
    b. The student reflects on the total information and decides on priorities of care.
    c. The student asks questions about the reasons for prescribed medications.
    d. The student tries to relate textbook information to client and chart information.
    e. The student plans for specific assessment information that will be needed in the initial morning assessment.
    f. The student tries to relate diagnostic findings to the client's pathophysiology.
    g. The student decides to wait until the clinical experience to review any procedures that he or she may need to complete.

BEST PRACTICES

12. The client is a 66-year-old man with terminal cancer of the colon. He is admitted with significant pain and in what appears to be a declining condition. He is very agitated and having difficulty focusing on any conversation. In addition, he tells you that his wife is at home and is ill and can't be with him at the hospital right now. Assess the client and list the priorities of immediate and long-term care. Give a rationale for your answer.

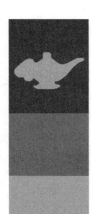

CHAPTER 4

Complementary and Alternative Therapies

CHAPTER OBJECTIVES

4.1   Define complementary and alternative medicine (CAM).
4.2   Relate the use of complementary medicine to conventional medicine.
4.3   Differentiate the practice of alternative and integrative medicine.
4.4   List the classifications of CAM therapies.
4.5   List examples of each class of CAM therapies.
4.6   Discuss the nurse's role in the use of CAM therapies.
4.7   Discuss standards for dietary and herbal supplement manufacturers including the DSHEA (1994) and the 2005 update to the Anabolic Steroid Act (1990).
4.8   Discuss drugs from plant derivatives.
4.9   Discuss the appropriate use of the word *antioxidant*.
4.10   Discuss the use of caution and potential or lack of benefits with alternative medicines.

UNDERSTANDING TERMINOLOGY

1.   Define *complementary and alternative medicine.*

2.   Define *integrative medicine.*

3.   Explain the term *placebo effect.*

4.   Relate antioxidants to "redox agents."

5.   Describe Reiki and therapeutic touch as CAM therapies.

THEORIES AND TRENDS

6.   Differentiate between complementary and alternative medicine as described by NCCAM.

7. List the five major domains of CAM therapies.
   a.

   b.

   c.

   d.

   e.

8. True or False

   _____ About 30% of all modern medicines come from plant sources.

   _____ About 80% of the population in the United States has used CAM at some point.

   _____ The most rapidly growing area of CAM is the use of dietary supplements.

   _____ A new ruling by the FDA will allow food companies to make health claims on labels if most of the scientific evidence supports a benefit.

REVIEWING YOUR KNOWLEDGE

9. True or False

   _____ Dietary and herbal supplement manufacturers are held to the same strict standards as manufacturers of pharmaceuticals.

10. State the main problem with the DSHEA ruling of 1994.

11. What dietary supplements have been demonstrated to have a positive effect on age-related macular degeneration?
    a.

    b.

    c.

12. An example of a CAM alternative medical system is:
    1. homeopathic medicine.
    2. shamanism.
    3. dietary supplements.
    4. massage.
    5. magnetic therapy.

13. An example of CAM mind-body intervention is:
    1. acupuncture.
    2. hypnosis.
    3. alternative diets.
    4. chiropractic medicine.
    5. Reiki.

APPLYING YOUR KNOWLEDGE

14. Explain what actions the nurse initiates to assess information about a client's use of CAM.

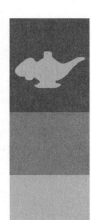

CHAPTER 5

Ambulatory Health Care

CHAPTER OBJECTIVES

5.1 Describe the magnitude of ambulatory health care in the United States.
5.2 Differentiate ambulatory health care from health care in a hospital setting.
5.3 Characterize ambulatory care nursing.
5.4 Differentiate models of ambulatory care nursing practice.
5.5 Discuss the various nursing roles illustrated in the conceptual framework for ambulatory care nurses.
5.6 Describe three major ambulatory care settings.
5.7 Describe the ambulatory care clientele and the various classifications.
5.8 Discuss aspects of nursing practice unique to the ambulatory care setting.
5.9 Discuss certification and multistate licensure related to ambulatory care nursing.
5.10 Discuss research and the lack of and need for research in the ambulatory care setting.

UNDERSTANDING TERMINOLOGY

1. Define *ambulatory care nursing* according to the AAACN definition.

2. Differentiate between primary health care and primary care.

3. Define *telehealth nursing practice.*

THEORIES AND TRENDS

4. The ambulatory setting is a major site for health care delivery because:
   1. the number of hours and days clients stay in hospital has increased.
   2. new technology for surgery and procedures is available.
   3. private insurance will not reimburse for in-hospital care.
   4. the acuity of clients in ambulatory settings is decreasing.

5. Describe the Levels of Prevention Model. Identify the three levels of prevention.

6. List seven challenges to ambulatory care nurses based on demographic and socioeconomic trends.
   a.

   b.

   c.

   d.

   e.

   f.

   g.

REVIEWING YOUR KNOWLEDGE

7. True or False

   _____ Autonomy is a characteristic of nursing practice in ambulatory care settings.

   _____ Ambulatory nursing care is episodic and lasts 24 to 48 hours.

   _____ Clinical services provided in the ambulatory care setting have traditionally been provided based on the medical model of care.

   _____ The major role of nurses in hospital outpatient departments is client and family education and case management.

   _____ Working with a multidisciplinary team in the ambulatory care setting is challenging because nurses may be asked to provide care beyond their scope of practice.

   _____ Nursing competence is based on knowledge, skill, and ability to effectively carry out a given role.

   _____ Nursing certification in ambulatory care nursing is a means of demonstrating competence.

8. Describe why nursing assessment is a challenge in the ambulatory care setting.

9. The three classifications of ambulatory care settings are _____, _____, and _____.

10. Describe the three means of classifying ambulatory clients.

11. Explain the nurse's role in telephone triage.

12. The two types of telephone surveillance (or monitoring) that are in common practice are _____ and _____.

13. Explain what should be included in the documentation of a telehealth encounter in the client's medical record.

14. Explain the purpose of accreditation of ambulatory care settings.

15. List the three organizations which provide accreditation for ambulatory care settings:
    a.

    b.

    c.

APPLYING YOUR KNOWLEDGE

16. Characteristics of clients seen for care in ambulatory care settings include: (Select all that apply.)
    1. men make more visits than women.
    2. older adults make more visits than children.
    3. African-Americans are more likely to use hospital outpatient departments.
    4. difficulty breathing is a common reason for visits.

17. Explain the rationale for the nurse to be culturally competent in the ambulatory care setting.

18. The benefits of the Nurse Licensure Compact for nursing licensure include: (Select all that apply.)
    1. reduced barriers to interstate practice.
    2. improved tracking for disciplinary purposes.
    3. cost-effectiveness.
    4. unduplicated counts of nurses in practice.
    5. decreased consumer access to nurses in their state.

BEST PRACTICES

19. An example of a primary prevention health promotion activity is:
    1. blood glucose screening.
    2. immunizations.
    3. cardiac rehabilitation.
    4. nutrition education.

20. An example of secondary prevention activity is:
    1. blood glucose screening.
    2. immunizations.
    3. cardiac rehabilitation.
    4. nutrition education.

21. An example of tertiary prevention activity is:
    1. blood glucose screening.
    2. immunizations.
    3. cardiac rehabilitation.
    4. nutrition education.

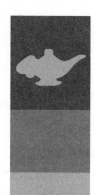

CHAPTER **6**

Acute Health Care

CHAPTER OBJECTIVES

6.1   Discuss acute health care and the changes that occurred in the 1980s and 1990s that affected the use of hospital care.

6.2   Distinguish the different types of hospitals.

6.3   Discuss the client admission process and the need for postacute care beyond an acute care stay.

6.4   Describe the role of hospitals and community preparedness for disasters.

6.5   Describe nursing's various roles in the hospital setting.

6.6   Distinguish care delivery models found in various acute care settings.

6.7   Describe the use of unlicensed assistive personnel (UAPs) as they are incorporated in a care delivery model.

6.8   Describe the aspects of quality client care including safety as a major client care concern.

6.9   Describe the regulations that assure the safety of the public in health care settings.

6.10   Discuss the future of nursing in the acute care setting.

UNDERSTANDING TERMINOLOGY

1.   Match each type of hospital admission to the appropriate description.

Type of Admission

_____   a.   Emergency

_____   b.   Direct

_____   c.   Scheduled

Description

1.   Client is seen in the physician's office and it is determined that the client needs nursing care and specialized monitoring.

2.   Client has elected to undergo a special diagnostic or surgical procedure.

3.   Client is seen in an outpatient department and it is determined that client needs surgery, nursing care, or monitoring and cannot manage the disease at home.

2.   Describe a physician hospitalist.

3.   Define *service lines*.

4. Match each type of care provided by nurses in acute care settings with the appropriate description.

Type of Care

_____ a. Interdependent

_____ b. Direct

_____ c. Indirect

Description

1. Processes that support actual bedside nursing

2. Provision of treatment or administration of medications

3. Assess, care for, educate, and comfort clients

5. Explain what is meant by *cross-training*.

6. Define *culturally competent care*.

7. Define *risk management*.

THEORIES AND TRENDS

8. True or False

_____ The expected outcome of using a nursing classification system for staffing according to patient acuity is a reduction in costs, improvement in care, and an increase in client satisfaction.

9. Explain the purpose of hospital surveys by regulating agencies.

10. A trend that will influence the delivery of care in hospitals is:
    1. technology will decrease the acuity of clients.
    2. health care will be directed at individuals.
    3. pandemic concerns.
    4. fewer health care workers will be immigrants.

REVIEWING YOUR KNOWLEDGE

11. The new prospective payment system implemented in 1983 to stem the rise in health care costs was _____ _____.

12. In the 1990s, hospitals changed from a _____-driven, fee-for-service system to a _____ _____-driven, capitated, and managed care system.

13. True or False

_____ As a consequence of cost-containment efforts, hospitals merged in the 1990s to become "health-care systems."

_____ A hospital is described as an institution whose function is to provide diagnostic and therapeutic client services for a variety of medical conditions.

_____ Voluntary/not-for-profit hospitals are only concerned about meeting expenses on an ongoing basis.

_____ The requirement for nursing care is the primary reason clients are hospitalized.

_____ Postacute care is designed to fill the gap between home care and long-term care.

_____ A certified lactation specialist is a formal nurse educator who teaches clients in the hospital and provides follow-up care in the community.

_____ Research of clinical practices contributes to efforts to contain costs.

_____ Most hospitals use one type of nursing care delivery.

_____ Today's client is submissive to suggestions for care.

_____ It is appropriate for incident reports to be used for punitive activity.

_____ Lawsuits rely upon information revealed in an incident report.

14. List the three types of hospitals.
   a.

   b.

   c.

15. List the three goals of case management.
   a.

   b.

   c.

16. Explain the purpose of work-redesign.

17. The purpose of skill-mix between RNs and other nonlicensed personnel is achieved when

   _____

   _____ .

18. _____ staff are used to make staffing adjustments caused by fluctuation of census data and acuity levels.

19. The nurse, as manager of client care, is primarily focused on the _____ of the care for the client.

20. Identify the federal legislation associated with each impact or purpose.

Impact or Purpose	Federal Legislation
a. Requires places of employment to be free from recognized hazards	
b. Laid the foundation for equal employment	
c. Take affirmative action to recruit, hire, and advance handicapped people	
d. Promote employment of older people	
e. Eliminate workplace discrimination against Americans with disabilities	

21. List the five categories of highest risk in a hospital setting.

    a.

    b.

    c.

    d.

    e.

APPLYING YOUR KNOWLEDGE

22. Nursing at the beginning of the 20th century is best characterized by which of the following? (Select all that apply.)
    1. Nurses worked in hospitals on a fee-for-service basis.
    2. Most nurses worked in private duty.
    3. Hospitalized clients were poor and generally had communicable diseases.
    4. It was desirable for affluent clients to be admitted to hospitals.

23. Following the Great Depression, the demand for hospital-based nurses increased due to:
    1. the increased demand for nurses to work in private duty.
    2. hospitals providing room and board instead of salary.
    3. the availability of hospital insurance through Blue Cross.
    4. a decrease in the number of nursing graduates.

24. Compare and contrast informal versus formal education provided to clients or groups.

25. Functional nursing requires that:
    1. care provided under this model is done solely by RNs.
    2. all caregivers are licensed.
    3. the RN provides basic, bedside care to the client.
    4. the RN coordinates care for an entire team or unit.

26. A major advantage of team nursing is:
    1. it is economical.
    2. the RN knows clients well.
    3. care is less fragmented.
    4. the team is comprised of multiple RNs.

BEST PRACTICES

27. List six characteristics that describe a *magnet hospital*.

    a.

    b.

    c.

    d.

    e.

    f.

28. True or False

    _____ Research has conclusively demonstrated that the use of unlicensed assistive personnel improves client outcomes.

    _____ Evidence-based practice uses research findings and client characteristics to guide clinical practice.

    _____ If something is not documented in the medical record, it is assumed that it was not done.

29. List eight factors that should be considered when developing a plan for quality client care.

   a.

   b.

   c.

   d.

   c.

   f.

   g.

   h.

30. The one indicator of quality of care that hospitals should always consider is _____ _____ _____.

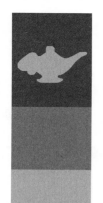

CHAPTER 7

Critical Care

CHAPTER OBJECTIVES

7.1 Define *critical care nursing*.
7.2 Identify the magnitude of critical care and the age and likely diagnoses of clients often admitted to a critical care unit.
7.3 Identify types of critical care units in the United States.
7.4 Describe aspects of critical care nursing that support healing or cause impaired healing for clients.
7.5 Discuss the role of the critical care nurse as an advocate for the client.
7.6 Relate the competencies essential to the practice of the critical care nurse and critical care certification to client outcomes.

THEORIES AND TRENDS

1. Critical care units have been evolving since the:
   1. 1940s.
   2. 1950s.
   3. 1960s.
   4. 1970s.

2. Which of the following can improve care delivered to the client in the critical care unit? (Select all that apply.)
   1. Certification by AACN.
   2. Using standard care plans or care maps.
   3. Having an intensivist lead a multidisciplinary team.
   4. Having one expert nurse oversee the care of all the clients in the unit.

REVIEWING YOUR KNOWLEDGE

3. True or False

   _____ The critical care unit provides care to clients who are unstable or potentially unstable.

   _____ Research has demonstrated that despite their beliefs, nurses and physicians caring for clients in the ICU underestimate family needs for information.

   _____ The physician is primarily responsible for coordinating the care of a client in the ICU.

   _____ Clients in the critical care unit need constant physiologic monitoring.

   _____ The American Association of Critical Care Nurses defines *critical care nursing* as the specialty that deals with human responses to life-threatening problems.

   _____ Most clients admitted to a critical care unit are under the age of 65.

APPLYING YOUR KNOWLEDGE

4. Explain why clients with each type of disorder might require nursing care in a critical care unit.
   a. Respiratory disorders:

   b. Circulatory disorders:

c. Neurologic changes:

d. Life-threatening infections:

e. Metabolic problems:

f. Major surgical procedures:

g. Postoperative with history of cardiac or pulmonary disease:

5. List two disorders under each body system that are commonly seen in the critical care unit.
   a. Brain:

   b. Pulmonary:

c. Cardiovascular:

d. Childbirth/reproductive:

e. Endocrine:

f. Multisystem:

6. List five types of critical care units.
   a.

   b.

   c.

   d.

   e.

7. Explain how the environment of the critical care unit can be disorienting to a client and offer one solution the nurse can provide to decrease the adverse effects of that stimulation.

8. Describe the role of the nurse as advocate for the client in the critical care unit.

9. Identify the two professional organizations that provide the ICU nurse with practice guidelines, educational programs, and professional publications among other benefits.
   a.

   b.

10. A possible consequence of inadequate sleep quantity and quality for the ICU client is:
    1. a decrease in oxygen consumption.
    2. a decrease in carbon dioxide production.
    3. a positive nitrogen balance.
    4. impaired immunity and delayed healing.

BEST PRACTICES

11. Explain why it is imperative that the ICU nurse engages in continuing education, obtains national certification, and uses standardized protocols for delivering client care.

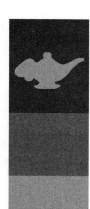

CHAPTER **8**

Home Health Care

CHAPTER OBJECTIVES

8.1   Distinguish home health care nursing as a service provided in community-oriented nursing.

8.2   Discuss trends in home health care nursing including the need for the service along with trends in aging.

8.3   Identify sources of payment for home health care services.

8.4   Define *seamless health care systems*.

8.5   Identify differences in the role of the community health nurse versus a nurse in a hospital or other inpatient agency.

8.6   Discuss the historical perspective of home health and community-oriented nursing.

8.7   Identify the client as the source of control in the home health nursing relationship.

8.8   Identify resources of the nurse to assist in providing care to the client.

8.9   Define the purpose and component parts of the Omaha System.

8.10   Discuss the use of the Omaha System within a clinical setting.

8.11   Discuss the use of information technology to facilitate nursing care in the home and community settings.

UNDERSTANDING TERMINOLOGY

1.   Define *home health care nursing*.

THEORIES AND TRENDS

2.   All of the following have contributed to the growth of home health services *except*:
    1.   shrinking health care costs.
    2.   aging of the population.
    3.   federal legislation.
    4.   the increase in managed care.

3.   List the four purposes of legislative and regulatory changes made in 1997 that reduced Medicare-Medicaid reimbursement to home health agencies.
    a.

    b.

    c.

    d.

4.   True or False

    _____   The practice of home health care nursing originated in the early 1900s.

    _____   Francis Root was the first known employed home visit nurse.

    _____   Clara Barton established the Henry Street Settlement in New York City.

    _____   Lillian Wald's vision included sending nurses into the home to provide care for new mothers, infants, and the sick.

    _____   By 1912, as many as 2500 nurses were employed by some kind of visiting nurse association.

    _____   Persons 65 and over constitute around 70% of all home health clients and this group is expected to continue growing significantly in the future.

REVIEWING YOUR KNOWLEDGE

5. Explain the primary role of the nurse case manager employed by home health agencies.

6. The Boy Scout motto that applies to home health care is _____ _____. Explain why this is critical for the nurse.

7. Invaluable resources that a nurse takes with her to a home visit that contribute to her ability to provide high-quality care are _____ _____, _____ _____, and _____.

8. The most important thing for a nurse to do during the initial visit with the home health client is to establish _____ _____.

9. List and explain the four levels of the Problem Classification Scheme in the Omaha System:
   a.

   b.

   c.

   d.

10. Describe the Problem Rating Scale for Outcomes of the Omaha System.

11. True or False

   _____ Community health nursing provides an umbrella under which all types of home health care are practiced.

   _____ Ideally, the shift of health care services from the hospital to the community decreases fragmentation of care, increases collaboration among health care team members, and increases accountability.

   _____ It is common practice for the home health nurse to be the individual to verify financial data and source of payment with the client during the initial intake.

   _____ A hospice team is comprised of representatives of multiple health care disciplines whose goal is to support end-of-life decisions made by clients and their families.

   _____ The client and nurse establish goals of care in home health nursing.

   _____ The Problem Rating Scale for Outcomes in the Omaha System provides the nurse with an opportunity to compare client status at different points in time to determine nursing effectiveness.

APPLYING YOUR KNOWLEDGE

12. Nursing activities that a nurse would implement during the initial client visit include: (Select all that apply.)
   1. gathering subjective data.
   2. assessing the physical environment.
   3. gathering objective data about the client only.
   4. interpretation of data and problem identification.

13. Explain the Intervention Scheme of the Omaha System.

BEST PRACTICES

14. Explain the importance of communication and collaboration among home health care staff.

15. Discuss the basic core values central to the community-oriented philosophy of care practiced in home health agencies.

16. Describe basic principles that nurses who practice in home health care can incorporate to maximize outcomes of care.

17. The ability of a client to remain at home despite medical problems rests mainly on the _____
_____
_____
_____
_____.

18. Discuss the client's role in the home health care setting.

19. Describe the role of each of the following pieces of information technology.
    1. Cell phone:

    2. Internet:

    3. Telehealth systems:

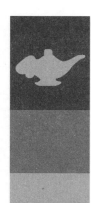

CHAPTER 9

Long-Term Care

CHAPTER OBJECTIVES
9.1   Describe the perception and reality of long-term care today.
9.2   Describe the complex nature of long-term care.
9.3   Identify significant historical developments of long-term care facilities (LTCFs).
9.4   Identify federally mandated staffing in long-term care facilities.
9.5   Describe nursing responsibilities for clients in the LTCF.
9.6   Identify the MDS as the tool to document nursing assessment of the client.
9.7   Describe the challenging nature of nursing assessment in the LTCF.
9.8   Describe the nature of the LTCF environment and the adjustments necessary for the resident.
9.9   Relate timely communication to the care of residents.
9.10 Describe the management role of the nurse in LTCFs.
9.11 Identify other forms of long-term care.

THEORIES AND TRENDS

1. Early long-term care facilities were characterized by: (Select all that apply.)
    1. adequate supplies to care for clients.
    2. sound nutritional food.
    3. residents being forced to sleep on floors.
    4. overcrowding.
    5. residents being forced to work for keep.
    6. open drunkenness and sexual relations.

2. True or False

    _____ Long-term care facilities historically had their origin in the tradition in European countries to segregate the aged and disabled from the rest of society.

    _____ Historically, the development of community institutions to care for individuals with long-term care needs was developed so that clients did not remain in hospital beds for extended periods of time.

REVIEWING YOUR KNOWLEDGE

3. The federal legislation which provided funds for the construction of nursing homes was the

    _____.

4. The federal legislation passed in 1987 which provided strict regulations and produced profound reform in nursing home care was the _____

    _____.

5. List the two specific nursing staffing requirements specified by federal regulations for long-term care facilities.
    a.

    b.

6. Residents of long-term care facilities must have an assessment completed within _____ days of admission. They must be reassessed at least _____ or whenever there is a _____

    _____.

7. The tool used to document the assessment and used as a basis for care planning is the _____ _____.

8. List seven skills that are essential for an effective manager in a long-term care facility.
   a.

   b.

   c.

   d.

   e.

   f.

   g.

9. True or False

   _____ The passage of the Social Security Act provided a means for older adults to purchase care through an informal system of care.

   _____ Medicare and Medicaid were developed to ensure a minimum level of health care for the aged and poor.

   _____ Lobbying efforts by the American Medical Association and owners of long-term care facilities ensured provisions for reimbursement for nursing home care in Medicare and Medicaid.

   _____ Long-term care facilities which do not meet required conditions and regulations may have Medicare and Medicaid reimbursement terminated.

   _____ Nurses and nursing organizations played an active role in the development of regulations and guidelines for long-term care facilities.

   _____ The role of nurses may vary in LTCF from performing selected roles such as medication administration to providing total care.

   _____ It is not uncommon for residents and their families to experience negative reactions when the resident transitions to living in a LTCF.

_____ Nurses working in long-term care facilities function in a variety of management roles which require them to be familiar with regulations, reimbursement programs, legal aspects of nursing practice, and employee-employer relations.

APPLYING YOUR KNOWLEDGE

10. A condition that long-term care facilities must meet to receive reimbursement through Medicare and/or Medicaid is that residents must:
    1. be totally dependent.
    2. have a comprehensive health assessment within the first 3 weeks of care.
    3. have personal funds managed by facility personnel.
    4. have nursing care consistent with level of care and needs.

11. Characteristics of residents of long-term care facilities include: (Select all that apply.)
    1. the risk of being in an LTCF decreases with age.
    2. women residents outnumber men.
    3. the majority of residents are African-American.
    4. most residents have some impairment of self-care.
    5. a medical diagnosis is a key criteria for admission.
    6. change in caregiver status often precipitates admission.

12. Describe problems with the MDS as an assessment tool which may impact nursing care planning.

BEST PRACTICES

13. Regulations specify components of the care plan used in a LTCF. List six characteristics of the care plan.

    a.

    b.

    c.

    d.

    e.

    f.

14. Explain the importance of effective communication and documentation for nursing caregivers of LTCF residents.

15. List six activities a nurse can implement to ensure safety in telephone orders from physicians for LTCF residents.

    a.

    b.

    c.

    d.

    e.

    f.

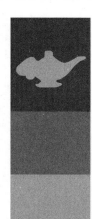

CHAPTER 10

Rehabilitation

CHAPTER OBJECTIVES

10.1 Explain rehabilitation care as part of the continuum of health care.

10.2 Compare and contrast rehabilitation care with acute care.

10.3 Define *rehabilitation nursing*.

10.4 Identify the World Health Organization's classification framework for those who qualify for rehabilitation care.

10.5 Define components of the International Classification Framework (ICF).

10.6 Relate the specific components of the ICF to a comprehensive assessment of the client.

10.7 Identify different rehabilitation settings.

10.8 List Medicare regulations for being admitted to rehabilitation.

10.9 Describe the fulfillment of the goals of rehabilitation nursing leading to self-management of a chronic illness.

10.10 Identify the unique principles of rehabilitation care.

10.11 Relate the process of rehabilitation care to potential client outcomes.

THEORIES AND TRENDS

1. List two factors that have contributed to an increased number of clients requiring rehabilitation services.

   a.

   b.

2. Describe the World Health Organization's International Classification System for clients requiring rehabilitation.

3. Describe the goal of rehabilitation nursing.

REVIEWING YOUR KNOWLEDGE

4. *Rehabilitation nursing* is defined as the diagnosis and treatment of human responses of individuals to actual or potential health problems relative to _____

   _____.

5. Using WHO International Classification of Functioning, Disability, and Health as a guide, match each term with the appropriate definition.

Term

_____ a. Body structure

_____ b. Activities

_____ c. Personal factors

_____ d. Participation
_____ e. Impairments
_____ f. Body functions
_____ g. Environmental factors

Definition

1. External physical, social, and attitudinal conditions that can influence an individual's capacity to perform functions
2. Problems that deviate significantly from the expected norm
3. Physiologic and psychological components of body systems
4. Organs, limbs, and their components
5. Involvement in life situations
6. Execution of a task or action by an individual
7. Non-health conditions of an individual's life

6. List the five different types of rehabilitation service settings.
    a.

    b.

    c.

    d.

    e.

7. Describe factors that are used to determine the most appropriate setting for a client's rehabilitation.

8. True or False
    _____ Ongoing evaluation of progress toward rehabilitation goals is achieved through team conferences.

    _____ Anticipatory guidance is an effective intervention to help clients transition successfully from one level of care to another.

    _____ Encouragement from a nurse for the client to achieve independence is viewed as poor quality of care.

    _____ Before discharge, clients and families are usually very competent in their ability to manage all aspects of client care at home.

APPLYING YOUR KNOWLEDGE

9. Medicare requires that a client must be able to participate actively in at least _____ hours of therapy a day and need at least _____ therapeutic modalities in addition to rehabilitation _____ _____ and _____ _____.

10. Explain each of the following key principles related to the focus of rehabilitation and the nurse's role for each.
    a. Client-centered:

    b. Goal-oriented:

    c. Focus on functional ability:

    d. Use of a team approach:

    e. Client finding acceptable quality of life:

f.   Wellness focus:

g.   Adapting to change:

h.   Coping and adjusting:

i.   Understanding role of culture:

j.   Client and family education:

11.   A factor that can interfere with an effective rehabilitation process is:
      1.   the attitude of the client.
      2.   the support of family members.
      3.   adequate financial resources.
      4.   available community resources.

12.   True or False

      _____   The most important reason for nurses to understand the rehabilitation component of the continuum of care is that it enables them to make appropriate referrals and to prepare clients for the rehabilitation experience.

BEST PRACTICES

13.   Explain why it is important for the nurse to make sure the client and family members understand the differences between acute care and rehabilitation settings.

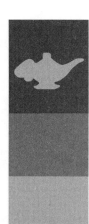

CHAPTER 11

Clients with Fluid Imbalances

CHAPTER OBJECTIVES

11.1 Define *dehydration, cellular dehydration, fluid overload, water intoxication, third spacing, hyponatremia,* and *hypernatremia.*

11.2 Identify the causes of each disorder.

11.3 Describe the pathophysiology of the disorders.

11.4 Identify the clinical manifestations and diagnostic measures significant to each disorder.

11.5 Describe outcomes of successful treatment of each disorder.

11.6 Assess, diagnose, intervene, and identify outcomes for the client with each disorder.

11.7 Educate clients about the specific self-care requirements to manage or prevent recurrence of disorders at home.

ANATOMY & PHYSIOLOGY REVIEW

1. Label the structures of the cell.

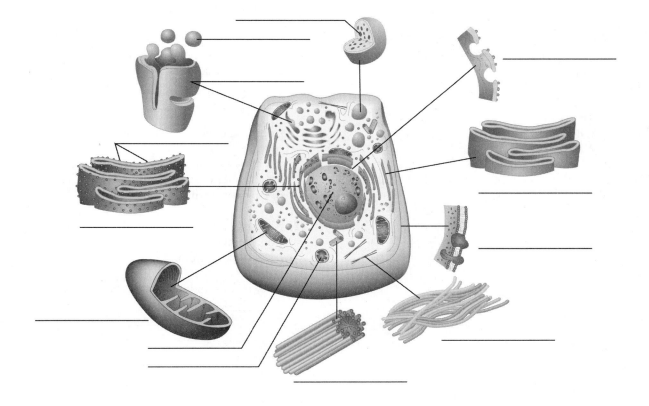

UNDERSTANDING PATHOPHYSIOLOGY

2.   Match the following terms with their definitions or descriptions.

Term

_____ a.   Dehydration

_____ b.   Cellular dehydration

_____ c.   Fluid overload

_____ d.   Water intoxication

_____ e.   Third spacing

_____ f.   Hyponatremia

_____ g.   Hypernatremia

Definition/Description

1.   Can be called ECFVE and is seen in both the vascular spaces and interstitial spaces

2.   Severe dehydration, seen in older adults and in those who have extreme fluid losses

3.   Physiologically useless fluids found in areas such as the pleural cavity, peritoneal cavity, or pericardial sac

4.   Severe manifestations can be seen at 115 mEq/L

5.   Associated with total body water deficit, this condition carries a high mortality rate

6.   Most often caused by overadministration of hypotonic IV solutions

7.   Also called extracellular fluid volume deficit (ECFVD)

3.   Thirst is inhibited by _____ _____.

4.   List the two types of fluid shifts.
     a.

     b.

5.   What hormone(s) is/are responsible for increasing water and sodium reabsorption? (Select all that apply.)
     1.   ADH
     2.   Estrogen
     3.   Thyroxin
     4.   Calcium
     5.   Aldosterone

6.   Identify the three types of extracellular fluid (ECF) volume deficits.
     a.

     b.

     c.

7.   Decreased urine output is a classic sign of _____.

8.   Clinical signs that a client is dehydrated include: (Select all that apply.)
     1.   dry mucous membranes.
     2.   sunken eyes.
     3.   decreased skin turgor.
     4.   elevated alkaline level.

9.   Oral rehydration is inhibited by cola drinks because they contain _____ and _____.

10.   The most common causes of hyponatremia are conditions that _____ _____ _____.

11.   Common conditions that can lead to hypernatremia are:
      1.   hypovolemic hypernatremia.
      2.   euvolemic hypernatremia.
      3.   hypervolemic hypernatremia.

12.   A serum sodium of below _____ indicates hyponatremia; a serum sodium above _____ indicates hypernatremia.

13.   Early manifestations of hyponatremia are _____ and _____ and are caused by _____ _____ _____.

14. No matter the cause, clients with hypernatremia are at risk for dysrhythmias because _____ _____ _____.

APPLYING YOUR KNOWLEDGE

15. The most common fluid and electrolyte disturbance in the United States is:
    1. hypokalemia.
    2. dehydration.
    3. sodium retention.
    4. obesity.

16. Physiologic regulators of fluid balance include: (Select all that apply.)
    1. thirst.
    2. hormones.
    3. the lymphatic system.
    4. the kidneys.

17. Clients with a high risk of developing fluid imbalances include clients with: (Select all that apply.)
    1. dysphagia.
    2. dementia.
    3. diabetes insipidus.
    4. renal failure.

18. Dehydration can be caused by: (Select all that apply.)
    1. unmonitored use of potent diuretics.
    2. severe vomiting.
    3. diarrhea.
    4. excessive exercise.

19. Older clients are at risk for excessive fluid loss for several reasons, including: (Select all that apply.)
    1. decreased renal concentration of urine.
    2. altered ADH response.
    3. increased body fat.
    4. diminished thirst.

20. A client with inadequate fluid volume would have which of the following clinical signs? (Select all that apply.)
    1. Decreased blood pressure
    2. Weak pulse
    3. Decreased central venous pressure
    4. Elevated respirations

21. The nurse should notify the team leader if a client has not had at least _____ of urine output for 8 consecutive hours.

22. Complications of too-rapid IV fluid infusion can result in _____ and _____.

23. In evaluating renal function in clients, which lab test is critical in maintaining adequate renal output?
    1. Creatinine
    2. CBC
    3. ADH level
    4. Lipase

BEST PRACTICES

24. Which conditions predispose clients to fluid loss? (Select all that apply.)
    1. Fever
    2. Hyperglycemia
    3. Gastrointestinal suctioning
    4. Ileostomy
    5. Burns
    6. Hyperventilation

25. A 78-year-old female is starting to experience cerebral anoxia due to fluid loss. What sign would indicate this and needs to be reported to the physician? (Select all that apply.)
    1. Restlessness
    2. Apprehension
    3. Headache
    4. Confusion

26. The goals of treatment for fluid volume deficit are to: (Select all that apply.)
    1. restore normal fluid volumes by using fluids similar in composition to those lost.
    2. replace ongoing losses.
    3. correct the underlying problems (such as vomiting or diarrhea).
    4. ensure replacement of magnesium to the system.

27. Which of the following assessment criteria are critical when managing patients with fluid volume deficits? (Select all that apply.)
    1. Urine output
    2. Body weight
    3. Sodium and potassium lab value
    4. Osmolality
    5. BUN

28. When weighing a client, it is important to: (Select all that apply.)
    1. rely on what the client tells you his or her weight is.
    2. weigh the client daily.
    3. use the same scale for each weight.
    4. weigh the client at the same time each day.
    5. have the patient void prior to weighing.

29. Respiratory assessments that would indicate fluid volume excess are: (Select all that apply.)
    1. diminished lung sounds.
    2. crackles, ronchi.
    3. coughing.
    4. dyspnea.

30. What intravenous fluid(s) are considered hypotonic?

31. What intravenous fluid(s) are considered isotonic?

32. What intravenous fluid(s) are considered hypertonic?

33. List appropriate outcomes and five nursing interventions with scientific rationale for the nursing diagnosis Fluid volume deficit related to vomiting and diarrhea.
    Outcomes:

    Intervention #1:

    Intervention #2:

Intervention #3:

Intervention #4:

Intervention #5:

34. List appropriate outcomes and five nursing interventions with scientific rationale for the nursing diagnosis Fluid volume excess related to ineffective cardiac pump secondary to congestive heart failure.
    Outcomes:

    Intervention #1:

    Intervention #2:

    Intervention #3:

    Intervention #4:

    Intervention #5:

35. List safety precautions the nurse should use when administering 3% saline infusions.

    a.

    b.

    c.

36. List appropriate outcomes and five nursing interventions with scientific rationale for the nursing diagnosis Impaired oral mucous membranes related to lack of body water secondary to hypernatremia.

    Outcomes:

    Intervention #1:

    Intervention #2:

    Intervention #3:

    Intervention #4:

    Intervention #5:

37. List teaching measures for self-care related to hypernatremia.

    a.

    b.

    c.

    d.

    e.

    f.

    g.

KEEPING DRUG SKILLS SHARP

38. Mild diuretics and digitalis promote _____ _____ and improve _____ _____.

39. Clients taking diuretics and digitalis need to be monitored for: (Select all that apply.)
    1. plasma electrolytes.
    2. digitalis toxicity.
    3. hypokalemia.
    4. hypernatremia.

40. True or False

    _____   Unmonitored use of potent diuretics can cause hyperkalemia.

    _____   Lemon and garlic are safe low-sodium salt substitutes.

    _____   Clients taking ACE inhibitors can use potassium salt substitutes sparingly.

    _____   Digitalis toxicity is common in older adults.

41. The nurse will administer albumin to a client to assist in:
    1. clotting of blood.
    2. formation of red blood cells.
    3. activation of white blood cells.
    4. development of oncotic pressure.

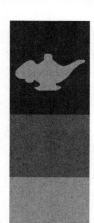

CHAPTER **12**

Clients with Electrolyte Imbalances

CHAPTER OBJECTIVES

12.1 Define *hypokalemia, hyperkalemia, hypocalcemia, hypercalcemia, hypophosphatemia, hyperphosphatemia, hypomagnesemia,* and *hypermagnesemia.*

12.2 Describe the cause, risk factors, and pathophysiology for each imbalance.

12.3 Describe the clinical manifestations of each imbalance.

12.4 Identify the specific medical and nursing outcomes for each imbalance using a collaborative problem format.

12.5 Describe specific interventions for each collaborative problem.

12.6 Educate the client on maintenance of electrolyte balance for self-care.

UNDERSTANDING PATHOPHYSIOLOGY

1. Anyone with decreased intake, decreased availability, or increased loss of electrolytes is at risk for _____.

2. Nursing diagnoses that may apply to clients with electrolyte imbalances include:
   a.

   b.

   c.

   d.

3. The most ominous result of hypocalcemia is _____.

4. *Hypokalemia* is defined as a plasma K$^+$ level less than _____.

5. Clinical manifestations of hypokalemia include: (Select all that apply.)
   1. abnormal findings on EKG.
   2. GI abnormalities.
   3. muscle weakness.
   4. leg cramps.

6. Dysrhythmias with hypokalemia are due to _____ _____ _____.

7. The underlying cause of hyperkalemia is often associated with _____ kidney function.

8. Define *Trousseau's sign.*

9. Define *Chvostek's sign.*

10. The three most common causes of hypercalcemia are: (Select all that apply.)
    1. metastatic malignancy.
    2. hyperparathyroidism.
    3. thiazide diuretics.
    4. corticosteroid-induced.

11. Normal calcium levels are _____ or _____.

12. Hypermagnesemia is a magnesium level above
_____.

13. Manifestations of hypermagnesemia are related
to the _____
which results in a decrease in _____
_____.

14. Options for treating hypermagnesemia include:
a.

b.

c.

d.

e.

15. Hypomagnesemia is a plasma level of _____.

16. Nursing interventions for the client with hypomagnesemia include: (Select all that apply.)
1. monitoring vital signs every 4-8 hours.
2. reviewing ECG strip hourly.
3. institute safety and seizure precautions.
4. assess deep tendon reflexes for early changes.

17. Hypomagnesemia is implicated in treatment-
refractory _____ and
_____.

18. Magnesium deficits are often seen in clients with:
a.

b.

c.

d.

e.

f.

19. GI losses from several problems account for
many cases of hypomagnesemia. What do these
GI problems have in common?

20. The normal range for phosphorus is _____
_____.

21. Major risk factors for hypophosphatemia are:
a.

b.

c.

22. Hypophosphatemia can affect every body system
because of _____
_____
_____.

23. Hyperphosphatemia is a serum phosphate level
above _____.

24. Mild or moderate cases of hyperphosphatemia
are managed by:
a.

b.

c.

APPLYING SKILLS

25. What EKG changes would a nurse expect to find in the client with hypokalemia? (Select all that apply.)
    1. Depressed and prolonged ST segment
    2. Depressed and inverted T waves
    3. Prominent U waves
    4. Wide QRS complexes

BEST PRACTICES

26. Oral potassium (chloride and gluconate) is extremely irritating to gastric mucosa and must be administered with: (Select all that apply.)
    1. juice.
    2. meals.
    3. milk.
    4. water.

27. Self-care measures the nurse should teach a client being discharged after an episode of hypokalemia include: (Select all that apply.)
    1. eating a well-balanced diet with foods low in potassium.
    2. trying alternative cooking methods or eating vegetables raw.
    3. drinking 30-60 ml/hour of an electrolyte-containing solution when sick.
    4. manifestations of hypokalemia the client should report.
    5. calling the health care provider if the client with chronic health problems is sick for more than 24 hours.

KEEPING DRUG SKILLS SHARP

28. Medications that commonly cause hypokalemia include: (Select all that apply.)
    1. thiazide diuretics.
    2. osmotic diuretics.
    3. steroids.
    4. digitalis preparations.

29. Clients who have acute hypocalcemia and develop tetany will be treated with: (Select all that apply.)
    1. IV calcium chloride.
    2. IV calcium gluconate.
    3. Lasix.
    4. vitamin D.

30. List the precautions the nurse takes when administering IV potassium.
    a.

    b.

    c.

    d.

    e.

    f.

    g.

    h.

    i.

    j.

    k.

31. Mild hyperkalemia can be treated with
    _____, _____, and
    _____.

32. Immediate treatment for severe hyperkalemia
    includes: (Select all that apply.)
    1. IV calcium gluconate.
    2. sodium bicarbonate.
    3. albuterol.
    4. insulin with glucose.
    5. Kayexalate.

33. Oral calcium supplements are best given:
    1. with a full glass of water.
    2. on an empty stomach.
    3. 30 minutes prior to other medications.
    4. with a glass of milk.

34. IV calcium should be diluted in which IV solution?
    1. D_5W
    2. 0.45% NS
    3. NS
    4. sodium bicarbonate

35. Clients with severe hypophosphatemia are often
    treated with _____.

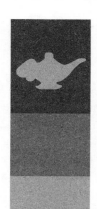

CHAPTER 13

Acid-Base Balance

CHAPTER OBJECTIVES

13.1 Describe the interdependence of buffers, excretion of acid by the lungs, and excretion of acid by the kidneys in the regulation of acid-base balance.

13.2 Describe the impact of electrolytes on acid-base balance.

13.3 Describe compensatory actions by the body that maintain acid-base balance.

13.4 Analyze the specific components of arterial blood gases to determine acid-base balance.

13.5 Describe each disorder of acid-base balance.

13.6 Identify the specific component, $Paco_2$ or HCO_3^-, that is primary in each disorder.

13.7 Identify the major causes, risk factors, pathophysiology, clinical manifestations, and outcome management of each disorder.

UNDERSTANDING PATHOPHYSIOLOGY

1. A normal serum pH is _____ _____.

2. An acidic solution has a pH of less than _____ _____.

3. An alkaline solution has a pH of greater than _____.

4. Acids that cannot be converted to gases must be eliminated in _____.

5. True or False

   _____ The kidneys regulate serum pH by secreting H^+ into the urine and by regenerating HCO_3^-.

6. The organ that regulates the electrolyte balance in the body is the:
   1. liver.
   2. kidney.
   3. heart.
   4. parathyroid.

7. Acid-base compensation acts to restore the normal ratio of _____ and normalize _____.

8. _____ refers to any pathologic process that causes a relative excess of acid.

9. _____ refers to excess acid in the blood.

10. _____ indicates a primary condition resulting in excess base in the body.

11. _____ refers more narrowly to elevation of serum pH.

12. Name the body's three buffering systems:
    a.

    b.

    c.

13. The _____ system can compensate for a metabolic problem.

14. The kidneys can compensate for a _____ _____ problem.

15. In hyperkalemia, renal tubular cells secrete more _____ but retain _____ for electroneutrality.

16. In a chloride deficiency, the kidney reabsorbs more _____ to maintain electroneutrality.

APPLYING SKILLS

17. No matter the type of acid-base derangement, treatment priorities focus on _____ _____.

18. True or False

    _____ Respiratory acidosis can be treated with increased oxygenation and ventilation.

    _____ Sodium bicarbonate is often used to treat acidosis.

    _____ Acetazolamide (Diamox) is a diuretic that promotes the loss of bicarbonate in the urine to treat metabolic alkalosis.

    _____ Alkali administration hastens recovery in diabetic ketoacidosis.

    _____ Rebreathing carbon dioxide by using a paper bag can temporarily treat respiratory alkalosis.

    _____ The problem in respiratory disorders is an alteration in the HCO_3^- level.

    _____ The $Paco_2$ is altered in respiratory disorders.

19. Match each blood gas value with its corresponding condition.

    Blood Gas Value

    _____ a. pH 7.53; $Paco_2$ 33 mm Hg; HCO_3^- 25 mEq/L

    _____ b. pH 7.4; $Paco_2$ 26 mm Hg; HCO_3^- 16 mEq/L

    _____ c. pH 7.31; $Paco_2$ 58 mm Hg; HCO_3^- 25 mEq/L

    _____ d. pH 7.64; $Paco_2$ 48 mm Hg; HCO_3^- 47 mEq/L

    Condition

    1. Respiratory alkalosis

    2. Respiratory acidosis

    3. Metabolic acidosis

    4. Metabolic alkalosis

20. Match each condition with its corresponding acid-base imbalance.

    Condition

    _____ a. Sedative or narcotic overdose
    _____ b. Mechanical overventilation
    _____ c. Diabetic ketosis
    _____ d. Respiratory failure
    _____ e. Renal failure
    _____ f. Prolonged vomiting

    Acid Base Disturbance

    1. Respiratory acidosis
    2. Respiratory alkalosis
    3. metabolic acidosis
    4. metabolic alkalosis

21. It is essential that nurses be alert for signs of acid-base imbalance in which of the following high-risk clients? (Select all that apply.)
    1. Pulmonary, cardiovascular, and renal system clients
    2. Clients receiving total parenteral nutrition or enteral tube feedings
    3. Clients receiving mechanical ventilation
    4. Clients with diabetes mellitus
    5. Clients with vomiting, diarrhea
    6. Older clients

BEST PRACTICES

22. _____ must be used to treat hypoxemia.

23. What test is performed to ensure adequate circulation in the hand prior to a radial artery puncture for an arterial blood gas?
    1. Allen's test
    2. Open hand draw
    3. Arterial compliant test
    4. CBC

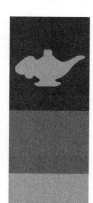

CHAPTER **14**

Clients Having Surgery

CHAPTER OBJECTIVES

14.1   Define *perioperative nursing*.
14.2   Identify the aspects of a preoperative assessment.
14.3   Relate the aspects of the medical history review to the surgical event.
14.4   Identify the purpose of the preoperative physical examination.
14.5   Describe important body system assessments necessary preoperatively.
14.6   Differentiate preoperative teaching for older adults.
14.7   Identify all aspects of informed consent essential prior to surgical procedures.
14.8   Identify important aspects of nursing care during the intraoperative period.
14.9   Describe the types of anesthesia.
14.10 Describe the important safety procedures prior to the incision.
14.11 Discuss nursing care in the postanesthesia care unit (PACU).
14.12 Describe the client assessment when the client is returned to the surgical unit.
14.13 Identify the potential for complications following surgery along with the nursing care of these clients.
14.14 Identify important discharge instructions for a client prior to discharge from the hospital.

UNDERSTANDING TERMINOLOGY

1.   Define *perioperative nursing*.

UNDERSTANDING PATHOPHYSIOLOGY

2.   Explain the additional surgical risks a client who smokes faces versus a client who does not smoke.

3.   Clients with diabetes are at increased risk for _____ and _____ _____.

4.   Describe the immediate assessment the PACU nurses make when a client arrives from the operating room.

5.   List the seven potential causes of postoperative hypotension.
    a.

    b.

    c.

    d.

    e.

    f.

    g.

6. Older adults with _____ or _____ impairments may take longer to regain orientation postoperatively.

7. Clinical manifestations of postoperative hypoxia include: (Select all that apply.)
   1. orientation.
   2. restlessness.
   3. pink, moist skin.
   4. pulse oximetry below 90%.
   5. warm skin.

8. The postoperative client at greatest risk for thrombus and devastating emboli is the client who had _____ surgery.

9. The three clinical manifestations which may alert the nurse to thrombus are:
   a.

   b.

   c.

10. Explain why obese clients have a delayed return to consciousness after anesthetic procedures.

11. True or False
   _____ Postoperatively, temporary deficits in memory and recall are considered normal.
   _____ For surgical wounds to heal effectively clients must be in a state of negative nitrogen balance.
   _____ Caudal anesthesia is commonly used with obstetric clients.
   _____ The purpose of reviewing the medical history preoperatively is to determine operative risk.
   _____ Informed consent is only needed once per hospitalization.
   _____ The nurse ensures the client receives accurate and honest information on what to expect during and after the surgical procedure.
   _____ To obtain informed consent, the nurse explains the surgical procedure, risks, and possible complications to the client and significant others.

APPLYING SKILLS

12. Explain each component of the ABCDE mnemonic used to gather information from the preoperative client.
   A.

   B.

   C.

   D.

   E.

13. Which assessment findings should be reported to surgeon and anesthesiologist immediately?
   1. Recent upper respiratory infection
   2. Failure of the client to stop smoking until 2 days ago
   3. Diminished breath sounds in both bases with expiratory wheezing
   4. Clear breath sounds

14. Identify the two laboratory studies performed before surgery to diagnose respiratory conditions and explain why they are performed.

15. List the three common preoperative tests ordered to assess renal function.
   a.

   b.

   c.

16. List the laboratory tests used to determine nutritional status in the preoperative client.
   a.

   b.

   c.

   d.

17. Of the following clients scheduled for surgery, which is at greatest risk for a poor surgical outcome?
    1. 19-year-old athlete
    2. 30-year-old obese housewife
    3. 45-year-old height and weight proportionate office manager
    4. 50-year-old running coach

18. Describe important precautions the intraoperative nurse takes to ensure client safety in the operating room.

19. Explain the role of each of the following members of the surgical team.
    a. Surgeon:

    b. Anesthesiologist/nurse anesthetist:

    c. Circulating nurse:

    d. Scrub personnel:

20. When using a unipolar electrosurgical unit (ESU), the OR nurse would: (Select all that apply.)
    1. inspect the plug and wires for intactness.
    2. place a ground pad under the thigh.
    3. place a ground pad under the shoulder.
    4. place a ground pad over a previous surgical scar.
    5. ensure that skin is intact before placing a ground pad.

21. List the three phases of the postoperative period.
    a.

    b.

    c.

22. List the two main types of anesthesia.
    a.

    b.

23. The minimum body temperature a client must have to be discharged from the PACU is _____ _____.

24. The three characteristics to include in assessment of postoperative drainage are:
    a.

    b.

    c.

BEST PRACTICES

25. The priority teaching implemented preoperatively to prevent hypoventilation with an obese client is _____ _____.

26. Which of the following methods for getting out of bed should the nurse teach a client having abdominal surgery to minimize pain and discomfort?
    1. Raise the HOB to 90 degrees and swing legs to the side of the bed.
    2. From a flat supine position, sit up in bed and swing legs to the side of the bed.
    3. Turn onto side, use arms to push self into an upright position.
    4. Raise HOB to 45 degrees and swing legs to the side of the bed.

27. Which of the following should the nurse teach the client about postoperative pain control?
    1. Pain medication will be provided and the client should ask for medication when the pain is becoming unbearable.
    2. Pain medication will be provided sparingly due to a high risk for addiction.
    3. Pain medication will be given when the client is participating in postoperative ambulation exercises.
    4. Pain medication will be available and the client should ask for medication when he or she begins to feel uncomfortable.

28. When providing preoperative teaching for the older client, the nurse should consider factors such as: (Select all that apply.)
    1. decreased sensory ability.
    2. difficulty hearing high-pitched sounds.
    3. glare from lights may bother the eyes.
    4. increased susceptibility to hypothermia.

29. Informed consent can be provided by:
    1. 10-year-old girl with written permission from an absent parent.
    2. 17-year-old high school senior.
    3. 16-year-old married boy.
    4. 18-year-old college freshman.

30. Explain safety measures the nurse provides for the client after preoperative medications are given.

31. A postoperative client who had spinal anesthesia complains of a headache. An appropriate nursing intervention would be to:
    1. place the client in Trendelenburg position.
    2. provide a warm compress.
    3. keep the client flat.
    4. restrict fluid intake.

32. Identify four factors the nurse considers when positioning a client on the operating table.
    a.

    b.

    c.

    d.

33. The circulating nurse notices a break in surgical asepsis by the surgical assistant when he touched his mask with a gloved hand. Which action should the nurse take?
    1. Record the break in technique on the OR record.
    2. Ask the assistant to leave the OR.
    3. Change the assistant's mask.
    4. Change the assistant's glove.

34. Which of the following actions are initiated to promote a smooth transport from the OR to the PACU? (Select all that apply.)
    1. Move the client rapidly from the OR table to the stretcher.
    2. Maintain the client's modesty.
    3. Avoid kinking the IV tubing.
    4. Provide warm blankets.
    5. Keep the side rails up on the stretcher.

35. The client is positioned in PACU to ensure _____ and the preferred position is _____ _____ .

36. A major complication in the PACU is airway obstruction. The primary nursing intervention to prevent this is:
    1. suctioning.
    2. use of an oral airway.
    3. use of a nasal airway.
    4. positioning of the head.

37. The nursing intervention for a client experiencing laryngospasm after endotrachial extubation is _____ _____ .

38. If shock is suspected, an appropriate nursing intervention for the PACU nurse to initiate would be to:
    1. place the client in a flat supine position.
    2. increase the rate of IV fluids.
    3. decrease the oxygen flow rate.
    4. raise the head of the bed.

39. Explain the nursing actions to be initiated if a client eviscerates a postoperative wound.

40. Explain the postoperative instructions that should be reviewed with a client and caregiver before discharge.

41. True or False
    _____ Alterations in skin integrity not due to the surgical procedure are preventable by the surgical nurse and operative team.
    _____ The nurse encourages family members of surgical clients to go home while the client is in surgery.
    _____ A client experiences a cardiac arrest in the OR and it is the circulating nurse's responsibility to call a "code blue."

KEEPING DRUG SKILLS SHARP

42. Preoperative medications are given in order to:
    (Select all that apply.)
    1. lower blood pressure.
    2. allay anxiety.
    3. increase oxygen availability.
    4. decrease pharyngeal secretions.
    5. reduce anesthesia side effects.
    6. promote urinary retention.

43. Match each medication with the correct desired effect or action (each answer may be used more than once).

Medication	**Desired Effect**
_____ a. midazolam (Versed)	1. Inhalation anesthetic
_____ b. nitrous oxide	2. Tranquilizing agent
_____ c. thiopental	3. Neuromuscular blocking agent
_____ d. fentanyl	4. IV anesthetic
_____ e. vecuronium	5. Opioid analgesic

44. It is important to monitor a client for malignant hyperthermia and shivering if he or she received:
    1. enflurane (Ethrane).
    2. fentanyl citrate–droperidol (Innovar).
    3. nitrous oxide.
    4. fluothane (Halothane).

45. List the eight methods for administering regional anesthesia.
    a.

    b.

    c.

    d.

    e.

    f.

    g.

    h.

46. A highly toxic topical anesthetic agent is:
    1. procaine.
    2. tetracaine.
    3. lidocaine.
    4. cocaine.

47. The PACU nurse best monitors the postoperative client for return to consciousness by: (Select all that apply.)
    1. asking the client for details related to time and place.
    2. seeing if the client can remember information he/she was told since being in the PACU.
    3. checking current status with baseline information obtained during the preoperative assessment.
    4. ascertaining if the client can recognize family members when they come into the PACU.

48. The nurse in the PACU notes that the client's surgical dressing has become saturated with blood. Appropriate actions include: (Select all that apply.)
    1. changing the dressing.
    2. reinforcing the dressing.
    3. notifying the surgeon.
    4. documenting this information.

49. Assessments the nurse working on the surgical floor makes on a new admission include:

a.

b.

c.

d.

e.

f.

g.

h.

50. List four complications of surgery and nursing interventions to either prevent or to treat them.

a.

b.

c.

d.

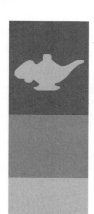

CHAPTER 15

Perspectives in Genetics

CHAPTER OBJECTIVES

15.1 Discuss areas of clinical practice affected by the Human Genome Project (HGP) identification of the human genome.

15.2 Describe the three primary categories of genetic conditions.

15.3 Explain the nature of two chromosomal abnormalities.

15.4 Define *single gene disorder*.

15.5 Discuss the occurrence of single gene disorders.

15.6 Differentiate the three single gene disorder types and give examples.

15.7 Describe multifactorial inheritance of diseases as Alzheimer's, diabetes, and cancer.

15.8 Discuss the role of the nurse in genetic clinical care including family assessment, pedigree interpretation, and an expanded family history.

15.9 Discuss ethical issues related to genetic testing.

TRENDS AND THEORIES

1. Describe the areas of nursing and health care affected by work on the HGP.

   a.

   b.

   c.

   d.

   e.

   f.

   g.

   h.

UNDERSTANDING PATHOPHYSIOLOGY

2. _____ are a basic unit of heredity.

3. Humans have _____ pairs of chromosomes.

4. Chromosome pairs 1-22 are called _____ _____.

5. Females have _____ chromosomes and males have _____ _____ chromosomes.

6. True or False

   _____ Single gene disorders are common.

   _____ Mutations or alterations in a single gene leads to a Mendelian pattern of inheritance for genetic disorders.

   _____ Cystic fibrosis is an example of an X-linked single gene disorder.

   _____ Each child of heterozygous parents who are carriers for an autosomal recessive disease has a 75% chance of being a carrier.

   _____ Males and females are equally affected by autosomal dominant disorders.

   _____ Neurofibromatosis is an example of an autosomal dominant disorder.

_____ A male with an X-linked mutation will always express the disorder.

_____ Duchenne's muscular dystrophy is an example of multifactorial inheritance.

7. List and describe the three primary patterns of inheritance for single gene disorders.

a.

b.

c.

8. Mature onset of diabetes of the young (MODY), a subset of NIDDM, can be inherited as an _____ trait.

9. Most cancers result from an accumulation of _____ that occur over time in somatic cells.

APPLYING SKILLS

10. Select the three primary categories of genetic conditions.
    1. Chromosomal
    2. Single gene (Mendelian)
    3. Multifactorial (complex trait)
    4. Direct trait line

11. Babies with Down syndrome have which chromosome disorder?
    1. Trisomy 21
    2. Trisomy 29
    3. United ALS
    4. CFR-88

12. True or False

_____ Cystic fibrosis (CF) is a common autosomal recessive genetic disorder in the Caucasian population.

_____ Parents of children with cystic fibrosis are heterozygous carriers for the CF gene.

BEST PRACTICES

13. During prenatal counseling, it is critical to explain to families with histories of X-linked conditions that: (Select all that apply.)
    1. the mother of a boy affected with an X-linked condition may be a carrier of the condition.
    2. the son may be affected as a result of a new mutation that occurred during periconceptual period.
    3. a male child inherits his X chromosome only from his mother.
    4. a male child inherits his Y chromosome only from his father.

14. Disorders for which carrier testing is recommended include: (Select all that apply.)
    1. Tay-Sachs disease.
    2. sickle cell.
    3. cystic fibrosis.
    4. thalassemia.
    5. fragile X syndrome.

15. State the primary goal of prenatal genetic testing.

16. Describe the role of the nurse in genetic clinical care.

17. Describe potential ethical issues related to genetic testing.

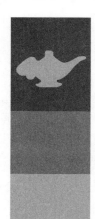

CHAPTER **16**

Perspectives in Oncology

CHAPTER OBJECTIVES

16.1   Define terms related to oncology.
16.2   Discuss the epidemiology of cancer.
16.3   Describe the factors associated with cancer causation.
16.4   Describe the transformation or carcinogenesis of normal cells to cancer cells.
16.5   Compare poorly differentiated cancer cells with well-differentiated cancer cells regarding prognosis.
16.6   Relate aneuploidy to prognosis.
16.7   Describe the importance of tumor-specific antigens in the diagnosis of cancer.
16.8   Compare neoplastic cell growth with normal cell growth.
16.9   Discuss the stages of metastasis and angiogenesis.
16.10   Discuss the impact of the immune system on cancer cells.
16.11   Discuss apoptosis as it relates to cell death, tumor necrosis factor, and the p53 protein.
16.12   Relate genetics to the potential for cancer treatment.
16.13   Compare benign and malignant neoplasms.
16.14   Classify neoplasms according to benign or malignant, tissue of origin, and TNM stage.

UNDERSTANDING TERMINOLOGY

1. The word *tumor* simply refers to a _____ _____.

2. A neoplasm is an abnormal _____ _____ that serves no useful purpose and may harm the host organism.

3. *Metastasis* refers to _____ _____ _____.

4. The term *oncology* refers to the:
   1. medical specialty that deals with the diagnosis, treatment, and study of cancer.
   2. study of regional lymph nodes and dissection of tumors.
   3. study of veins and graphs of nodes.
   4. medical study of epidemiology.

5. A person with expertise in treating cancer with chemotherapy or biotherapy and in handling general medical problems is referred to as a

   _____.

6. _____ is the study of distribution and determinants of diseases and health.

7. Match each term with the appropriate definition.

_____ a. Incidence rates for cancer

_____ b. Prevalence of cancer

_____ c. Mortality rates

1. Total number of people with cancer alive today
2. Reflects the number of new cases of cancer occurring in a specified population during a year
3. Number of deaths caused by cancer that occur in the specified population in a given year

8. Match each term with the appropriate definition or description.

_____ a. Fibromas

_____ b. Lipomas

_____ c. Leiomyomas

_____ d. Benign tumor

_____ e. Malignant neoplasms

_____ f. Carcinoma in situ

_____ g. Apoptosis

1. Common benign neoplasm that arises in adipose tissue
2. May grow anywhere in the body, but are frequently found in the uterus
3. Expands in size as it grows, but does not infiltrate or metastasize
4. Represent a serious threat to the life and well-being of the host
5. Benign neoplasm of smooth muscle origin, most common benign tumor in women
6. Neoplasm of epithelial tissue that remains confined to the site of origin
7. Part of the process of carcinogenesis when cell death does not occur

THEORIES AND TRENDS

9. Identify the process through which normal cells are transformed into malignant or cancer cells and the stages and their definitions.

a.

b.

c.

d.

e.

10. Briefly describe the three stages of a metastatic cascade.

Stage 1:

Stage 2:

Stage 3:

11. The _____ usually defends against bacterial or viral invaders and plays a key role in controlling the growth of cancer cells.

12. True or False

_____ Cancer is a genetic disease.

REVIEWING YOUR KNOWLEDGE

13. _____ causes more cancer in the U.S. than do all other known causes combined.

14. True or False

    _____ Certain viruses are strongly associated with cancer.

15. Some host characteristics that influence cancer susceptibility include: (Select all that apply.)
    1. age.
    2. sex.
    3. genetic predisposition.
    4. ethnicity or race.

16. A specific tumor marker for prostate cancer can be detected by an elevated result on which blood test?
    1. Prostate-specific antigen (PSA)
    2. Alpha-fetoprotein (AFP)
    3. EAS
    4. RNA factor

17. Cancer can be associated with: (Select all that apply.)
    1. radiation.
    2. chemicals.
    3. viruses.
    4. other physical agents

APPLYING YOUR KNOWLEDGE

18. Health promotion programs that defend against cell transformation include: (Select all that apply.)
    a. smoking cessation.
    b. Pap smears.
    c. colonoscopy.
    d. monitoring of moles.

19. When cancers cells are graded, the report might say "tumor cells are well-differentiated." What does this mean?

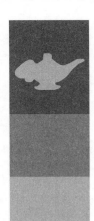

CHAPTER 17

Clients with Cancer

CHAPTER OBJECTIVES

17.1   Define *primary* and *secondary prevention* as they relate to cancer prevention.
17.2   Describe primary and secondary prevention activities.
17.3   Differentiate cancer prevention and cancer screening.
17.4   Describe cancer prevention and screening activities for specific cancer conditions.
17.5   Discuss the ability to achieve wellness, or tertiary prevention, during cancer treatment.
17.6   Identify aspects of the medical outcomes management of cancer.
17.7   Discuss surgery, radiation therapy, chemotherapy, biotherapy, and other treatment modalities for cancer.
17.8   Discuss myelosuppression, GI effects, skin effects, and reproductive effects of treatment modalities on the cancer patient.
17.9   Describe the urgency of oncologic emergencies that can result in death if not detected early.
17.10 Discuss the need for support for the client and family during cancer diagnosis and treatment.

UNDERSTANDING PATHOPHYSIOLOGY

1. Risk factors associated with many cancers include: (Select all that apply.)
    1. smoking.
    2. dietary habits.
    3. alcohol consumption.
    4. ingestion of proteins.

2. The American Cancer Society recommends that women perform monthly breast self-examination beginning at age _____.

3. True or False

    _____ Lung cancer is the leading cause of cancer deaths among Americans.

    _____ Colorectal cancer has a higher incidence in men.

    _____ African-American men have the highest incidence of prostate cancer in the world.

    _____ Women are at greater risk of head and neck cancer than men.

4. The main objective of chemotherapy is to _____ _____ _____.

5. Clinical manifestations of an immediate hypersensitivity reaction include: (Select all that apply.)
    1. dyspnea.
    2. chest tightness.
    3. pruritus.
    4. urticaria.
    5. tachycardia, dizziness.

6. Cancer staging is the process of determining the extent of disease as the basis for treatment decisions. It is called _____ and is defined as ____ = _____, ____ = _____ _____, and ____ = _____ _____.

APPLYING SKILLS

7. Tests and procedures used in early detection of cancers include: (Select all that apply.)
   1. mammograms.
   2. Pap smears.
   3. endoscopy.
   4. radiologic imaging studies.

8. True or False

   _____ The Pap smear detects cancer in a pre-malignant stage.

9. Side effects of radiation therapy include: (Select all that apply.)
   1. skin reactions.
   2. fatigue.
   3. diarrhea.
   4. nausea and vomiting.
   5. esophagitis and dysphagia.

10. _____ is the cardinal sign of an infection in a client with cancer.

BEST PRACTICES

11. True or False

    _____ The American Cancer Society recommends that cervical cancer screening begin 3 years after the onset of vaginal intercourse, but no later than the age of 21.

    _____ The U.S. Nuclear Regulatory Commission requires that radiation exposure of people be kept as low as reasonably achievable.

12. The first actions taken by the nurse when a hypersensitivity reaction occurs after drug administration include: (Select all that apply.)
    1. immediately stopping drug administration.
    2. maintaining IV access with 0.9% normal saline.
    3. maintaining airway.
    4. taking the client's temperature.

13. The three key principles that the nurse should follow to protect him- or herself and others from excessive radiation exposure are _____ _____, _____, and _____.

14. The physician may prescribe _____ _____ to elevate or maintain the erythrocyte level and decrease the need for transfusions.

15. Decisions made at the time of first diagnosis of cancer are crucial because _____ _____ _____.

16. Cytological specimens are best obtained _____ _____ _____ _____.

17. Surgery is not always the first phase of treatment for cancer clients. Many treatment protocols begin with _____ _____ or _____ _____.

18. Vascular access devices (VAD) are used during initial treatment of cancer clients who require: (Select all that apply.)
    1. continuous chemotherapy.
    2. multiple access.
    3. parenteral fluids.
    4. antibiotics.
    5. frequent blood testing.

KEEPING DRUG SKILLS SHARP

19. Combination chemotherapeutic agents are used to: (Select all that apply.)
    1. destroy more malignant cells.
    2. produce fewer side effects.
    3. strike cancer cells at different points in the cell cycle.
    4. individualize complex regimens.

20. When administering chemotherapeutic agents, which of the following steps are critical? (Select all that apply.)
    1. Verification of the drug
    2. Verification of the dose of drug
    3. Verification of schedule of drug
    4. Verification by two nurses against written orders

21. The most common complications of vascular access devices for use with chemotherapy are _____ and _____.

22. Medication administration during chemotherapy has greatly improved with advent of: (Select all that apply.)
    1. serotonin receptor antagonists.
    2. Zofran.
    3. Kytril.
    4. Anzemet.

23. Radiation therapy is frequently employed to kill residual cancer cells left behind after _____ _____.

24. Chemotherapy doses are usually based on: (Select all that apply.)
    1. body surface area in square meters (m²).
    2. client's height and weight.
    3. client's last hemoglobin.
    4. previous chemotherapy orders.

25. _____ is the term used for when some of the drug escapes from the vein.

26. True or False

    _____ Corticosteroids used in many treatment protocols can leave a client vulnerable to cancer-associated infections because they suppress immune functions.

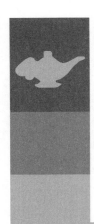

CHAPTER 18

Clients with Wounds

CHAPTER OBJECTIVES

18.1   Describe wound healing including necessary components of the healing process.
18.2   Relate the phases of the wound healing process to the outcome of the healing process.
18.3   Distinguish primary, secondary, and tertiary wound healing intention.
18.4   Relate intrinsic and extrinsic factors of wound healing to wound healing intention.
18.5   Describe the desired outcomes of medical, surgical, and nursing management of acute or chronic inflammation, incisions, open wounds, delayed wound healing, wound infections, wound dehiscence, or other nonhealing wounds.
18.6   Identify compartment syndrome as an emergent condition requiring immediate treatment.

UNDERSTANDING PATHOPHYSIOLOGY

1.   The first component necessary for proper wound healing to occur is: (Select all that apply.)
    1.   vascular response.
    2.   nutrition.
    3.   antibiotic therapy.
    4.   oxygen.

2.   Compare and contrast the activities that occur in each of the four phases of wound healing.

Phase	Activity
Vascular	
Inflammation	
Proliferative	
Maturation	

3. Capillary dilation increases blood flow to the site of injury and: (Select all that apply.)
   1. delivers more carbon dioxide to the area.
   2. delivers more nutrients to the area.
   3. carries phagocytes away from the area.
   4. dilutes toxins secreted by invading organisms.

4. Increased numbers of _____ _____ indicate a bacterial invasion as the bone marrow releases immature cells to combat the infection.

5. Chronic wounds that do not heal are said to have an imbalance of _____ _____.

6. True or False

   _____ Wound remodeling can take over a year to complete.

   _____ Scar tissue is stronger than original tissue because it is thicker.

   _____ Eosinophils secrete antihistamine and basophils secrete histamine.

   _____ Kinins decrease vascular permeability to control excessive bleeding at the site of injury.

   _____ Neutrophils can squeeze through the lining of a capillary wall through a process called diapedesis.

   _____ "No inflammation, no healing."

   _____ Platelets release growth factors to stimulate healing.

   _____ Inflammation does not occur when dead cells are present.

   _____ Neutrophils can handle up to 100,000 bacteria invading a wound.

   _____ Angiogenesis is a process which assists platelets to stop bleeding.

   _____ An obese client with a large wound should have carbohydrate calorie restrictions but sufficient protein intake.

   _____ Autolytic debridement can be used with infected wounds less than 5 cm.

   _____ Hyperalimentation is sometimes used to facilitate wound healing.

   _____ The key to prevention of pressure ulcers is turning and repositioning.

   _____ Clean sandwich baggies can be used as alternative gloves by clients doing dressing changes in their homes.

   _____ To obtain appropriate wound culture specimens, remove the exudate and then swab the wound bed.

7. Identify each type of wound healing as primary, secondary, or tertiary intention.

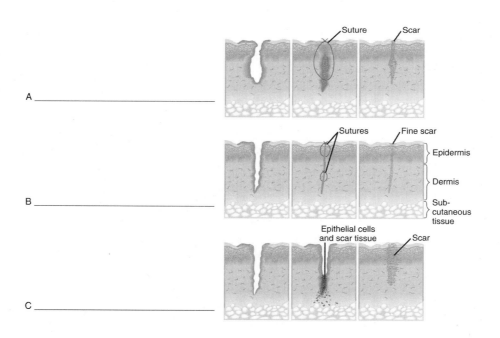

A _____

B _____

C _____

8. Identify the pathologic effects of each factor on wound healing.

Factor	Effect
Diabetes mellitus	
Lack of vitamin C	
Neuropathy	
Foreign bodies	
Protein malnutrition	
Smoking	

9. Why is inflammatory exudate from a wound considered helpful?

10. Nutritional impairment can delay wound healing. The lab value indicative of the nutritional status of the client is the _____ _____.

APPLYING SKILLS

11. Purulent exudate from a wound is a manifestation of _____.

12. A nurse must check for an edematous area on a client's leg to monitor for increased swelling. Identify the appropriate action to ensure accurate measurements.

13. Prior to beginning a dressing change, the nurse should assess the client's _____ _____.

14. True or False

_____ Exudate from a wound can help in the healing process.

_____ A blister is an example of a serous exudate.

_____ Low-grade fever should be treated with antipyretics.

_____ When assessing edema, the nurse should use the uninvolved side as a baseline.

_____ Surgical incisions normally appear pink and swollen.

_____ Proper wound healing includes an internal scar known as a "healing ridge."

_____ Eschar helps to protect wound during the healing process.

15. Compare and/or contrast the types of wound appearance and the clinical significance of these assessment findings.

Wound Appearance	Clinical Significance
Edges approximated	
Open wound, edges apart	
Healing ridge under skin	
Serous exudates	
Purulent exudates	
Eschar	
Granuloma	

BEST PRACTICES

16. State the rationale for applying ice only for the first 24 to 72 hours to the site of an injury, then following it with heat.

17. When teaching a client how to care for a surgical incision, the nurse should emphasize all of the following *except*:
    1. clinical manifestations of infection.
    2. how to care for and empty the drain reservoir.
    3. use of water to cleanse a suture line.
    4. when to return for suture removal.

18. Define the methods of debridement.

Method	Procedure
Sharp	
Mechanical	
Enzymatic	
Autolytic	

19. A _____ solution is recommended as safe for wound care.

20. Identify the action the nurse would perform to enhance the effect of enzymatic ointment on dry, thick eschar over a wound.

KEEPING DRUG SKILLS SHARP

21. A client who is taking steroids is at risk for developing infections. Identify the mechanism for the increased risk.

22. True or False

_____ Diabetic clients with wounds should maintain blood glucose levels below 200 mg/dl to promote proper wound healing.

_____ Glucocorticoids help reduce inflammation and speed wound healing.

_____ Carbon monoxide is a vasoconstrictive agent that slows blood supply to the wound site and delays healing.

_____ Vitamin C in high doses is harmful to a wound due to its acidic content.

_____ NSAIDs can be used to reduce inflammation in wounds.

CONCEPT MAP EXERCISES

The following questions are based on the concept map *Understanding Inflammation and Its Treatment* in your textbook.

23. How does the "RICE" treatment affect the inflammatory process?

24. How do NSAIDs reduce inflammation?

25. Steroids are given to block the release of _____ from mast cells.

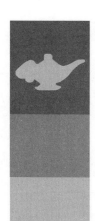

CHAPTER **19**

Perspectives on Infectious Disease and Bioterrorism

CHAPTER OBJECTIVES

19.1   Examine the historical perspective on infectious disease and bioterrorism.

19.2   Identify terminology related to the infectious process.

19.3   Describe the infectious process including a discussion on the agent, environment, and host.

19.4   Discuss the meaning of being a carrier of the pathogen.

19.5   Describe the different routes of transmission of pathogens.

19.6   Identify the lines of defense of the host.

19.7   Discuss the occurrence of the most common nosocomial infections.

19.8   Identify the most common pathogens in nosocomial infections.

19.9   Discuss additional pathogens that cause nosocomial infections.

19.10   Discuss the concept of drug resistance related to nosocomial infections.

19.11   Examine strategies of handwashing and alcohol-based hand rubs for prevention of infections in hospitals.

19.12   Examine strategies such as disinfection, sterilization, or anti-infective drugs to control transmission of pathogens.

19.13   Discuss immunization and its impact on infectious disease transmission.

19.14   Differentiate Standard Precautions from transmission-based infection control precautions.

19.15   Describe the OHSA blood-borne pathogens standard.

19.16   Discuss infection control in long-term care and community-based settings.

19.17   Describe the events that have led to concerns about bioterrorism.

19.18   Describe the specific agents that might be used in biologic warfare.

19.19   Discuss the pandemic influenza plan.

UNDERSTANDING PATHOPHYSIOLOGY

1.   Factors that resulted in the dramatic decrease of infectious diseases during the period from 1950 to 1980 include: (Select all that apply.)
   1. social, public health, and medical control efforts.
   2. environmental sanitation.
   3. international vaccination programs.
   4. restraint in prescribing antibiotics.
   5. development of new anti-infectives.

2.   Factors that have resulted in a steady increase in infectious diseases since the 1980s include: (Select all that apply.)
   1. new infectious agents.
   2. decreasing vaccination rates.
   3. increasing populations of chronically ill, malnourished, and immunocompromised clients.
   4. restraint in prescribing antibiotics.

3. List the common reservoirs for infection.
   a.

   b.

   c.

   d.

   e.

   f.

4. Explain why the identification of a "carrier" is of critical importance in controlling infection.

5. Portals of entry for a pathogen into a new host include: (Select all that apply.)
   1. ingestion.
   2. exhalation.
   3. contact with mucous membranes.
   4. the percutaneous route.
   5. the transplacental route.

6. How can ethnicity be considered a factor which might increase the susceptibility of a client to disease?

7. First-line defenses against infection include all of the following *except*:
   1. gag and cough reflexes.
   2. inflammatory response.
   3. peristalsis in GI tract.
   4. flushing action by tears and saliva.

8. Invasion of an organism that allows replication without clinical manifestation or detectable immune response is referred to as _____ _____.

9. The period of time during which a pathogen is replicating but before it is shed from the host is called the _____.

10. The _____ is the period of time from invasion of the disease to appearance of clinical manifestations.

11. Common nosocomial infections that health care workers are at particular risk for contracting include: (Select all that apply.)
    1. HIV.
    2. hepatitis B.
    3. pneumonia.
    4. tuberculosis.

12. True or False
    _____ The entire population needs to be immune to prevent disease epidemic.
    _____ Herd immunity decreases the likelihood of disease transmission.

13. Common portals of exit for infectious diseases include: (Select all that apply.)
    1. bodily secretions.
    2. body fluids.
    3. exhaled air.
    4. excretions (urine and feces).
    5. open lesions.
    6. exudates from wounds.

APPLYING SKILLS

14. Describe for each category of clients how their risk for developing nosocomial respiratory infections occurs.

Category	Etiology
Postoperative	
Diminished consciousness	
Impaired gag reflex	
Intubation	
Tracheostomy	
Old age	
Chronic lung disease	
Cardiac disease	
Renal insufficiency	
Malignancies	

15. True or False

_____ Bioterrorism is the intentional use of viruses, bacteria, and other germs as weapons in war or other conflicts.

_____ Bioterrorism preparedness includes assuring that the public health system can respond to biologic warfare emergencies.

_____ Category A agents pose the least risk to national security if used in biologic warfare.

_____ Inhalation anthrax is at the top of the terrorism threat list.

_____ Anthrax symptoms include fever and cough and are difficult to diagnose.

_____ Smallpox and the plague are completely treatable and less threatening as biologic warfare agents.

_____ Botulism causes muscle paralysis of the respiratory muscles.

_____ Hemorrhagic fever viruses can be disseminated by aerosols and produce clinical manifestations in 2 to 21 days.

BEST PRACTICES

16. Explain why it is important for the nurse to recognize subclinical infectious states when caring for clients.

17. State the rationale for discontinuing the practice of preoperative shaving of the surgical site.

18. A _____ dressing placed over an insertion site may contribute to the development of an infection because it allows for growth of normal skin flora.

19. _____ and the use of _____ hand rubs are the most effective ways to prevent the spread of infection.

20. List the common protective barriers used by health care workers to prevent transmission of infection.

    a.

    b.

    c.

    d.

21. List three transmission-based client care precautions for clients with known infections to contain transmission.

    a.

    b.

    c.

22. Health care institutions are required by JCAHO to reduce the risk of institutionally acquired infections. Select from the following list the JCAHO requirements.
    1. Following CDC hand hygiene guidelines
    2. Administering flu and pneumococcus vaccines to those who have not had them previously
    3. Reporting fatal infections
    4. Denying admission to those with communicable disease

KEEPING DRUG SKILLS SHARP

23. The mechanisms that allow bacteria to develop resistance to antibiotics include all of the following *except*:
    1. producing an enzyme that will inactivate or destroy the antibiotic.
    2. altering the target site to evade action of the antibiotic.
    3. overprescribing penicillin.
    4. preventing antibiotic access to the target site on bacterium.

24. Measures to reduce the incidence of antimicrobial resistance include: (Select all that apply.)
    1. obtaining appropriate specimens for culture before starting antibiotics.
    2. checking sensitivity reports to ensure antibiotic is appropriate.
    3. thorough handwashing.
    4. strict aseptic techniques.
    5. use of barrier precautions.

25. True or False

    _____ Tetanus boosters are due every 10 years after the primary series.

    _____ Women of childbearing age should avoid immunizations for rubella.

    _____ A child who has had a varicella infection does not need the immunization.

    _____ Influenza vaccine is recommended for people older than 65, nursing home residents, and people with chronic cardiac or pulmonary disorders.

    _____ Pertussis vaccine is given only after age 60 to prevent complications.

    _____ People born before 1957 have natural immunity to measles, mumps, and rubella.

    _____ Older people need vaccinations because of a decline in their immune system function.

    _____ OSHA requires all employers to provide hepatitis B vaccination to at-risk employees at the employer's expense.

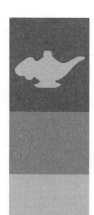

CHAPTER 20

Clients with Pain

CHAPTER OBJECTIVES

20.1　Define *pain*.
20.2　Identify sources of nociceptive stimuli.
20.3　Distinguish acute and chronic pain, including characteristics, descriptors, and physical responses.
20.4　Identify types of chronic pain.
20.5　Compare cutaneous, somatic, and visceral pain.
20.6　Describe other types of pain such as neuropathic, breakthrough, psychogenic, and phantom limb sensation.
20.7　Identify factors that will affect a client's perception of pain.
20.8　Describe the desired outcomes of medical management of pain.
20.9　Identify medications to control pain including administration methods, factors related to administration, and important assessments during medication administration.
20.10　Describe the desired outcomes of nursing management of pain.
20.11　Distinguish administration of medications for pain and assessment of response in older clients.
20.12　Identify nonpharmacologic interventions for pain.
20.13　Identify important evaluation and documentation information related to pain management.

UNDERSTANDING PATHOPHYSIOLOGY

1.　Explain how pain can be beneficial to the client.

2.　Describe nociception and relate it to the pain mechanism.

3.　Compare and contrast the characteristics of acute pain and chronic pain.

Type	Characteristics
Acute pain	
Chronic pain	

4. Identify examples of each type of chronic pain.
   a. Persistent:

   b. Intermittent:

   c. Malignant:

5. Identify the three classifications for sources of pain in the body and give examples of each.
   a.

   b.

   c.

6. True or False

   _____ Cutaneous pain tends to be diffuse, poorly localized, and vague.

   _____ Somatic pain is poorly localized and may cause nausea.

   _____ Skeletal muscle is sensitive to stretching and ischemia which will cause pain.

   _____ Pain from deep structures may radiate from the primary site, such as lumbar disk pain radiating to the sciatic nerve.

   _____ Pain in the GI tract is the result of inflammation, ulcers, or muscle spasms.

7. _____ pain is a form of visceral pain that is felt in an area distal to the site of the pain stimulus, such as myocardial ischemia.

8. List the factors that affect how pain is perceived.
   a.

   b.

   c.

   d.

   e.

   f.

   g.

   h.

9. Differentiate between pain threshold and pain tolerance.

10. Factors that affect the duration of action of pain medications include: (Select all that apply.)
    1. pain intensity.
    2. route of administration.
    3. dose size.
    4. the client's ability to absorb, biotransform, and eliminate medication.

11. The _____ provides pain relief by delivering electrical bursts through the skin which mask the pain signals to the brain.

APPLYING YOUR KNOWLEDGE

12. Margo McCaffery's definition of pain is "whatever the experiencing person says it is and existing whenever the person says it does." Explain how this definition affects a nurse's assessment of a client in pain.

13. Clients can undergo behavioral changes when experiencing pain for prolonged periods of time. Common characteristics of clients experiencing chronic pain syndrome include: (Select all that apply.)
    1. depression.
    2. fatigue.
    3. limited function.
    4. poor sleep.
    5. drastically increased activity level.

14. Clients may exhibit which of the following behaviors in an attempt to adapt to pain? (Select all that apply.)
    1. Guarding the painful area
    2. Showing a blank expression
    3. Exhibiting decreased activity
    4. Reporting pain frequently
    5. Increased physical activity
    6. Exhibiting sleepiness
    7. Reporting pain only if asked
    8. Showing painful expressions

15. List five standards for pain management as stated by various policy and accrediting organizations (e.g., the Joint Commission).
    a.

    b.

    c.

    d.

    e.

16. Identify the single most important indicator of pain intensity.

17. The _____ scale is more appropriate for assessing pain in children than numerical or visual descriptor scales.

18. Critical factors to determine when assessing pain in clients include: (Select all that apply.)
    1. location.
    2. quality.
    3. duration.
    4. distress.

BEST PRACTICES

19. State the nurse's role as part of the health care team in addressing pain relief needs for the client.

20. List two responsibilities of the nurse to correct misinformation about pain.
    a.

    b.

21. True or False

    _____ The health care team can determine a person's pain tolerance level.

    _____ Past experience with pain can alter a client's perception of pain.

_____ Many health care providers believe that the amount of pain can be based on a medical condition.

_____ Pain perception does not depend exclusively on the degree of physical damage.

22. Identify four nursing interventions to assist the client in pain in addition to providing pain medication.
    a.

    b.

    c.

    d.

23. The nurse should not identify complete pain relief as a realistic outcome for a client with _____ pain.

24. Identify an independent action the nurse can implement to relieve pain.

KEEPING DRUG SKILLS SHARP

25. List the three steps of the "pain ladder" developed by the World Health Organization.
    a.

    b.

    c.

26. Neurolytic agents are used for nerve blocks typically only for extreme unrelieved pain of a _____ _____.

27. _____ are only used with caution for HIV clients because of reports of cross-reaction with acetaminophen drugs used to treat the HIV infection.

28. The ceiling for maximum dosage of morphine that can be administered to clients with pain is

_____

_____.

29. Describe the characteristics of the common anesthetic agents lidocaine and bupivacaine.

Agent	Characteristics
Lidocaine	
Bupivacaine	

30. Application of _____ 45 minutes to 1 hour prior to the site of venipuncture, injection, or heel sticks will reduce pain by providing local anesthesia.

31. True or False

_____ Side effects of opioid analgesics such as nausea and vomiting subside with increased use of the analgesics.

32. List three interventions used to treat constipation as a side effect of opioid analgesics.
a.

b.

c.

33. Morphine is a powerful opioid that can cause respiratory depression. Identify the time frames for the nurse to assess respiratory status after administering morphine via the following routes:

IV:

IM:

SC:

Epidural:

34. For each type of adjuvant medication, identify the medication category and indication for use.

Medication	Category	Indication
Tegretol		
Dilantin		
Neurontin		
Decadron		
Lioresal		

35. List the two nontraditional routes of administration that have been developed for fentanyl (long-acting morphine).

    a.

    b.

36. Explain the advantage of patient-controlled analgesia (PCA) over PRN administration of pain medication by the nurse.

37. Oral and subcutaneous doses must be _____ IV preparations.
    1. less than
    2. the same as
    3. higher than

38. Explain how peak analgesic effect impacts nursing care for the client in pain.

39. Factors to be assessed before analgesic administration include:
    a.

    b.

    c.

    d.

    e.

40. True or False

    _____ All of the medications to treat pain can be used with older clients.

    _____ Confusion and delirium as adverse effects of opioids may occur quickly in the older client and are best prevented with oral opioids or nonopioids.

    _____ Smaller doses of analgesic drugs may produce adverse effects in older clients.

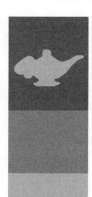

CHAPTER **21**

Perspectives in Palliative Care

CHAPTER OBJECTIVES

21.1 Examine American perspectives on dying.
21.2 Discuss palliative care as well as hospice care as a model.
21.3 Discuss quality of life as it relates to palliative care.
21.4 Relate the concept of disease trajectory to diseases at the end of life.
21.5 Discuss symptoms at the end of life and the appropriate nursing care and drug therapy to alleviate the symptoms.
21.6 Discuss the concept of dehydration at the end of life.
21.7 Discuss signs of imminent death.
21.8 Describe communication with clients and families during the dying process.
21.9 Describe how the nurse cares for caregivers and supports a grieving family.

UNDERSTANDING PATHOPHYSIOLOGY

1. List the five phases of the normal death and dying experience as identified and defined by Elizabeth Kübler-Ross.

   a.

   b.

   c.

   d.

   e.

2. State the focus of palliative care.

3. The chronic diseases that are major causes of death in the United States include: (Select all that apply.)
   1. heart disease.
   2. cancer.
   3. stroke.
   4. COPD.
   5. dementia.

4. Identify four factors that contribute to a definition of quality of life.

   a.

   b.

   c.

   d.

5. Possible *reversible* causes for delirium are: (Select all that apply.)
   1. medications (especially opioids), sedatives.
   2. hypoxia.
   3. dehydration.
   4. metabolic causes (hyponatremia).
   5. sepsis.
   6. polypharmacy.
   7. increased ICP from metastatic disease.

6. Provide examples of the common causes of fatigue in the hospice client.

Problem	Example
Disease/treatment-related	
Physiologic	
Psycho-emotional	
Spiritual	

APPLYING SKILLS

7. A client's _____ is determined by a thorough history and physical evaluation of the client's status and wants/desires.

8. The most effective instrument for assessing changes in cognitive status is the _____
_____
_____.

9. Clinical manifestations that occur during the active dying process include: (Select all that apply.)
   1. decrease in urinary output; urinary retention or incontinence.
   2. increase in anxiety.
   3. mottling of skin color with peripheral cyanosis.
   4. tachypnea or Cheyne-Stokes respirations.
   5. impaired swallowing, loss of gag reflex.
   6. delirium, altered cognition.
   7. acute confusion, anxiety.

10. The sense of _____ remains intact throughout the dying process.

11. A 72-year-old grandmother has been diagnosed with metastatic breast cancer and has been told her prognosis is less than 6 months. Her family is concerned with her increasing fatigue and wants to reduce her pain medication dosages to allow her to interact more with the family when they visit. Explain how can the nurse differentiate between effects of medications and true fatigue

to help maintain the client's comfort level and improve the quality of family interactions.

12. A client has been battling liver cancer for over a year and has begun to show clinical manifestations of an active dying process. Identify the clinical presentations the hospice nurse would observe to indicate an active dying process rather than a stable chronic condition.

BEST PRACTICES

13. Nursing interventions to assist the client with dyspnea include: (Select all that apply.)
   1. calming presence.
   2. breathing exercises.
   3. a fan blowing in room.
   4. relaxation therapy.
   5. offering cold fluids.
   6. incentive spirometer therapy.
   7. massage.
   8. pursed-lip breathing.

14. Nursing interventions to correct reversible causes of fatigue include all of the following *except*:
    1. administering prescribed transfusions or erythropoietin to correct anemia.
    2. counseling, education, and relaxation and massage to address stress.
    3. limiting fluid intake.
    4. modifying activity and rest patterns.
    5. administering prescribed corticosteroids to lessen effects of tumor-induced substances and increase appetite.
    6. administering prescribed psychostimulants to increase energy.

15. Identify nursing interventions to assist the client and his or her family cope with the last days of life.
    a.

    b.

    c.

    d.

16. List the four tasks of mourning for conclusion of bereavement.
    a.

    b.

    c.

    d.

KEEPING DRUG SKILLS SHARP

17. Common opioids used to provide pain relief include: (Select all that apply.)
    1. morphine.
    2. amitriptyline.
    3. hydromorphone.
    4. fentanyl.

18. The maximum amount of opioid that can be administered to a hospice client is _____ _____.

19. Compare and contrast common adjuvant medications used in hospice care.

Medication	Action	Indication
NSAIDs		
Tricyclic antidepressants and anticonvulsants		
Anticholinergics		
Benzodiazepines		

20. True or False

_____ Therapeutic levels of analgesics must be maintained at all times for clients with persistent or chronic pain.

_____ Around-the-clock scheduling of medications is the most appropriate for hospice clients.

_____ Immediate-release oral morphine should be given every 5–6 hours as needed.

_____ Controlled-release medications may be given every 8, 12, or 24 hours.

_____ Short-acting medications should be given to cover a spike in the client's pain.

_____ A client experiencing pain 2 hours after a rescue dose should wait until the next scheduled dose to prevent oversedation and respiratory depression.

_____ Morphine is used to relieve dyspnea (difficulty breathing).

21. _____ is the drug of choice for hallucinations.

22. Medications used for sleep disturbances include all of the following *except*:
    1. zolpidem (Ambien).
    2. flurazepam (Dalmane).
    3. oxazepam (Serax).
    4. oxycontin (Oxycodone).
    5. temazepam (Restoril).

23. _____ are effective medications for treating smooth muscle spasms.

24. Clients with neuropathic pain described as "shooting," "burning," or "shock-like" can be treated with _____ medications.

25. If an intracranial tumor causes increased pressure, _____ would be effective in reducing the edema.

26. Occasionally, because of agitation from morphine metabolites or other reasons, morphine will need to be changed to another medication. To assure the same or better pain control, the dosage must be _____ .

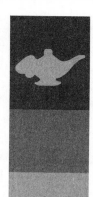

CHAPTER **22**

Clients with Sleep and Rest Disorders and Fatigue

CHAPTER OBJECTIVES

22.1 Describe the impact of sleep disorders on the general population.
22.2 Differentiate the two major classifications of sleep disorders.
22.3 Define *sleep pattern disturbance*.
22.4 Discuss chronobiology as it relates to sleep alterations and drug administration.
22.5 Describe outcomes management for the sleep disorders.
22.6 Relate various medication use for sleep disorders.
22.7 Discuss disorders that contribute to sleep alterations.
22.8 Identify the diagnostic assessment for sleep disorders.
22.9 Discuss nursing assessment, diagnoses, outcomes, and interventions for sleep disorders.
22.10 Explain sleep hygiene to clients with sleep disorders.
22.11 Describe chronic fatigue and chronic fatigue syndrome, including the clinical manifestations and nursing interventions.

UNDERSTANDING PATHOPHYSIOLOGY

1. True or False

    _____ Sleep is a normal state of altered consciousness during which the body rests.

    _____ Inadequate sleep hygiene can contribute to transitory periods of insomnia.

    _____ Narcolepsy is characterized by excessive daytime sleepiness and is not associated with disturbed nocturnal sleep.

    _____ Nightmares are parasomnias associated with REM sleep.

    _____ Fatigue is a subjective state in which the client feels a sense of physical exhaustion but is mentally rested.

2. Characteristics of sleep and sleep pattern disturbances include: (Select all that apply.)
    1. during a given year, approximately half of the population has some problem.
    2. sleep disturbances may be secondary to environmental stressors.
    3. sleep disturbances have a reciprocal relationship to underlying illness and disorders.
    4. sleep pattern disturbance is always transitory.

3. All of the following are polysomnography parameters of sleep *except*:
    1. brain wave activity.
    2. eye movements.
    3. respiratory rate and depth.
    4. muscle tone.

4. Psychophysiologic insomnia is associated with increased physiologic response to _____
    _____.

5. Cataplexy is best described as:
   1. excessive daytime sleepiness.
   2. a circadian rhythm in the sleep cycle.
   3. the time it takes to fully awaken from a sleep cycle.
   4. a loss of muscle tone at times of unexpected emotion.

6. List the three associated factors with obstructive sleep apnea syndrome in adults.
   a.

   b.

   c.

7. List and briefly describe the three circadian rhythm sleep disorders.
   a.

   b.

   c.

8. Sleep disorders are often secondary to other medical or psychological problems. List the three primary neurotransmitter imbalances associated with sleep disorders and briefly discuss each.
   a.

   b.

   c.

9. Match each hormonal imbalance with the appropriate description of the sleep pattern disturbance associated with it.

Hormonal Imbalance

_____ a. Hyperthyroidism
_____ b. Hypothyroidism
_____ c. Diabetes mellitus
_____ d. Premenstrual syndrome
_____ e. Menopause
_____ f. Postmenopausal

Description

1. Less slow-wave sleep
2. Nightmares and early morning headaches
3. Snoring and obstructive sleep apnea
4. Fragmented, short sleep periods
5. Excessive sleepiness
6. Poor sleep quality and mood changes

10. An internal stimuli that contributes to sleep fragmentation is:
    1. nocturnal temperature.
    2. bruxism.
    3. the urge to void.
    4. room light.

11. State the factors that contribute to sleep deprivation in clients in a critical care unit.

12. Defining characteristics of chronic fatigue include: (Select all that apply.)
    1. verbalization of a lack of energy.
    2. disruption of usual routines.
    3. emotional stability.
    4. increased libido.
    5. accident-proneness.

APPLYING SKILLS

13. True or False

    _____ Chronobiology is the study of biologic changes as they occur in relation to time.

14. A nurse who is planning care would anticipate a sleep pattern disturbance during hospitalization in which of the following clients because of altered circadian rhythms?
    1. 20-year-old male
    2. 35-year-old female
    3. 45-year-old female
    4. 75-year-old male

15. What factors that influence sleep patterns in older adults should the nurse consider when planning care?

16. Clients who experience early morning awakenings should be screened for _____ _____.

17. The primary diagnostic test for sleep disorders is _____.

18. What visible signs of sleep disorder should the nurse observe for during the physical assessment?

Case Study

A client is being evaluated for a possible sleep disorder. The client is a male, age 49 years, height 5'10", weight 254 lbs. His chief complaint is that he feels tired in the morning when he wakes up, "Like I haven't been to sleep at all. But my wife says I had to have been sleeping because my snoring is keeping her awake." The client states that he had seen a physician about 6 months ago and was given a prescription for a benzodiazepine for "anxiety." When questioned further, the client states that he doesn't think the medicine has helped; if anything, he feels worse. When asked if there were other things the client was concerned about, he stated that he was having trouble maintaining an erection during intercourse. The client's history and physical exam is unremarkable, although the nurse notes that his neck is short and thick and that he drinks 1 or 2 beers 3 or 4 nights a week.

19. What factors place this client at risk for obstructive sleep apnea syndrome?

20. What clinical manifestations does the client present which suggest obstructive sleep apnea syndrome?

21. What in the client's history should the nurse report to the physician immediately and why?

A diagnosis of Obstructive sleep apnea syndrome is made. The client is encouraged to lose weight, reduce or cease consumption of alcohol, and use CPAP during sleep.

22. What is the rationale for encouraging the client to decrease alcohol consumption?

23. What should the nurse teach the client about CPAP?

BEST PRACTICES

24. Based on an understanding of external stimuli that cause sleep disturbance, a nurse working the night shift would plan to awaken clients (if necessary) not any more frequently than every _____ minutes.

25. The nurse is caring for a client with psychophysiologic insomnia. Which of the following nursing interventions should the nurse implement to promote sleep?
    1. Introduce the client to relaxation exercises and have him or her initially practice them at bedtime.
    2. Allow the client to vary time of rising to accommodate periods of unrest.
    3. Allow the client to take short power naps during the day.
    4. Combine sleep hygiene education and cognitive restructuring of beliefs about sleep.

26. Appropriate interventions for a client with narcolepsy include: (Select all that apply.)
    1. emphasize good sleep hygiene.
    2. allow variation in the sleep schedule.
    3. provide naps at preset times in the awake cycle.
    4. plan naps for periods associated with sleepiness.
    5. develop a safety plan to cope with potential disruptions.

27. A client with seasonal affective disorder (SAD) asks the nurse to explain why she needs to buy a special light and can't use the floor lamp. What explanation should the nurse provide?

28. Explain what precautions the nurse should take with clients who experience REM-associated erections and also have an indwelling catheter.

29. List the nursing interventions the nurse can implement to assist hospitalized clients with sleep onset difficulty.
    a.

    b.

    c.

    d.

30. Explain why the client with chronic fatigue syndrome should be taught to balance periods of gentle activity with frequent rest periods.

KEEPING DRUG SKILLS SHARP

31. Based on an understanding of chronopharmacology, a nurse would anticipate that clients receiving continuous intravenous heparin would have a greater risk of bleeding in the _____ _____.

32. Explain why antidepressants are part of the treatment for narcolepsy.

33. Explain the rationale for prescribing skeletal muscle relaxants for clients with periodic limb movement disorder.

34. Initial pharmacotherapy for clients with chronic fatigue syndrome who are experiencing pain would be:
    1. antihistamines.
    2. sedatives.
    3. antidepressants.
    4. anti-inflammatory agents.

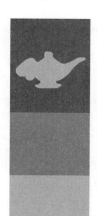

CHAPTER 23

Clients with Psychosocial and Mental Health Concerns

CHAPTER OBJECTIVES

23.1 Relate psychosocial and mental health concerns to clients in all nursing care settings.

23.2 Relate anxiety, schizophrenia, and mood disorders to patients with medical-surgical conditions.

23.3 Explain reasons that anxiety, stress, coping, and self-esteem affect all clients.

23.4 Describe the biologic and psychological etiology of mental disorders.

23.5 Explain outcomes management for medical-surgical clients with anxiety, schizophrenia, and mood disorders.

23.6 Apply assessment, communication, education, and referral strategies as interventions in the care of the medical-surgical client.

UNDERSTANDING PATHOPHYSIOLOGY

1. It is important for the nurse to understand the psychological and social aspects of a client's health because: (Select all that apply.)
   1. physical health may be altered by underlying psychological processes.
   2. the stress of physical illness may alter a client's normal emotional response.
   3. social abilities may alter a client's ability to negotiate the health care delivery system.
   4. the manner in which clients respond psychologically to physical illness may vary.

2. List the four universal psychosocial concepts and related factors which influence response to stressors.
   a.

   b.

   c.

   d.

3. Anxiety is:
   1. a strong feeling of fear or dread with an unknown cause.
   2. a phenomenon occurring between a person and the environment which endangers well-being.
   3. a response to a stressor that is emotion-focused.
   4. an unconscious response to a stressor.

4. Compare and contrast emotion-focused and problem-focused coping behavior.

5. Match each type of self-esteem with the typical client response.

Type of Self-Esteem

_____ a. High self-esteem

_____ b. Low self-esteem

Typical Response

1. Consistently pessimistic
2. Positive expectations

6. Identify the two causes of psychiatric disorders and briefly explain each.

7. A positive clinical manifestation of schizophrenia is:
   1. blunted affect.
   2. avoidance of social contact.
   3. auditory hallucination.
   4. lack of attention to hygiene.

8. Match each clinical manifestation associated with mood disorders with the appropriate type of disorder (answers may be used more than once).

Clinical Manifestation

_____ a. Sad mood

_____ b. Decreased sexual interest

_____ c. Negative thinking

_____ d. Change in sleep pattern

_____ e. Rapid speech

_____ f. Crying spells

_____ g. Increased energy

_____ h. Impulsive behavior

Type of Disorder

1. Depressive mood disorder
2. Mania

9. A typical manifestation of a client with a depressive-type mood disorder is:
   1. an overabundance of energy.
   2. an optimistic attitude.
   3. increased motivation.
   4. hopelessness.

10. Major depressive disorders are characterized by: (Select all that apply.)
    1. occurrence of onset between 20 and 50 years of age.
    2. prevalence in adolescents and adult men.
    3. concurrence with other psychiatric and medical illness.
    4. suicide.

11. True or False

    _____ Clients who experience the same event will have the same stress response.

    _____ When verbal and nonverbal communication is incongruent, the verbal communication reflects the true meaning.

_____ Anxiety disorders are the most common psychiatric disorder in the United States.

_____ The key element in mood disorders is that the person cannot control the severity of the feeling.

APPLYING SKILLS

12. The ego defense mechanism most frequently used by clients with a serious illness is _____ _____.

13. Which of the following have a high risk for suicide?
    1. Young adults and school-age children
    2. A person just before a psychiatric hospitalization
    3. A person with a history of a previous attempt
    4. A person with a signed safety contract

14. True or False

_____ Ego defense mechanisms operate at the conscious level to disguise a real threat and protect the person from feeling anxious.

BEST PRACTICES

15. A nurse is providing care to a client with anxiety about a recent diagnosis. A nursing intervention to help to decrease the client's anxiety would be to:
    1. refer all questions the client has to the physician.
    2. provide a brightly lit environment with noise for distraction.
    3. avoid looking directly at the client during communication.
    4. acknowledge the client's feelings and help the client to explore them.

16. List the four components of basic client and family teaching for a client with a psychiatric disorder.
    a.

    b.

    c.

    d.

17. When providing health teaching to a client with a pre-existing mental illness, the nurse should always include a _____ in the teaching.

18. An appropriate intervention for interacting with a client with an anxiety disorder would be to:
    1. establish a pattern of making eye contact, looking away, and reestablishing eye contact.
    2. speak in a loud, firm voice.
    3. avoid using touch when talking.
    4. answer questions honestly.

19. True or False

_____ Mood disorders can almost always be managed with a combination of medication and psychotherapy.

KEEPING DRUG SKILLS SHARP

20. Match each description with the type of side effect associated with antipsychotic agents used in the treatment of schizophrenia. (The type of side effect may be used more than once.)

Description	**Type of Side Effect**
_____ a. Requires emergency hospitalization	1. Extrapyramidal symptoms
_____ b. Drooling and acute muscle spasms of the tongue	2. Tardive dyskinesia
_____ c. Occurs in one-third of clients	3. Neuroleptic malignant syndrome
_____ d. Extreme muscle rigidity, high fever, sweating, and fluctuations in consciousness	
_____ e. Involuntary movements of the tongue, face, hands, and legs	
_____ f. Treated with anticholinergic agents	

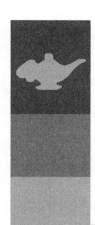

CHAPTER 24

Clients with Substance Abuse Disorders

CHAPTER OBJECTIVES

24.1   Comprehend the complexity and impact of substance abuse disorders on lives of individuals and families.

24.2   Describe the conceptual explanations for addiction.

24.3   Apply the terminology associated with substance abuse to discussions of substance abuse behavior.

24.4   Identify common nursing diagnoses related to substance abuse.

24.5   Assess own attitudes toward substance abuse and addiction.

24.6   Assess clients for potential misuse of substances using specific instruments.

24.7   Understand the use of the blood alcohol content test.

24.8   Examine pharmacologic and nonpharmacologic concepts of management of a substance abuse client regarding alcohol withdrawal.

24.9   Describe commonly abused drugs and the related effects of intoxication.

24.10 Describe the importance of education in the management of substance abuse clients and families.

24.11 Examine confrontation, treatment options, preventing relapse, and impact of surgery with the substance abuse client.

24.12 Examine the implications of substance abuse on the professional nurse.

UNDERSTANDING PATHOPHYSIOLOGY

1. A biologic theory of substance abuse would maintain that:
    1. biochemical abnormalities predispose individuals to alcoholism.
    2. Native Americans experience tachycardia, a sensation of warmth, flushing, and generalized discomfort when they consume alcohol.
    3. Asian-Americans have the highest rate of alcohol consumption.
    4. acetaldehyde, a metabolic by-product, provides a sense of well-being when alcohol is consumed.

2. Compare and contrast the psychoanalytic, psychodynamic, behavioral, and family system theories that predispose individuals to substance abuse.

3. Match each substance abuse term with the appropriate definition.

Term

_____ a. Substance abuse

_____ b. Substance dependence

_____ c. Addiction

_____ d. Intoxication

_____ e. Tolerance

_____ f. Predisposition

_____ g. Withdrawal

_____ h. Recovery

Definition

1. Any factor that increases the likelihood of an event occurring
2. Return to a normal state of health
3. Discontinuation of a substance by a dependent person
4. Continued use of a psychoactive substance despite accompanying problems
5. A compulsion, loss of control, and progressive pattern of drug use
6. A range of symptoms indicating that a person persists in using a substance
7. An altered physiologic state resulting from the use of a psychoactive drug
8. Person needs to increase amounts of a drug to achieve the same effects

4. Which statements accurately characterize polysubstance abuse? (Select all that apply.)
   1. Polysubstance abuse may be a coping strategy for clients with a chronic illness.
   2. Polysubstance abuse applies to multiple use of illegal substances only.
   3. Clients with polysubstance abuse require special care during withdrawal.
   4. Use of alcohol and nicotine is polysubstance abuse.

5. The immediate result of overconsumption of any psychoactive substance is _____ _____.

6. Factors which influence the withdrawal process in persons who sharply reduce or stop using psychoactive substances include: (Select all that apply.)
   1. overall physical health.
   2. the reason for use.
   3. the type of drug used.
   4. the method of intake.

7. A client is withdrawing from alcohol. Which of the following clinical manifestations would the nurse expect to see 2 to 3 days after the last drink was ingested?
   1. Below-normal body temperature
   2. Hypotension
   3. Disorientation
   4. Chest pain

8. The two body systems most directly affected by cocaine use are _____ and _____.

9. Which statements accurately characterize the physiologic effects of inhalants? (Select all that apply.)
   1. Inhalants cause CNS excitement within minutes of use.
   2. Inhalants increase heart rate, respirations, and overall mental activity.
   3. Continuous use may result in bone marrow dysfunction.
   4. Sudden death is a potential outcome.

10. The human body produces a natural opioid called _____, which facilitates a feeling of well-being.

11. A manifestation associated with marijuana intoxication is:
    1. improved memory capacity.
    2. precise hand-eye coordination.
    3. decreased body temperature.
    4. lower heart rate.

12. Select correct descriptions of phencyclidine (PCP) and the body's response to it. (Select all that apply.)
    1. Increased production of dopamine
    2. Papillary dilation
    3. Diplopia
    4. Excreted in the urine
    5. Hypotensive
    6. Psychosis-like state

13. The classic symptom associated with caffeine withdrawal is _____
_____ .

14. The most commonly used illegal drug in the United States is _____ .

15. True or False

_____ Alcoholism, as evidenced by research, has a genetic component.

_____ According to the sociocultural framework of addiction, the societal environment contributes to drug use, treatment, and recovery.

_____ Alcohol is a CNS stimulant that affects all levels of the brain.

_____ Marijuana residues in the lungs are more carcinogenic than tobacco residue.

_____ Nicotine use is the leading cause of preventable death in the United States.

_____ The most common health consequences of abusing drugs and alcohol are disorders of the cardiovascular system.

_____ Nurses have a higher prevalence of substance abuse than other health care professionals such as physicians.

_____ Clients who abuse hallucinogens are at high risk for acts of violence.

_____ The effects of hallucinogens on individuals are predictable.

APPLYING SKILLS

16. When conducting a drug and alcohol assessment, the nurse needs to consider that: (Select all that apply.)
    1. one of the purposes is to determine the relationship between the abuse and other health problems.
    2. clients who abuse drugs or alcohol are forthcoming about their problem.
    3. the ability to conduct a comprehensive assessment may be influenced by the nurse's personal beliefs and feelings.
    4. all clients need to be assessed for drug and alcohol abuse.

17. Explain the rationale for the nurse to monitor the respiratory status of clients experiencing acute intoxication.

18. The purpose of the blood alcohol level test is to detect and estimate the level of alcohol in the _____ . The legal limit in most states is _____%.

19. A nurse in the emergency department is caring for a client 4 hours after ingesting a hallucinogen. Assessment findings would reveal:
    1. pinpoint pupils.
    2. hypotension.
    3. eupnea.
    4. tachycardia.

20. A client who has abused a CNS depressant such as a sedative may require gastric lavage if the substance was taken within the last _____ to _____ hours.

21. Signs of chemical dependence in a professional colleague include: (Select all that apply.)
    1. mood changes.
    2. pale complexion.
    3. impeccable appearance.
    4. wearing a sweater constantly.
    5. frequent breaks in the nurse's lounge.
    6. recurrent unfinished assignments.

22. True or False

_____ A nurse caring for a client who abuses cocaine and was admitted from the emergency department 8 hours ago should assess the client for cocaine intoxication.

BEST PRACTICES

23. Prior to being effective in establishing a therapeutic relationship and providing treatment to substance abusers, the nurse must first engage in _____ .

24. The nursing intervention with the highest priority in a client experiencing an opioid overdose is to:
    1. monitor cardiac status.
    2. maintain airway.
    3. establish IV access.
    4. administer naloxone (Narcan).

25. The safe treatment for opioid addiction is

_____

and _____

_____.

26. When providing nursing care for clients who have taken an overdose of a sedative, hypnotic, or anxiolytic, the focus of nursing care is on:

a.

b.

c.

27. A "therapeutic intervention" for a substance abuse client:
    1. is used with clients who agree with the family that drug and alcohol treatment is needed.
    2. requires involvement of family and friends to be effective.
    3. follows a loosely constructed script to allow for flexibility.
    4. is implemented with firm, abrasive communication to emphasize the seriousness of the problem.

28. Identify the primary, secondary, and tertiary treatment options for a substance-abusing client.

a.

b.

c.

29. Interventions implemented to prevent relapse in a substance abuser include: (Select all that apply.)
    1. build on the client's coping skills.
    2. keep environmental variables constant.
    3. discuss measures to handle craving.
    4. encourage support group participation.
    5. teach strategies for a healthy lifestyle.

30. True or False

    _____ A key component of education for the substance abusing client and family concerns the role the family plays in the addiction.

    _____ The major nursing intervention for a client experiencing withdrawal from alcohol is to promote a safe, calm, and comfortable environment.

    _____ In the client who abuses caffeine, nursing intervention begins with recognizing manifestations of excessive use and withdrawal.

KEEPING DRUG SKILLS SHARP

31. Explain the rationale for using benzodiazepines in clients withdrawing from alcohol.

32. Alcoholics Anonymous (AA) opposes the use of naltrexone hydrochloride (ReVia) for the treatment of alcoholism because: (Select all that apply.)
    1. use of this drug is not consistent with a total abstinence model.
    2. its use is seen as a crutch.
    3. clinical evidence does not support the drug's effectiveness.
    4. clients who use the drug have a higher relapse rate.

33. List the four areas of focus for nursing care of the client who abuses amphetamines.

a.

b.

c.

d.

34. Which statements accurately characterize cocaine and cocaine use? (Select all that apply.)
    1. Cocaine may be used intravenously, snorted, or chewed.
    2. Cocaine prevents dopamine reuptake.
    3. Cocaine is metabolized in the liver and excreted in the urine.
    4. Cocaine use can lead to cardiac failure.
    5. Upon withdrawal, clients may experience euphoria.

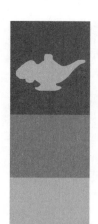

C H A P T E R 25

Assessment of the Musculoskeletal System

CHAPTER OBJECTIVES

25.1 Examine the aspects of musculoskeletal assessment including an accurate analysis of clinical manifestations.

25.2 Describe specific data to collect during the review of systems in a musculoskeletal assessment.

25.3 Discuss the aspects of a physical examination during a musculoskeletal assessment.

25.4 Describe specific diagnostic tests that support a musculoskeletal assessment.

ANATOMY & PHYSIOLOGY REVIEW

1. Label the principal muscles of the body.

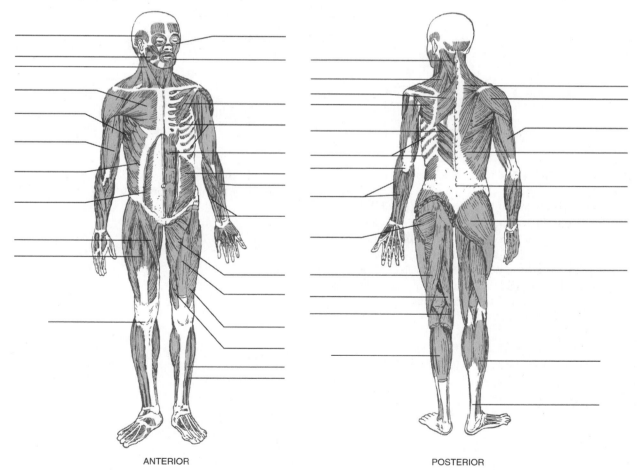

ANTERIOR   POSTERIOR

2. Label the principal bones of the adult human skeleton.

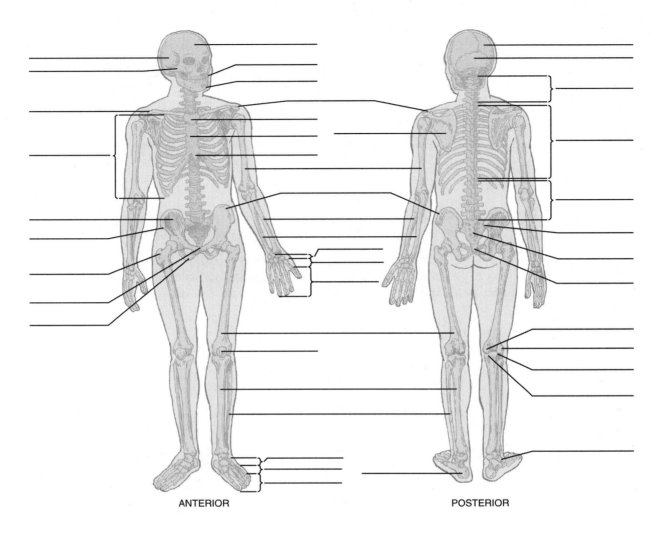

ANTERIOR   POSTERIOR

APPLYING SKILLS

3. The nurse is examining a client with painful, limited range of motion in the fingers and swelling in the right wrist, present over the last 4 weeks. The client plays golf 4 days a week and says that the pain has gotten progressively worse. Which parts of the client's health history are important for the nurse to ascertain? (Select all that apply.)
   1. Chief complaint
   2. Health history
   3. Lifestyle data
   4. Medications taken

4. When assessing musculoskeletal injuries, what assessments are important to make?
   a.

   b.

   c.

   d.

   e.

   f.

   g.

5. Match the appropriate diagnostic exam to the correct description.

Diagnostic Exam

_____ a. Arthrogram

_____ b. Radiography

_____ c. Bone scan

_____ d. MRI

_____ e. Indium imaging

_____ f. Arthrocentesis

_____ g. Arthroscopy

_____ h. Electromyography

_____ i. DEXA scan

Description

1. "Gold standard" for diagnosing osteoporosis
2. Fiberoptic arthroscope allows endoscopic examination of various joints
3. Used to assess problems such as muscle weakness, altered gait
4. Use of a substance connected to leukocytes to detect infections in bone or joint implants
5. Aspirating fluid, blood, or pus via a needle inserted into a joint cavity
6. Images of entire skeleton are obtained to detect malignancies, stress fractures, and osteomyelitis
7. Usually used to produce detailed pictures of soft tissue like tendons, ligaments, and muscles
8. Most often used noninvasive test to detect bony abnormalities
9. Radiographic examination of soft tissue joint structures after dye injection

6. The nurse evaluated the laboratory results of a client with arthritis. Which results, if elevated, would indicate bone and joint disease and cause the nurse to notify the physician?
   1. SGOT
   2. ESR
   3. hemoglobin
   4. INR

7. When performing a neurovascular assessment of clients with musculoskeletal injuries, which clinical signs and indications should be noted and documented?
   a.

   b.

   c.

   d.

   e.

   f.

   g.

8. Pallor, coolness, and cyanosis of an extremity due to an injury can indicate _____ _____ in that the particular limb.

9. The nurse is examining a client with a fractured left ankle. Checking pulses and capillary refill bilaterally will help determine the:
   1. function of knee joints above the injury.
   2. adequacy of blood supply to the lower leg.
   3. rotation of muscle mass to extremity.
   4. joint range of motion extension.

10. Laboratory studies that would be helpful when assessing a client for a musculoskeletal problem include:
    a.

    b.

    c.

    d.

    e.

    f.

    g.

    h.

    i.

    j.

    k.

11. Describe the usual cause of these differing types of pain.
    a. Aches:

    b. Sharp pain:

    c. Throbbing pain:

KEEPING DRUG SKILLS SHARP

12. List herbal preparations that may have an effect on musculoskeletal problems and their possible use.
    a.

    b.

    c.

    d.

    e.

    f.

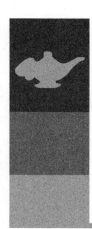

CHAPTER **26**

Management of Clients with Musculoskeletal Disorders

CHAPTER OBJECTIVES

26.1 Identify the various types of bone disorders.
26.2 Identify the causes and risk factors for bone disorders.
26.3 Relate the pathophysiology and clinical manifestations of bone disorders.
26.4 Describe the medical, surgical, and nursing management of the client with bone disorders.
26.5 Identify the medications for clients with bone disorders.
26.6 Identify specific surgical procedures and postoperative care for clients with bone disorders.
26.7 Discuss the risk of deep vein thrombosis for surgical clients with bone disorders.
26.8 Describe education for self-care of clients following surgery for bone disorders.

UNDERSTANDING PATHOPHYSIOLOGY

1. True or False

_____ Osteoarthritis is now recognized as a chronic, progressive process in which new tissue is produced in response to joint insults and cartilage deterioration.

_____ Osteoarthritis has no systemic involvement and inflammation is not typical.

_____ Osteoporosis becomes apparent when the bone structure is so weakened it can't withstand even normal stress.

_____ Interventions to increase peak bone mass can be effective up until about age 45.

_____ Drugs like corticosteroids can cause osteoporosis when taken long-term.

_____ An erythrocyte sedimentation rate (ESR) is useful only if systemic manifestations are present.

2. Osteoarthritis accounts for substantial disability in the lower extremities as a result of its effects on _____.

3. Studies have shown that overweight people have higher rates of osteoarthritis of the _____ _____ than people of normal weight.

4. Match the following descriptions and definitions with the correct disorder (answers may be used more than once).

Descriptions/Definitions

_____ a. Most often treated with braces or corsets to straighten the spine

_____ b. Common in bones of spine, hip, and wrist

_____ c. Deformity caused by flexion contracture of PIP joint

_____ d. Loss of total bone mass substance

_____ e. Pain when walking and change in gait pattern

_____ f. Replacement of normal marrow with vascular connective tissue

_____ g. May occur as a result of local irritation of restrictive foot-wear

_____ h. Bowed legs and cranial enlargement

_____ i. Occurs most frequently in femur, tibia, sacrum, and heels

_____ j. Results from vitamin D deficiency

_____ k. Generalized bone decalcification with bone deformity

_____ l. Idiopathic blood disorder/abnormal accelerated bone reab-sorption

_____ m. Produces painful deformities of femur, tibia, lower spine

_____ n. Posterior rounding of the thoracic spine

_____ o. Severe pyogenic infection of bone and surrounding tissue

_____ p. Common foot deformity involving first metatarsal and great toe

Disorder

1. Osteoporosis

2. Paget's disease

3. Osteomalacia

4. Kyphosis

5. Osteomyelitis

6. Bunions

7. Hammer toe

APPLYING SKILLS

5. Diagnosis of osteoarthritis may be confirmed by: (Select all that apply.)
   1. radiographic changes.
   2. absence of osteophytes.
   3. narrowed joint space on x-ray.
   4. erosion of articular cartilage.

6. What symptoms would likely be prominent in a 68-year-old male with osteoarthritis? (Select all that apply.)
   1. Worsening pain, stiffness increase with activity
   2. Crepitus, joint enlargement
   3. Mild tenderness in area of joint
   4. Deficits in range of motion
   5. Rough, reddened skin over joints

7. An 80-year-old female is scheduled for a total hip replacement due to osteoarthritis. The most common serious complication would be:
   1. venous thrombus embolism.
   2. crepitus of the hip.
   3. gastrointestinal bleeding.
   4. osteomyelitis.

8. Surgery on any joint carries a risk for neurologic or vascular impairment. What assessment finding would cause the nurse to report possible nerve damage to the physician?
   1. Pallor
   2. Numbness
   3. Bleeding
   4. Dislocation

9. What laboratory test will be ordered to confirm the diagnosis of gout?
   1. Serum calcium
   2. Serum uric acid
   3. BUN
   4. Bilirubin

BEST PRACTICES

10. When developing a teaching plan for a client with osteoarthritis, the nurse must include: (Select all that apply.)
    1. pain management.
    2. strenuous exercise program.
    3. nutrition and weight loss.
    4. self-care strategies.

11. A client with osteoarthritis can minimize stress on a painful joint by:
    1. becoming less physically active.
    2. eating green and yellow vegetables.
    3. maintaining normal weight.
    4. increasing intake of fruits and bread.

12. A 58-year-old female with osteoarthritis is scheduled for an arthroplasty with insertion of an artificial knee joint. The physician has ordered a continuous passive motion (CPM) machine during the postoperative period in order to:
    1. strengthen leg and calf muscle.
    2. reduce foot and toe swelling.
    3. restore joint function and range of motion with good muscle control.
    4. reduce knee swelling.

13. What beverage should the clients with gout avoid even in small amounts?
    1. Soda
    2. Alcohol
    3. Coffee
    4. Tea

14. Self-care measures to promote bone health and possibly prevent osteoporosis include: (Select all that apply.)
    1. adequate intake of vitamin D and calcium.
    2. regular weight-bearing exercise.
    3. avoiding tobacco and alcohol abuse.
    4. frequent stretching and flexibility exercises.

15. A client is worried about her mother who is confused and lives in a nursing home. The mother is not cooperative about taking medications, but fortunately she likes dairy products. What activity could the nurse suggest to the daughter that might help reduce the risk of the mother developing osteoporosis?
    1. Try to disguise medications in food.
    2. Ask the physician to order a vitamin D patch.
    3. Make sure the mother has 15 minutes of sun exposure daily.
    4. Encourage the mother to attend "bend-n-stretch" activities.

KEEPING DRUG SKILLS SHARP

16. The client with osteoarthritis has been prescribed 1 gram of acetaminophen PO every 6 hours for pain because acetaminophen: (Select all that apply.)
    1. is the drug of choice for hip and knee osteoarthritis.
    2. is effective, safe, and low-cost.
    3. is less likely to cause gastrointestinal, hepatic, or renal damage over nonsteroidal anti-inflammatory drugs.
    4. improves circulation to the bone and reduces RBC formation.

17. Pharmacologic agents routinely given to decrease risk of DVT include all of the following *except*:
    1. aspirin.
    2. low-dose heparin.
    3. low-molecular–weight heparin.
    4. warfarin.
    5. chlormycetin.

18. What laboratory tests do clients taking warfarin undergo to monitor its effects?
    1. Platelet count
    2. Prothrombin time (reported as INR)
    3. CBC
    4. ESR

19. Medications used to treat gout by reducing uric acid include: (Select all that apply.)
    1. mercurial diuretics.
    2. allopurinol.
    3. probenecid.
    4. salicylates.

20. A 58-year-old male is being treated for an acute inflammation of gout. What body part or structure is most likely to be affected?
    1. Great toe
    2. Index finger
    3. Temporomandibular joint (TMJ)
    4. Vertebral coccyx

21. During an acute attack of gout, the physician prescribes colchicines to reduce pain and inflammation. What sign indicates toxicity from this drug?
    1. Headaches
    2. Elevated temperature
    3. Vomiting
    4. Dizziness

22. Which medications might be prescribed to treat osteoporosis? (Select all that apply.)
    1. Hormone replacement therapy
    2. Alendronate
    3. Raloxifene
    4. Lovenox

23. The key to successful pain management for the client who had surgery for a bone tumor is to:
    1. decrease the interval between PRN doses of opioid analgesics.
    2. give pain medications around the clock.
    3. respond promptly when a client requests pain medication.
    4. combine an opioid with a nonopioid medication like acetaminophen.

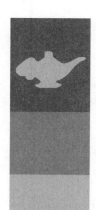

C H A P T E R 27

Management of Clients with Musculoskeletal Trauma or Overuse

CHAPTER OBJECTIVES

27.1 Describe fracture and its contribution to life changes and causes of death.
27.2 Discuss the etiology and risk factors for fractures.
27.3 Relate the pathophysiology of fractures to subsequent clinical manifestations.
27.4 Identify classifications of fractures.
27.5 Identify grading of tissue damage with open fractures.
27.6 Identify specific areas of the body prone to fracture such as the hip and upper and lower extremities.
27.7 Relate the stages of bone healing to subsequent weight-bearing of the client.
27.8 Describe the desired outcomes of medical and surgical management for fractures.
27.9 Distinguish immediate and long-term complications of fracture.
27.10 Discuss desired outcomes of nursing management for clients with casts, external fixation, or traction.
27.11 Identify assessments necessary to detect compartment syndrome, deep vein thrombosis (DVT), and pulmonary embolism (PE).
27.12 Distinguish dislocations and subluxations.
27.13 Describe common shoulder and knee sports-related injuries.

TRENDS AND THEORIES

1. True or False

   _____ Trauma is the leading cause of death for all age groups.

   _____ Fractures make up a large number of traumatic injuries.

   _____ Osteoporosis is a known risk factor for fractures.

   _____ Environmental factors may increase an older person's risk of falls.

   _____ Hip fractures require significant trauma because the hip is very stable.

   _____ Classic manifestations of hip fracture make them easy to diagnose.

   _____ A grade III open fracture is larger than 6–8 cm and has significant contamination.

UNDERSTANDING PATHOPHYSIOLOGY

2. Which of the following conditions would slow the rate of healing in an older patient with a lower leg fracture?
   1. Osteoporosis
   2. Thyroid
   3. Scleroderma
   4. Gastroenteritis

3. Nerve damage to an extremity due to injury or fracture may result in which of the following clinical signs and manifestations? (Select all that apply.)
   1. Pallor
   2. Coolness of affected extremity
   3. Changes in client's ability to move digits/extremity
   4. Paresthesia
   5. Increasing complaints of pain

APPLYING SKILLS

4.   Match the type of injury with correct description or definition.

Type of Injury

_____ a.   Impacted

_____ b.   Burst

_____ c.   Comminuted

_____ d.   Meniscus injury

_____ e.   Linear

_____ f.   Sprain

_____ g.   Displaced

_____ h.   Oblique

_____ i.   ACL tear

_____ j.   Spiral

_____ k.   Strain

_____ l.   Transverse

_____ m.   Stellate

_____ n.   Avulsion

_____ o.   Compression

_____ p.   Impingement

Description/Definition

1.   Multiple pieces of bones, occurs at bone ends
2.   Often results from rotation of the foot in a fixed position while bearing weight on the affected side
3.   Often caused by hyperextension, internal rotation, extremes of external rotation, and deceleration
4.   Fragments out of normal position at fracture site
5.   Fracture line intact, caused by force to bone
6.   Telescoped fracture with one fragment forced into another
7.   Stretch and/or tear of a ligament
8.   Fracture line from twisting force, spiral encircling bone
9.   Multiple fracture lines, two bone fragments, splintered
10.   Fracture line at 45-degree angle/long axis of bone
11.   Caused by repeatedly working with the arm over the head, throwing, or other repetitive actions of the arm
12.   Bone fragments torn from body/site ligament/tendon
13.   Bone buckles due to unusual force to long axis
14.   Fracture line at 90-degree angle to long axis
15.   Fracture lines radiate from one central point
16.   A twist/pull/tear of a muscle or tendon

5.   Which of the following best describes a greenstick fracture of the right ulna?
1.   Incomplete fracture of bone with one side flexed and splintered
2.   Bone fractured at different sites
3.   Complete dislocation of the bone
4.   Fracture across the child's growth plate

6.   A _____ is a possible early complication of a compound or crushing fracture of a long bone.

7.   True or False

_____ Skeletal traction uses pulleys/ropes attached to bones with weights.

_____ A complication of a fracture or a surgery on long bones is fat embolus.

_____ Arthroplasty is fusion of a bone.

_____ The nurse should check traction equipment each shift and as needed.

_____ Traction weights must hang clear of the bed and floor.

_____ Touch-down weight-bearing means the client can put as much weight as desired on the toes which are touching down on the floor.

_____ To maintain non-weight–bearing status, the client should be instructed to not allow the foot to touch the floor.

8.   The greatest swelling to an extremity with a cast is likely to be evident in the first _____ to _____ hours.

9.   _____ is a late sign of compartment syndrome.

10.   The nurse can best assess circulation to an extremity of a patient with a lower leg fracture by:
1.   asking the patient to wiggle his toes.
2.   checking skin color.
3.   checking skin temperature.
4.   examining the leg for deformity.

11. While assessing a lower leg cast of a 12-year-old boy, the nurse detects an unusual odor. This is a sign of:
    1. limited areas for healing.
    2. infection under the cast.
    3. the skin being dirty and in need of washing.
    4. the cast drying to the skin.

12. When fracture fragments heal in improper alignment, the nurse would expect to see:
    1. external deformity of involved extremity.
    2. the fracture healing has not occurred.
    3. the client complains of bone pain and tenderness.
    4. enlarged bone fragments.

BEST PRACTICES

13. What details are helpful in determining the type of fracture and associated injuries to clients with musculoskeletal injuries? (Select all that apply.)
    1. Was the patient in an MVA?
    2. Did the patient have a seatbelt on?
    3. What was the angle of impact?
    4. Was the patient pulled from car postcollision?
    5. Did the injury occur as result of a fall?

14. A client recently had a left hip fracture repair with an ORIF (open reduction internal fixation). The affected extremity should be maintained in a position of:
    1. abduction.
    2. internal rotation.
    3. external rotation.
    4. adduction.

15. Following hip surgery, the nurse is instructed to ambulate the patient. These patients must: (Select all that apply.)
    1. use a walker for balance.
    2. not bear weight on affected side.
    3. not dangle legs or sit in a chair.
    4. avoid flexion on the hips.
    5. avoid positions with 60- to 90-degree flexion.

16. To prevent or relieve swelling in clients with casts, the nurse should elevate the extremity with the cast _____ for the first 24 to 48 hours.

17. The nurse preparing to assist with casting would do which of the following? (Select all that apply.)
    1. Cut the stockinette several inches longer than the cast is expected to be.
    2. Make sure the skin to be covered is clean and free from debris.
    3. Use fingertips to hold the cast so the area touched is minimal.
    4. Cover the wet cast with a blanket or towel to keep the client warm while it dries.

18. _____ a cast means cutting it along each side and splitting it open to relieve pressure on underlying tissue or to allow the nurse to inspect a wound.

19. A client in the emergency department has an injury the physician describes as the opposing joint surfaces no longer in contact. This is called _____.

20. A subluxation occurs when joint surfaces_____ _____ _____ _____.

21. The client has just returned from surgery where a cast has been applied to the right lower leg. In assessing his neurovascular status, the nurse must be aware of: (Select all that apply.)
    1. circulation/color of affected extremity, pulse, capillary refill.
    2. movement of affected extremity.
    3. sensations of affected extremity.
    4. edema.
    5. pain (rate on pain scale 0–10).

KEEPING DRUG SKILLS SHARP

22. The client with orthopedic injuries is at high risk for thromboembolic conditions such as DVT and PE. Given the patient's condition, what pharmacologic agents will be used during treatment? (Select all that apply.)
    1. Oral anticoagulants
    2. Subcutaneous or IV heparin (fixed dose)
    3. Antibiotics
    4. Steroids

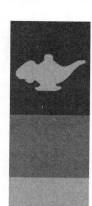

CHAPTER **28**

Assessment of Nutrition and the Digestive System

CHAPTER OBJECTIVES

28.1   Describe the aspects of nutritional health including dietary habits, caloric intake, and activity levels.

28.2   Define *primary and secondary starvation, micronutrient malnutrition,* and *obesity* as forms of malnutrition.

28.3   Distinguish the need for nutritional screening versus nutritional assessment.

28.4   Discuss the components of a nutritional history.

28.5   Identify the clinical manifestations often associated with nutrition or upper GI function.

28.6   List the specific questions to ask the client to elicit information about the clinical manifestations.

28.7   Discuss appropriate questions for the client in the review of systems.

28.8   Identify client nutrition risks based on medical and surgical history.

28.9   Distinguish food allergies from food intolerances.

28.10   Discuss interactions of medications and dietary supplements.

28.11   Determine desirable body weight for self and clients using the body mass index (BMI), frame size, and circumference measurements.

28.12   Perform a physical assessment on the mouth and abdomen to detect any interference with adequate nutrition.

28.13   Describe diagnostic testing including the appropriate use for each test regarding nutrition and digestive system.

     117

ANATOMY & PHYSIOLOGY REVIEW

1. Label the structures of the digestive system.

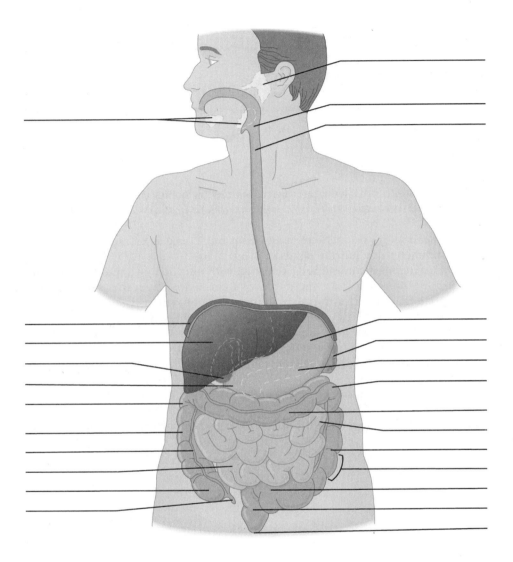

UNDERSTANDING PATHOPHYSIOLOGY

2. To meet the body's nutrient requirements, nutrients must be metabolized and used at the _____ level.

3. Identify the alterations in RDA that must be made for the following disease processes, and state the rationale for each.
    a. Kidney or liver failure:

    b. Pancreatic exocrine dysfunction:

    c. Pancreatic endocrine dysfunction:

4. Identify the two main causes for the epidemic of obesity in America.

   a.

   b.

5. Differentiate between primary and secondary starvation.

6. Conditions that can place clients at high risk for malnutrition and potential nutritional deficit include: (Select all that apply.)
   1. fat malabsorption.
   2. short-bowel syndrome.
   3. pressure ulcers.
   4. cancer.
   5. AIDS.
   6. gastric surgery.

7. Identify diseases that have a familial or genetic link.

APPLYING SKILLS

8. Identify the quickest way to begin collecting information about dietary intake.

9. In addition to the types of foods consumed, factors the nurse should consider when evaluating nutritional status include all of the following *except*:
   1. the amount of food or drink consumed.
   2. how the food was prepared.
   3. where the food was obtained.
   4. the time of day food or drink was consumed.

10. Explain how evaluation of albumin and prealbumin can determine nutritional status of the client.

11. List the components of an anthropometric measurement of a client.

   a.

   b.

   c.

   d.

   e.

12. The _____ is a better standard for determining ideal body weight than conventional tables because it standardizes weight for the height of the individual.

13. True or False

   _____ A client with a BMI of 18.5 is in the acceptable range for weight.

   _____ Calculations for BMI are the same for males and females.

   _____ Bone and muscle are less dense than fat and count less in BMI.

   _____ Frame size of the client can be determined by measuring wrist circumference.

   _____ A muscular client can have a high BMI and not be considered overweight.

14. Upon assessment of a client's mouth, the nurse notes an oral lesion. The client says that the lesion has been present for some time and is not causing any pain. Identify the appropriate nursing action for this situation and state the rationale.

15. Pain at _____ may suggest acute appendicitis.

16. True or False

   _____ Sitting at eye level with the abdomen, the nurse should see peristaltic movements.

   _____ Diastasis recti is a true herniation just below the diaphragm and will require surgical correction.

_____ The nurse should apply the diaphragm of the stethoscope over the abdomen to listen for bowel sounds.

_____ Normal bowel sounds occur irregularly at a rate of 5–35 per minute.

17. Turbulent blood causes a _____ _____ sound, which may indicate an aneurysm or partial obstruction of a blood vessel.

18. State the rationale for the nurse asking the client to take a sip of water and then observing the client swallowing.

19. Noninvasive diagnostic testing that helps evaluate upper GI function and nutritional status include:
    a.

    b.

    c.

    d.

    e.

20. Endoscopy allows _____ _____ _____.

21. Esophageal manometry is used to assess and diagnose:
    a.

    b.

    c.

    d.

    e.

BEST PRACTICES

22. Describe the differences between a nutrition screening and a nutrition assessment and the rationale for each.

23. After collecting data from the client's 24-hour diet recall, the nurse can assess the client's nutritional status further by: (Select all that apply.)
    1. comparing the client's intake with a standardized reference such as the Food Pyramid.
    2. consult with a registered dietitian and the DRI to assess intake of specific nutrients.
    3. calculate the amount of calories and protein consumed by the client in a typical day.
    4. ask about daily physical activity and other medical problems like diabetes.

24. When assessing clients, the nurse should assess for common complaints related to GI function or nutritional status, such as:
    a.

    b.

    c.

    d.

    e.

25. Questions the nurse should ask related to abdominal pain include: (Select all that apply.)
    1. was the onset rapid or gradual?
    2. is the pain associated with food in any way?
    3. does the pain radiate?
    4. what is the intensity of the pain?

26. When a client complains about diarrhea, what question should the nurse specifically ask?

27. When a client presents with non-specific complaints such as nausea, vomiting, and diarrhea, questions the nurse should ask include
    a.

    b.

    c.

28. List some items from a client's past medical and surgical history that could affect nutritional status.
    a.

    b.

    c.

    d.

    e.

    f.

    g.

    h.

    i.

    j.

29. Differentiate between a food allergy and a food intolerance.

30. Nutrients in addition to iron that are needed for normal hematologic functioning include: (Select all that apply.)
    1. protein.
    2. vitamin B_{12}.
    3. zinc.
    4. copper.

KEEPING DRUG SKILLS SHARP

31. Explain how medications affect the older client's nutritional status.

32. List four common over-the-counter (OTC) medications which can interfere with GI function or cause complications.
    a.

    b.

    c.

    d.

33. Explain the hidden danger for clients using OTC supplements or herbs.

34. _____ medications are given to a client scheduled for an endoscopy because they decrease oropharyngeal secretions and prevent reflex bradycardia.

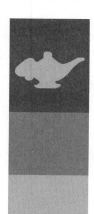

CHAPTER 29

Management of Clients with Malnutrition

CHAPTER OBJECTIVES

29.1 Define *malnutrition, undernutrition,* and *overnutrition.*
29.2 Identify causes and risk factors for under- and overnutrition disorders.
29.3 Relate the pathophysiology and clinical manifestations of malnutrition disorders.
29.4 Describe the desired outcomes of medical, surgical, and nursing management of malnutrition disorders.
29.5 Describe education for self-care for malnutrition disorders.

UNDERSTANDING PATHOPHYSIOLOGY

1. Differentiate between malnutrition and protein-energy malnutrition (PEM).

2. Explain why each category of client is at risk for PEM.
   a. Infants:

   b. Pregnant/lactating women:

   c. Older adults:

3. Secondary malnutrition is caused by all of the following *except*:
   1. decreased food intake.
   2. decreased nutrient absorption.
   3. increased nutrient losses.
   4. decreased nutrient requirements.

4. Socioeconomic factors that have a negative effect on nutrition include: (Select all that apply.)
   1. social isolation.
   2. limited access to food.
   3. emotional depression.
   4. substance abuse.
   5. poverty.

5. True or False

   _____ The functional status of the GI tract determines the site of the enteral feeding tube placement.

   _____ The larger the diameter of the tube, the more likely the problems with infusing formulas and medications.

   _____ Jejunostomy and gastrostomy tubes are used for long-term enteral feedings.

   _____ Percutaneous endoscopic gastrostomy tubes must be placed surgically and require the client to receive anesthesia.

6. List four factors that increase the incidence of obesity.
   a.

   b.

   c.

   d.

7. Health risks associated with obesity include all of the following *except*:
   1. type I diabetes.
   2. cardiovascular disease.
   3. hypertension.
   4. hyperlipidemia.
   5. stroke.
   6. sleep apnea.
   7. arthritis.
   8. some cancers.

APPLYING SKILLS

8. True or False

   _____ A BMI of over 25 is considered obese.

   _____ By the year 2010, obesity-related ailments will be the leading cause of death in developing countries.

   _____ Currently 66% of Americans are considered overweight.

   _____ The criteria for diagnosing anorexia nervosa include preoccupation with personal body weight and appearance, behaviors directed at thinness, and the physical results of these behaviors.

   _____ In anorexia nervosa, alterations in the metabolism of insulin, thyroid hormone, and catecholamines explain common clinical manifestations.

   _____ Clients with bulimia nervosa typically stay very thin through purging behavior.

9. State the rationale for the nurse to assess nutritional status of any client, rather than other types of health care workers.

10. Identify a possible physical diagnosis that could cause of each common manifestation that may lead to the nursing diagnosis of Self-care deficit, feeding.
    a. Impaired motor function:

    b. Impaired cognitive function:

    c. Sensory-perceptual alterations:

    d. Decreased appetite:

11. Compare and contrast between marasmus and kwashiorkor.

	Protein Intake	Calorie Intake	Appearance
Marasmus			
Kwashiorkor			

12. Upon assessment of an older client admitted from a long-term care facility, the nurse would note which of the following clinical manifestations of protein malnutrition? (Select all that apply.)
    1. Hair loss
    2. Oily skin
    3. Brittle nails
    4. Pale skin tone
    5. Periodontal disease or bleeding gums
    6. Muscle wasting/weight loss

BEST PRACTICES

13. Provide examples of the three phases of nursing interventions to help the client prevent or restore nutritional status.
    a. Health promotion:

    b. Health maintenance:

    c. Health restoration:

14. Nursing strategies to improve client nutritional status include: (Select all that apply.)
    1. allowing the client to choose from a menu.
    2. reducing noxious odors.
    3. consistently offering the same foods/beverages.
    4. oral care.

15. The nurse can assist the blind client to ensure adequate food intake by: (Select all that apply.)
    1. maximizing use of other senses: smell and taste.
    2. describing food to a visually impaired client.
    3. arranging food in clock-face pattern and describing positions to the client.
    4. not placing food on the client's blind side.
    5. making sure the client is wearing corrective lenses.
    6. using a highly patterned set of food dishes.

16. The nurse can assist the client with neuromuscular impairments to obtain adequate nutrition and maintain independence by: (Select all that apply.)
    1. positioning the client at 45-degree angle.
    2. consulting with occupational therapy for assistive devices.
    3. ensuring privacy to avoid embarrassment.
    4. allowing adequate time for eating.

17. _____ equipment must be kept available when feeding a client with impaired swallowing function.

18. True or False

    _____ If the client has an obstruction in the GI tract, the enteral feeding tube can be placed proximal to the site.

19. List four nursing responsibilities when administering enteral feedings to a client and state the rationale for each.
    a.

    b.

    c.

    d.

20. Teaching topics for the client who will perform enteral feedings at home include: (Select all that apply.)
    1. flushing the feeding tube.
    2. adding enteral formula to the feeding bag or feeding syringe.
    3. monitoring for complications.
    4. where to obtain formula and related supplies.

KEEPING DRUG SKILLS SHARP

21. The main components of TPN include all of the following *except*:
    1. carbohydrates: 50–70% caloric supply.
    2. fat emulsion: 30–50% caloric supply.
    3. amino acids: 3–15%: source of protein.
    4. fluids, electrolytes, vitamins, trace elements.

22. List the three types of FDA approved weight loss medications with an example of each.
    a.

    b.

    c.

23. Identify examples for each classification of enteral nutrition products.

Classification	Example Product
Semi-elemental, predigested	
Standard protein	
Fiber supplemented	
High protein	
Calorie dense	
Diabetes	
Renal failure	

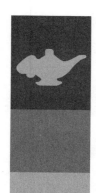

CHAPTER **30**

Management of Clients with Ingestive Disorders

CHAPTER OBJECTIVES
30.1   Identify nursing diagnoses appropriate for disorders of ingestion.
30.2   Describe causes of benign and malignant oral, salivary, and esophageal disorders.
30.3   Describe the desired outcomes of medical, surgical, and nursing management of the disorders.

UNDERSTANDING PATHOPHYSIOLOGY

1.   How does periodontal disease lead to tooth loss?

Plaque formation + bacterial colonization results in gingival inflammation if plaque not removed c̄ brushing. Inflammation destroys the underlying tissues + separates the gingiva from the tooth. Inflammation extends from gum O to the alveolar bone + periodontal ligament, destroying supporting structures of the teeth. Teeth loosen + fall out.

2.   List the two mechanisms for developing stomatitis.
   a.   *Mechanical – injury*
   b.   *Chemical –*

3.   Compare and contrast primary and secondary stomatitis.

Classification	Etiology	Examples
Primary	*Direct infection of tissues*	*aphthous ulcer (canker sore) herpes simplex Vincent's angina*
Secondary	*Client's lowered resistance allows an opportunistic infection to develop*	*Candidiasis*

4.   Common precipitating factors for Vincent's angina include: (Select all that apply.)
   (1.)   poor oral hygiene.
   (2.)   increased age.
   (3.)   nutritional deficiencies.
   (4.)   lack of rest/sleep.

5.   Only a ___*biopsy*___ can positively confirm oral cancer.

6.   The pain that occurs with difficulty swallowing is called ___*odynophagia*___.

7.   Differentiate between the pain of "heartburn" and the pain of cardiac origin (angina).

HB – substernal, midline burning tends to radiate toward the neck. Cramping or constricting. Cardiac – heavy, crushing, or tightening sensation in the chest that radiates to O arm.

8.   ___*Achalasia*___ develops when the lower esophageal sphincter (LES) fails to relax normally with swallowing, resulting in a buildup of food and fluid in the lower esophagus.

9. Compare and contrast the three surgical procedures to correct GERD.

Name	Procedure	Result
Nissen fundoplication	Suturing the fundus around the esophagus	An increase in pressure or volume in the stomach closes the cardia & blocks reflux into the esophagus.
Hill operation	Narrows the esophageal opening.	Narrows the esophagus & anchors the stomach & distal esophagus to the median arcuate ligament. Reinforces the sphincter & recreates the gastroesophageal valve.
Belsey (Mark IV) repair	Plication of the anterior & lateral aspects of the stomach onto the distal esophagus	Creates the esophagogastric angle without opening the esophagus or the diaphragm

10. Explain why esophageal cancer metastasizes so quickly. The rich lymphatic supply to the mucosa allows the cancer to spread widely & quickly.

11. Differentiate between leukoplakia and erythroplakia. Leukoplakia – potentially precancerous, yellow-white or gray-white lesion, may occur in region of the mouth. Usually elevated & have a roughened or leathery surface & clearly defined borders. Common disorder. Erythroplakia – red, velvety appearing patch that commonly indicates early squamous cell carcinoma

APPLYING SKILLS

12. Describe the difference in clinical manifestations between a hiatal hernia and a rolling hernia.
Sliding hiatal hernia – client may experience heartburn 30-60 min ? meals. Reflux may result in substernal pain.
Rolling hiatal hernia – client may complain of a feeling of fullness, eating or may have difficulty breathing. Client may experience chest pain similar to angina. Pain usually worse when the client lies down.

13. A client has undergone surgery to remove a cancerous lesion from the oral cavity. In addition to monitoring nutritional and fluid intake, what other changes within the oral cavity should the nurse be alert to?

venous drainage cause darker coloration to the skin.

14. True or False

___T___ Hemorrhage is a critical postoperative concern for the oral surgery client due to the large blood vessels that supply the mouth and oral area.

___F___ Esophageal diverticuli are common in Caucasian women. They are rare

___T___ Squamous cell carcinoma is more common in African-Americans than in Caucasians.

___F___ The greatest risk factor for esophageal cancer is tobacco use.
a major risk factor

BEST PRACTICES

15. State the rationales for each of the following nursing actions to provide postoperative care to the client following a tooth extraction.
    a. Instruct client to bite down gently on gauze pad: *put pressure on extraction site to reduce bleeding*

    b. Apply ice over jaw: *Reduce swelling*

    c. Monitoring bleeding from site: *Some bleeding expected. watch for bleeding last > 1 hr.*

    d. Avoid hot/cold foods for several days: *Extraction site is sensitive to temp. extremese.*

    e. Gentle mouth rinses/avoid tooth brushing: *to prevent recurrence of bleeding @ extraction site*

    f. Medicate for pain: *for pt. comfort & to encourage oral intake*

    g. Maintain fluid intake: *prevent dehydration*

16. Prior to discharge, the nurse should instruct the client with oral lesions to: (Select all that apply.)
    1. use gauze or sponge pads instead of a tooth-brush.
    2. use cold saline mouth rinses.
    3. swish antifungal medications around mouth and then swallow; do not drink fluids or rinse mouth afterwards.
    4. drink plenty of orange juice.
    5. report any signs of infection to physician promptly.

17. Nursing interventions for the diagnosis Impaired oral mucosa related to irritants include teaching the client to: (Select all that apply.)
    1. avoid oral irritants (tobacco, alcohol).
    2. notify physician of lesion that does not heal in 2–3 days. *weeks*
    3. perform careful oral hygiene daily. *– 3x a day*
    4. request medications if needed for nausea secondary to chemotherapy or radiation.
    5. see dentist about ill-fitting dentures.

18. True or False
    _F_ After local excisions of oral tumors, the client should rinse gently with ½ saline − ½ peroxide solution. *Saline + H₂O 94%*
    _F_ Oral suctioning may be done 48 hours after oral surgery if there is no bleeding noted.
    _F_ Clients who undergo oral surgery may begin tube feedings after 48 hours if no nausea or vomiting is present.

19. Treatment goals for achalasia include all of the following *except*:
    1. restoring normal esophageal function.
    2. relieving manifestations.
    3. providing nutritional support.
    4. modifying diet for ease of eating.

20. List appropriate diagnoses for the client being treated for esophageal cancer.
    a. *Imbalanced nutrition: less then Body Requirements related to the client's inability to swallow.*
    b. *Impaired swallowing r/t esophageal obstruction from tumor.*
    c. *Risk for ineffective coping r/t changes in body image & potentially terminal prognosis.*
    d. *Risk for injury r/t surgical procedure.*

21. List self-care measures for the client being discharged from the hospital after surgery for esophageal cancer.
    a. *wound healing*
    b. *nutritional support*
    c. *respiratory care*
    d. *medications*
    e. *wound care*
    f. *what manifestations to report.*
    g. *contact information*
    h. *date/time of f/u appt.*

KEEPING DRUG SKILLS SHARP

22. Treatment of the herpes does not include
    ___antimicrobial___ medications.

23. Medications used to treat stomatitis include: (Select all that apply.)
    1. fluconazole.
    2. nystatin troches.
    3. acetaminophen.
    4. hydrourea (Hydraea).

24. Common chemotherapeutic agents used in treatment of oral cancer include which of the following? (Select all that apply.)
    1. Taxanes (Taxol, Taxotere)
    2. Cisplatin (Platinol).
    3. Cyclophosphamide (Cytoxan).
    4. Doxorubicin (Adriamycin).
    5. 5-fluorouracil (5-FU).
    6. Methotrexate (Folex).

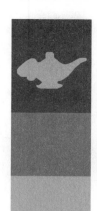

CHAPTER **31**

Management of Clients with Digestive Disorders

CHAPTER OBJECTIVES

31.1 Identify nursing diagnoses and general clinical manifestations for the client with gastrointestinal (GI) disorders.

31.2 Describe the reasons for gastrointestinal intubation.

31.3 Identify types of tubes and procedures for GI intubation.

31.4 Describe nursing management of the client with a GI tube.

31.5 Describe gastrointestinal disorders including the causes and risks.

31.6 Relate the pathophysiology and clinical manifestations of GI disorders.

31.7 Describe the desired outcomes of medical, surgical, and nursing management of the client with GI disorders.

31.8 Discuss complications of gastric surgery.

31.9 Discuss dumping syndrome and its management.

UNDERSTANDING PATHOPHYSIOLOGY

1. Identify two common causes of gastric pain.
   a. _Chemical irritation of nerve endings._
   b. _stretching + contracting of the stomach, caused in turn by ↑ motility & ↑ smooth muscle tension, is found in obstruction_

2. _Esophagogastric varices._ are the major cause of upper GI bleeding.

3. The major electrolyte lost through NG tube suctioning is _potassium_.

4. Dietary habits that can lead to acute gastritis include consumption of excessive amounts of: (Select all that apply.)
   1. tea or coffee.
   2. mustard.
   3. ketchup.
   4. paprika.
   5. cloves.

5. Chronic gastritis leads to an increased risk for _gastric cancer._ by causing a decrease in the production of stomach acid.

6. Chronic gastritis can cause _pernicious anemia_ by decreasing acid secretion, resulting in the loss of intrinsic factor and reducing the ability to absorb vitamin B_{12}. _malabsorption of B_{12}_

7. Explain the difference in etiology between duodenal ulcers and gastric ulcers.
   ↑ gastric acid secretions + rapid emptying of food from the stomach into the duodenum characterizes duodenal ulcers.
   gastric ulcers are caused by a break in the mucosal barrier exposing the stomach to hydrochloric acid.

8. A serious complication that can develop secondary to stress ulcers is _upper GI Bleeding_.

9. Compare and contrast common gastric surgical procedures and the indications for each procedure.

Procedure	Indication
Vagotomy	eliminates acid-secreting stimulus to the gastric cells.
Vagotomy with pyloroplasty	prevents gastric stasis + enhances gastric emptying
Gastroenterostomy	permits regurgitation of alkaline duodenal contents, thereby neutralizing gastric acid. / drains acid away from ulcerative area, promoting healing
Antrectomy	reduce acid-secreting portions of the stomach
Subtotal gastrectomy	tx. for duodenal ulcers.
Total gastrectomy	tx. for extensive cancer (gastric)

10. _____alkalosis_____ develops secondary to pyloric obstruction because the persistent vomiting causes the loss of large quantities of acid gastric juice, altering the acid-base balance.

11. Causative factors in the development of gastric cancer include: (Select all that apply.)
    1. cigarette smoking.
    2. *E. coli.*
    3. pernicious anemia.
    4. chronic atrophic gastritis.
    5. a diet of raw fish or meats.
    6. achlorhydria.
    7. metalcraft worker, coal miner, baker (dusty, smoky environment).

APPLYING SKILLS

12. Common clinical manifestations of gastric disorders include: (Select all that apply.)
    1. nausea and vomiting.
    2. acute pain.
    3. acid reflux.
    4. anorexia.
    5. indigestion.
    6. bleeding.
    7. diarrhea.
    8. belching/flatulence.

13. Identify the clinical significance of vomiting coffee ground-like material.

    Indicates a GI Bleed

14. Explain how the nurse would assess electrolyte losses for the client with an NG tube set to low suction.

    Assess for clinical manifestations, review labs, report any sign of electrolyte imbalance to the physician.

15. True or False

    __T__ Clients with duodenal ulcers have pain with an empty stomach.

    __F__ Gastric ulcer pain usually radiates toward the right side of the abdomen and upward toward the neck.

    __T__ Vomiting occurs more often with gastric ulcers than with uncomplicated duodenal ulcers.

    __T__ The major diagnostic test for gastric ulcers is an esophagogastroduodenoscopy (EGD) with an upper GI tract x-ray series.

16. Complications resulting from a gastric ulcer perforation include all of the following *except*:
    1. chemical peritonitis.
    2. bacterial septicemia.
    3. septic shock.
    4. paralytic ileus.

17. A client recovering from gastrojejunostomy is not tolerating her diet due to the increased rate of food emptying into the jejunum without mixing and duodenal digestive processing. When should the nurse assess for problems and what clinical manifestations would be present?

    manifestations occur 5-30min. p eating + involve vasomotor disturbances such as vertigo, tachycardia, syncope, sweating, palpitations, diarrhea + nausea.

18. List the rationales for GI intubation.
    a. *decompression*
    b. *lavage*
    c. *gastric analysis*
    d. *tube feedings*

19. Match the type of tube on the left with the purpose or description on the right.

    Type of Tube
    _4_ a. Short tube
    _1_ b. Cantor tube
    _5_ c. Dobhoff tube
    _2_ d. Medium tube
    _b_ e. Long tube
    _3_ f. Salem sump

    Purpose or Description
    1. Example of a long tube
    2. These tubes extend into the duodenum and are used for short-term feeding.
    3. This short tube has an air vent and is good for suctioning
    4. These can only extend into the stomach
    5. Example of a medium tube; placement is verified by x-ray
    6. These prevent gas and fluid accumulation in the intestine

BEST PRACTICES

20. Important client teaching points for management of dumping syndrome include: (Select all that apply.)
    1. decreasing the amount of food taken at one time.
    2. maintaining a low-protein, low-fat, high-carbohydrate, dry diet.
    3. delaying gastric emptying by eating in a recumbent or semi-recumbent position.
    4. avoiding fluids 1 hour before, with, or 2 hours after meals.

21. To facilitate insertion of intestinal tubes through the pylorus, the nurse should instruct the client to lie on his or her ____*right*____ side.

22. True or False
    _F_ Dietary alterations remain one of the basic interventions to help clients with gastric ulcers.

23. Identify the nursing action for a client who is experiencing melena.

    Report finding + take vitals.

24. A nurse caring for a client with an NG tube notices that the tube is not draining properly. The nurse irrigates the tube with 30 ml of normal saline solution and then connects the tube back to suction. Is the 30 ml of saline added to the intake amount for that shift? Why or why not?

    Yes, It is part of the fluid intake into the body, you need to keep accurate I + O's.

25. State the rationale for instilling room-temperature saline through an NG tube into a client who is experiencing gastric hemorrhage.

    Room temp. saline is cooler than body temp. so promotes mild vasoconstriction.

26. Identify the critical nursing observation in addition to monitoring vital signs that must be made in the client with severe hemorrhage due to gastric ulcers.

    Urine output should be recorded hourly. kidney perfusion is vital to client stability.

27. Explain why the nurse should avoid repositioning the NG tube in a client who has had gastric surgery.

    tube could be positioned by the suture line + moving could cause trauma.

28. Nursing diagnoses that are applicable to clients experiencing GI tract dysfunction include:
    a. *Imbalanced nutrition: less than Body requirements.*
    b. *Acute pain*
    c. *Ineffective therapeutic regimen management.*
    d. *fear*
    e. *Risk for injury*

KEEPING DRUG SKILLS SHARP

29. The phenothiazine derivative _____*Compazine*_____ _____ reduces vomiting by depressing chemoreceptor stimulation of the emetic center in the brain.

30. Describe how NSAIDs contribute to the development of stress ulcers in a client.

    Loss of prostaglandins expose gastric mucosa to acid secretions resulting in ulcers.

31. True or False
    __*F*__ Heptavax is a new vaccine being tested to prevent infection with *H. pylori,* a major cause of gastric ulcers.

32. Explain why a client with gastric ulcers must be cautious in using over-the-counter cold remedies.

    They may contain NSAID's or aspirin.

33. Identify the indications for use for each the following common medications for treatment of gastric problems.

Medication	Indication for Use
Enteric-coated aspirin	*protects against irritation from lost mucosa*
Cytotec	*protects against irritation from lost mucosa.*
Histamine receptor antagonists	*↓ gastric acidity*
Proton pump inhibitors	*block gastric acid secretions.*

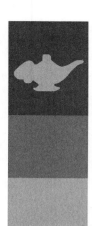

C H A P T E R **32**

Assessment of Elimination

CHAPTER OBJECTIVES

32.1 Describe the aspects of bowel and urinary elimination assessment.

32.2 Describe the health history for bowel and urinary elimination including biographic and demographic data.

32.3 Describe a thorough review of clinical manifestations with clients based on their description of current health status.

32.4 List the specific questions to ask the client to elicit information about the clinical manifestations.

32.5 Discuss appropriate questions for the client in the review of systems.

32.6 Identify client risk for bowel or urinary disease based on medical and surgical history.

32.7 Relate food allergies to clinical manifestations after ingestion of food.

32.8 Discuss interactions of medications and dietary supplements.

32.9 Identify benefits of dietary supplements for the genitourinary (GU) tract.

32.10 Identify medications that have GU side effects.

32.11 Discuss dietary habits related to clinical manifestations of the bowel or urinary tract.

32.12 Determine desirable body weight as it relates to possible body image problems.

32.13 Discuss social and family history as they relate to the client's clinical manifestations of the bowel or urinary tract.

32.14 Perform a physical assessment of the abdomen and genitalia.

32.15 Discuss the importance of abdominal palpation as the final step in the bowel elimination assessment.

32.16 Describe diagnostic test purposes related to examination of the bowel and urinary tract.

32.17 Relate diagnostic testing to specific clinical manifestations and subsequent need to treat the client.

UNDERSTANDING PATHOPHYSIOLOGY

1. When reviewing systems and symptoms for GI tract pathophysiology, identify three questions that should be asked of the client.

2. When reviewing systems for urinary tract pathophysiology, identify three questions that should be asked of the client.

3. High levels of carcinoembryonic antigen (CEA) are detected with which conditions? (Select all that apply.)
    1. Proctitis
    2. Colon cancer
    3. Lung cancer
    4. Breast cancer
    5. Liver disease
    6. Cirrhosis
    7. Appendicitis
    8. Inflammatory bowel disease

4. Compare and contrast the differences in urinary volume and their associated conditions and/or diseases.

Urine Output	Associated Conditions
Anuria	
Oliguria	
Polyuria	

5. Discuss the etiology, manifestations, and treatment of acute urinary retention.
   a. Etiology:

   b. Manifestations:

   c. Treatment:

6. Define *urinary incontinence* and list causes.

7. Identify potential GI clinical manifestations and list one condition that each manifestations could indicate.
   a.

   b.

   c.

   d.

   e.

   f.

8. True or False

   _____ Urinary tract disease does not always cause pain.

   _____ Acute, agonizing pain is due to an enlarged prostate gland.

   _____ The highest prevalence of urinary incontinence is in the older female population.

   _____ Prostate pain is not common in men.

   _____ Manifestations such as nausea, vomiting, and fever can signal urologic disease.

   _____ Benign prostatic hypertropy (BPH) is a common cause of both irritative and obstructive voiding complaints.

   _____ Microscopic urinalysis quantifies white and red blood cells.

   _____ Urine cultures are particularly important for recurrent urinary tract infections (UTIs).

   _____ Serum creatinine level is less specific for renal function than other studies.

9. Creatinine level in the urine is equivalent to the _____ filtration rate of the kidneys.

APPLYING SKILLS

10. When reviewing the chief complaint of someone with a potential GI disorder, it is important to discuss _____ manifestations since a GI health problem does not usually occur in the absence of other manifestations.

11. True or False

    _____ With abdominal pain, the area of pain should be examined first.

    _____ The diaphragm of the stethoscope is used to listen to bowel sounds.

    _____ If a client's bladder is full, a dull sound will be heard with percussion.

    _____ The client should be positioned supine for examination of the abdomen.

12. When assessing bowel sounds, they are normally heard every _____ seconds.

13. If bowel sounds are not heard for _____ minutes in _____ quadrant(s), they are considered absent.

14. Incidents reported in a client's history that may have caused injury to the urinary system include: (Select all that apply.)
    1. history of MVA.
    2. falls.
    3. straddle injuries.
    4. penetrating abdominal injury.
    5. contact sports injury.

15. Areas of the client's psychosocial history significant in relation to urinary problems include: (Select all that apply.)
    1. impairments in vision.
    2. level of mobility.
    3. marital status.
    4. living and work environment.
    5. wetness of clothing/odor/overall hygiene.
    6. access to toilets.
    7. positive or negative childhood experiences with toilet training.
    8. variables in daily life; stressors.

16. When taking a history for urinary problems, the nurse includes which of the following areas to form a basis for assessment? (Select all that apply.)
    1. Occupation
    2. Allergies
    3. Geographic location
    4. Nutrition
    5. Exercise habits
    6. Alcohol and tobacco use

17. When assessing a client with suspected renal enlargement masses, the advanced practitioner nurse should use which technique?
    1. Auscultation
    2. Deep palpation
    3. Inspection
    4. Percussion

18. Describe each of the diagnostic tests used for evaluating bowel function and the implication for their use.
    a. Computed tomography:

    b. Ultrasonography:

    c. Proctosigmoidoscopy:

    d. Colonoscopy:

    e. Flat plate of the abdomen:

    f. Fecal occult blood:

    g. Video capsule endoscopy:

BEST PRACTICES

19. True or False

_____ Palpation of the abdomen before percussion is recommended when clients have pain.

_____ Abdominal palpation proceeds from deep to light, and closest to any area of pain.

_____ Abdominal aortic bruits may be assessed with the diaphragm of the stethoscope placed 2 inches above the umbilicus.

_____ Rebound tenderness is assessed with slow and deep palpation away from the area of suspected inflammation.

20. True or False

_____ Renal artery bruits are heard just above and slightly left of the umbilicus.

_____ Avoid deep palpation if a renal artery bruit is heard.

_____ Palpation is the assessment skill that helps to identify a full bladder.

_____ Each of the four quadrants should be palpated lightly for areas of muscle resistance.

21. Identify the purpose of diagnostic tests for the urinary tract. Provide one reason for the use of the test.
    a. KUB:

    b. IVP:

    c. CT:

    d. Cystourethroscopy:

    e. Urinalysis:

    f. Creatinine clearance:

    g. Serum creatinine:

    h. BUN:

22. Questions about dietary habits are important to the assessment of the GI tract. Select specific factors that should be included in the assessment. (Select all that apply.)
    1. Fluid intake
    2. Amount of food eaten
    3. Typical day of eating
    4. Perceived ideal body weight
    5. Food tolerance or intolerance

23. True or False

_____ Traditional alternative and complementary therapies are used by 30% of the Western population for about $5 billion annually.

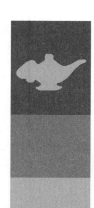

CHAPTER 33

Management of Clients with Intestinal Disorders

CHAPTER OBJECTIVES

33.1   Identify common nursing diagnoses for intestinal disorders.

33.2   Describe general clinical manifestations of gastrointestinal (GI) tract disorders.

33.3   Describe causes and risk factors for specific disorders of the GI tract.

33.4   Relate the pathophysiology and clinical manifestations of GI tract disorders.

33.5   Describe the desired outcomes of medical, surgical, and nursing management for GI tract disorders.

33.6   Distinguish peritonitis as a potential complication of surgical intervention.

33.7   Discuss care of the client with an ostomy, including type of ostomy, therapeutic regimen, psychosocial concerns, and stoma assessment.

33.8   Discuss education needs and teaching of the client with an ostomy.

33.9   Describe staging, tumor markers, and prognosis in colorectal cancer.

33.10   Distinguish types of hernias and their management.

33.11   Identify blunt or penetrating trauma as an accidental disorder of the GI tract requiring immediate medical, surgical, and nursing intervention.

UNDERSTANDING PATHOPHYSIOLOGY

1.   Compare and contrast the etiology for each of the major clinical manifestations of intestinal disorders.

Disorder	Etiology
Hemorrhage	trauma, ulceration or inflammation or growth that erodes thru a blood vessel.
Pain	mechanical, inflammatory or ischemic Δ's
Visceral	stimulus acting on the involved portion of the bowel.
Somatic	irritation of the parietal peritoneum
Referred	pain felt at a distance from the affected organ.
Nausea/vomiting	nausea results from distention of the duodenum. vomiting from Δ's in the integrity of the intestinal wall or from Δ's in the motility of the bowel.
Distention	excessive gas or trapped gas in the intestines, blockage
Diarrhea	Rapid propulsion of intestinal contents thru the small bowel
Constipation	infrequent or difficult passage of stools or the passage of hard or pellet stools.

2. Clinical manifestations of gastroenteritis relate directly to antibiotic therapy and loss of normal bowel bacteria and include which of the following? (Select all that apply.)
   1. Nausea and vomiting
   2. Abdominal pain
   3. Borborygmi
   4. Fever
   5. Bowel distention

3. True or False
   ___T___ *Clostridium difficile* is the most common cause of nosocomial infections in the hospitalized client.

   ___F___ Cooked foods are a source of *E. coli* bacteria.

   ___T___ Outbreaks of food-borne *viral* infections are almost always caused by contaminated shellfish.

   ___T___ Food can be a vehicle for transmitting actively growing microbes.

   ___T___ The incubation period for ALL viral and bacterial infections is 6 hours to 4–5 days.

4. Common causes of appendicitis include: (Select all that apply.)
   1. fecalith.
   2. kinking of the appendix.
   3. swelling of bowel wall.
   4. perforation of bowel wall.
   5. adhesions.

5. Common causes for the development of peritonitis include: (Select all that apply.)
   1. ruptured or gangrenous gallbladder.
   2. fibrous condition of bowel wall.
   3. perforated peptic ulcer.
   4. perforated stomach.
   5. penetrating wounds.

6. Inflammatory bowel disease (IBD) includes two chronic disorders: Crohn's disease and ulcerative colitis. Using the chart below, compare and contrast the two diseases:

	Crohn's Disease	Ulcerative Colitis
Area affected	Entire GI tract. All layers of bowel	Entire colon mucosa, submucosa
Age of client	15-30 yrs. of age	15-30 y/o
Amount of diarrhea	urgency @ night	10-20 stools/day
Appearance of stool	liquid, & blood	Bloody, mucus
Systemic symptoms	fever, fatigue, weight loss, pallor.	fever, fatigue, weight loss, pallor.
Nutritional deficiencies	Malabsorption	Malabsorption
Medical treatment	Antidiarrheals, Anti-inflammatory, Corticosteroids, Salicylates, Mesalamine, Flagyl, antibiotics.	Antidiarrheals, corticosteroids, Salicylates.
Surgical intervention	Not curative, only if complications	Remove colon, cure
Prognosis	Chronic, recurrent.	Chronic, recurrent.

7. _____*polyps*_____ are the most commonly found benign tumors in the bowel.

8. Explain the difference between *diverticulosis* and *diverticulitis*.

   diverticulosis is noninflammed diverticula, diverticulitis inflammed diverticula.

9. Causes of obstruction in the small bowel include all of the following *except*:
   1. inflammation.
   2. neoplasms.
   3. adhesions.
   4. hernias.
   5. aneurysms.
   6. volvulus.
   7. intussusception.
   8. food blockage.
   9. compression from outside intestines.

10. Compare and contrast *blunt* and *penetrating* trauma to abdomen.

	Cause	Injuries	Treatment
Blunt trauma	Steering wheel pedestrian accidents	Shearing Crushing Compressing Ruptured bowel	Observation
Penetrating injury	gunshot wounds stabbing	Damage all structures Perforations Peritonitis/ sepsis	Surgery IV antibiotics.

APPLYING SKILLS

11. Physical assessment of the client who is experiencing diarrhea should focus on all of the following *except*:
    1. the abdomen.
    2. muscle weakness/signs of fatigue.
    3. mucous membranes.
    4. the skin (especially in the perineal area).

12. True or False
    _F_ The confirmation of appendicitis is pain at the costovertebral angle.

13. State the rationale for assessing the following areas in the postoperative peritonitis client.
    a. Temperature: *An increase signifies a complication.*

    b. Blood pressure: *↓ can be shock*

    c. Respiratory rate: *Monitor for adult resp. distress syndrome.*

    d. Bowel sounds: *monitor for return to normal functioning*

    e. Urine output: *evaluate fluid status of client*

    f. Skin turgor/mucous membranes: *assess hydration status*

    g. Laboratory tests (CBC, electrolytes): *prevent complications, return levels to baseline.*

14. The nurse will assess for all of the following in a client who has returned from colon surgery *except*:
    1. return of peristalsis.
    2. colostomy output.
    3. stoma appearance.
    4. bowel sounds. *(circled)*
    5. dressings/drains.

15. Following surgery where an ostomy is created, the nurse assesses the stoma. Which of the following indicates a stoma that is healthy?
    1. Pale or dusky stoma
    2. Pressure on the stoma
    3. Pink and moist stoma *(circled)*
    4. Cyanotic stoma

BEST PRACTICES

16. State the rationale for the following treatment interventions for the client with gastroenteritis.
    a. Rest: *reduce energy demands on pt.*

    b. NPO status: *rest the bowel & reduce diarrhea*

    c. Fluids: *replace losses from diarrhea + vomiting*

    d. Electrolytes in fluids/IV: *return balance to vascular system*

    e. Perineal/skin care: *remove irritating fluids; prevent breakdown.*

17. To prevent the spread of disease from infectious diarrhea, the nurse should: (Select all that apply.)
    1. isolate the patient in a private room. *(circled)*
    2. observe contact isolation precautions. *(circled)*
    3. provide separate equipment (BP cuff, thermometer).
    4. follow facility protocol for cleaning surfaces/ equipment. *(circled)*

18. For each of the following nursing diagnoses for the client with appendicitis, identify an appropriate outcome and two interventions.

    a. Acute pain related to inflammation
       Outcome: *Client describes ↓ post operative pain.*

       Intervention #1: *Medicate as ordered evaluate effectiveness.*

       Intervention #2: *Teach client splinting of abdomen.*

    b. Risk for infection related to rupture of appendix
       Outcome: *Infection will not develop / rupture will be diagnosed early.*

       Intervention #1: *Monitor vitals closely.*

       Intervention #2: *Monitor pain closely for rigid & board-like.*

19. State the rationale for each of the following procedures to prepare the client for surgery to remove cancerous growths in the colon.

    a. Diet high in calories, protein, and carbohydrates:

    to provide nutrients to help pts. coping c̄ the stress of surgery + to ensure proper wound healing postoperatively.

    b. Diet low in residue/liquid diet:

    Reduce peristalsis + rest bowel

    c. Cathartics, such as GoLYTELY or Fleet Prep Kit:

    Clean out bowel + reduce bacterial growth in bowel.

    d. Administration of antibiotics:

    Reduce bacterial growth + prevent infection postoperatively

    e. Administration of enemas:

    Clean out inside (lumens) of bowel. Remove bacterial growth.

    f. Blood transfusions (if needed):

    Correct severe anemia; + enhance wound healing

    g. Enterostomal nurse consult:

    Provide emotional support + info. prior to surgery.

20. State the rationale for each nursing intervention for care of the client with an intestinal obstruction.

    a. Insertion of a nasogastric tube:

    Decompress; Remove fluid/gas

    b. NPO status:

    Rest the bowel

    c. IV fluids with electrolytes:

    Replace losses; maintain balance

    d. Monitor vital signs frequently:

    Signifies complications; infection

KEEPING DRUG SKILLS SHARP

21. Antidiarrheal medications are used for clients with Crohn's disease and ulcerative colitis but *not* clients with ___gastroenteritis___ _____.

22. Morphine is *not* used for pain control with diverticulitis because ___it has been shown to cause spasms of the colon___.

23. Compare and contrast common medications used to treat inflammatory bowel disease (IBD).

Medication	Indication for Use	Action
5-ASA Azulfidine Asacol/Rowasa Dipentum	Ulcerative colitis (UC) & Crohn's	Block production of prostaglandins leukotrienes ↓ inflammatory process.
Steroids	UC & Crohn's Inflam. Bowel Disease IBD doesn't respond to saliglates	↓ Inflammation.
Antacids Antihistamines	Steroid use for UC & Crohn's	Prevent gastric ulceration
Budesenide	Crohn's	New, nonsythetic steroid
Purinethol	UC & Crohn's	Immuno Suppression
Methotrexate Imuran Sandimmune	IBD fails to saliglates/ Steroids	Immunoregulatory
Remicade	Crohn's	Block action of tumor necrosis factor.
Antegren	IBD	Immune modulator Attach to immune cells & prevent them from leaving bloodstream to go to site of inflammation
Anticholinergics	UC & Crohn's	Relieve Abd. cramps
Antidiarrheals	UC & Crohn's	Relieve diarrhea
Antispasmodics	UC & Crohn's	Reduce spasms, rest colon
Flagyl	UC & Crohn's	Prevent / control infection
Cipro	Infection	Treat anal fistulas / perianal disease.

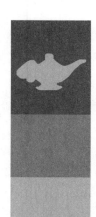

C H A P T E R **34**

Management of Clients with Urinary Disorders

CHAPTER OBJECTIVES

34.1 Identify common nursing diagnoses for clients with disorders of the urinary tract.
34.2 Describe causes and risks for disorders of the urinary tract.
34.3 Relate the pathophysiology and clinical manifestations of urinary tract disorders.
34.4 Describe desired outcomes of medical, surgical, and nursing management of the client with urinary tract disorders.
34.5 Identify education for health promotion and self-care activities for clients with urinary tract disorders.
34.6 Modify plans of care for older clients with urinary tract disorders.

UNDERSTANDING PATHOPHYSIOLOGY

1. A urinary tract infection (UTI) is confirmed on the basis of _____ in the urinary system, usually at a count greater than _____.

2. Identify two reasons why urinary tract infections are uncommon in men.
    a.

    b.

3. Common causes for urinary tract infections in female clients include: (Select all that apply.)
    1. sexual intercourse.
    2. poorly fitting contraceptive diaphragm.
    3. spermicides.
    4. synthetic hormones.
    5. tight jeans/wet bathing suits.
    6. feminine hygiene sprays/bubble baths.
    7. perfumed toilet paper/sanitary napkins.

4. The most accurate diagnostic tool for a UTI is a _____.

5. A serious complication that can develop from cystitis is _____ _____ from an ascending infection.

6. _____ is commonly associated with sexually transmitted disease.

7. Identify the two main causes of urolithiasis.
    a.

    b.

8. Compare and contrast the etiologies of the different types of calculi.

Type of Calculi	Etiology
Calcium	
Oxalate	
Struvite	
Uric acid	
Cystine	
Xanthine	

9. True or False

    _____ Visceral pain from renal calculi can be manifested with nausea and vomiting.

    _____ Stones smaller than 4–5 mm can pass through the urethra.

10. After age 50, the incidence of urinary reflux increases in male clients due to _____ _____.

11. Common causes of urinary retention include all of the following *except*:
    1. detrusor failure in women.
    2. enlarged prostate in men.
    3. urethral strictures.
    4. medications.
    5. calculi.
    6. aneurysms.
    7. tumors.
    8. neuropathies from diabetes, stroke.

APPLYING SKILLS

12. Clinical manifestations of urinary tract infection include: (Select all that apply.)
    1. dysuria.
    2. cloudy urine.
    3. complete emptying of bladder.
    4. hematuria.
    5. abdominal distention.
    6. frequency.
    7. urgency.
    8. inability to void.
    9. rebound tenderness in right lower quadrant.
    10. nausea/diarrhea.

13. Other complaints from female clients that may be confused with urinary tract infections include: (Select all that apply.)
    1. vaginal candidiasis.
    2. Chlamydia.
    3. trichomonas.
    4. gonorrhea.
    5. herpes simplex.

14. Interstitial cystitis is often mistaken for bacterial cystitis prior to an accurate diagnosis. Specific diagnostic criteria recommended include: (Select all that apply.)
    1. detailed client history and physical.
    2. complete bladder diary.
    3. bladder capacity evaluation.
    4. urine cytology.
    5. bladder biopsy.
    6. cystoscopy.

15. Clinical manifestations that would be noted for a client who is developing septic shock from urosepsis include: (Select all that apply.)
    1. fever.
    2. altered mental status.
    3. increased blood pressure.
    4. hyperventilation.

16. True or False
    _____ Peristalsis will return soon after bladder reconstruction surgery as the bowel is not involved in the process.
    _____ Urine never stops after surgery is done to remove bladder cancer.
    _____ A new stoma must be assessed every hour for the first 24 hours postoperatively.
    _____ The site for a stoma must be clearly visible to the client and avoid the umbilicus, pubis, and iliac crests.
    _____ A client with bladder cancer must complete a bowel prep before surgery.
    _____ Pain of kidney stones will be intermittent, meaning the renal stone may have moved.

BEST PRACTICES

17. To successfully treat a urinary tract infection, the nurse should instruct the client to discontinue antibiotics after:
    1. 10 days.
    2. 2 weeks.
    3. manifestations disappear.
    4. the full antibiotic course is completed.

18. State the rationales for each of the health promotion interventions to prevent further urinary tract infections.
    a. Encourage fluid intake of at least 3 liters per day:

    b. Avoid caffeinated beverages/alcohol:

    c. Learn risks associated with spermicides:

    d. Remind client to void every 2–3 hours:

    e. Instruct female clients to void before and after coitus:

19. Identify an appropriate outcome and two interventions for a client with the nursing diagnosis Impaired urinary elimination related to irritation and inflammation of the bladder mucosa.
    Outcome:

    Intervention #1:

    Intervention #2:

20. Identify an appropriate outcome and three interventions for a client with the nursing diagnosis Risk for injury from bacille Calmette-Guérin (BCG) instillation and/or radiation therapy related to side effects.
Outcome:

Intervention #1:

Intervention #2:

Intervention #3:

21. Following urinary diversion, ureteral catheters may be present. A major safety issue involves rules about _____ of the ureteral catheters.

22. Critical nursing interventions for the treatment of autonomic dysreflexia include: (Select all that apply.)
    1. removing triggering stimuli.
    2. re-establishing urine flow.
    3. removing fecal impaction.
    4. inserting urinary catheter or irrigating existing catheter.
    5. monitoring vital signs every hour.
    6. raising head of bed to semi-Fowler's position.

KEEPING DRUG SKILLS SHARP

23. _____ is often prescribed with antibiotics for the acute pain associated with cystitis.

24. Identify two considerations for administering medications to older clients with UTIs.
    a.

    b.

25. Nursing management of the medical client with cystitis includes teaching the client about _____.

26. Explain how the chemotherapeutic agent BCG is used in treating the client with bladder cancer.

27. Identify therapies for treating the different types of urinary incontinence.
    a.

    b.

    c.

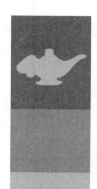

C H A P T E R **35**

Management of Clients with Renal Disorders

CHAPTER OBJECTIVES

35.1 Relate extrarenal systemic conditions to renal disease.

35.2 Describe causes and risk factors for acquired renal disorders and renal vascular disorders.

35.3 Relate pathophysiology and clinical manifestations of acquired renal disorders, renal vascular disorders, and congenital disorders.

35.4 Describe desired outcomes of medical, surgical, and nursing management of acquired renal disorders, renal vascular disorders, and congenital disorders.

35.5 Discuss teaching for self-care to prevent recurrent infectious processes.

35.6 Relate prescribed medications to specific disorders.

35.7 Related laboratory diagnostic testing to specific renal disorders.

35.8 Identify modifications of care plans for older clients experiencing treatment for renal disease.

UNDERSTANDING PATHOPHYSIOLOGY

1. Kidneys regulate which of the following functions in the body? (Select all that apply.)
   1. Body's fluid levels
   2. Electrolyte levels
   3. Acid-base balance
   4. Removal of toxic substances
   5. Erythropoietin synthesis
   6. Prostaglandin production
   7. Renin-angiotensin-aldosterone system

2. Decreased renal function causes _____ _____ due to retained excess sodium and water causing increased vascular volume.

3. Compare and contrast acute and chronic pyelonephritis.

	Acute	Chronic
Etiology		
Manifestations		
Testing		
Medical treatment		

4. An older client has undergone a procedure to relieve urinary obstruction with the placement of a ureteral stent. Explain how correcting this problem can result in fluid and electrolyte imbalance.

5. True or False

_____ Hypertension can cause or be affected by renal disease.

_____ Clients with type 1 diabetes mellitus have a greater likelihood to develop end-stage renal disease (ESRD).

_____ Hypotension is a classic symptom of glomerulosclerosis.

_____ The damage caused by rhabdomyolysis is irreversible and fatal.

_____ Blood flow to the kidneys decreases with normal aging.

_____ Most renal tumors are benign.

_____ There is a probable association between renal cancer and smoking.

_____ After undergoing a nephrectomy to remove renal cancer, the remaining kidney can meet the body's needs.

_____ The lungs and mediastinum are the most frequent sites for metastasis for renal cancer.

_____ Adenocarcinoma is the most common tumor type of renal cancer.

6. List the classic triad of manifestations of renal cancer.

a.

b.

c.

7. Compare and contrast acute and chronic tubulointerstitial disease.

	Acute	Chronic
Cause		
Onset		
Manifestations		
Prognosis		

8. Compare and contrast acute and chronic glomerulonephritis.

	Acute	Chronic
Onset		
Manifestations		

9. Identify the five categories of traumatic injury to the kidney.

a.

b.

c.

d.

e.

10. _____ is a cardinal manifestation of renal injury and found in approximately 80% of cases.

11. Identify six anomalies involving the kidney and describe the effect on renal function.

Disorder	Effect on Renal Function
a.	
b.	
c.	
d.	
e.	
f.	

12. List nephrotoxic agents in each category.
    a. Heavy metals:

    b. Poisons:

    c. Solvents:

    d. Other agents:

APPLYING SKILLS

13. Assessment of the client with hydronephrosis includes: (Select all that apply.)
    1. monitor for presence, location, and intensity of pain.
    2. urine output.
    3. CVA tenderness.
    4. reports of renal failure (oliguria, anorexia, lethargy).

14. _____ may occur after nephrectomy, observable as sudden shortness of breath and loss of breath sounds on the affected side.

15. When obtaining a history from a client with glomerulonephritis, why is a history of upper respiratory infections, skin infections, or recent invasive procedures of particular concern?

16. List teaching needed for self-care to prevent recurrent pyelonephritis.

BEST PRACTICES

17. Explain the rationale for each of the following nursing interventions for clients with altered renal function.
    Rhabdomyolysis: IV fluids and bedrest

    Hypertension: medication and diet changes

18. Nursing interventions to reduce renal damage when contrast x-ray studies are ordered include all of the following *except*:
    1. thorough history and physical before procedure.
    2. use non-dye studies whenever possible.
    3. limit client fluid intake.
    4. monitor client's urine output after study.

19. Identify an appropriate outcome and two interventions for a client with the nursing diagnosis Fluid volume deficit related to fever, nausea, vomiting, and possible diarrhea.
    Outcome:

    Intervention #1:

    Intervention #2:

20. Identify an appropriate outcome and two interventions for a client with the nursing diagnosis Acute pain related to an inflammatory process in the kidney and possible colic.
    Outcome:

    Intervention #1:

    Intervention #2:

21. State the rationale for each of the following nursing interventions for a postoperative nephrectomy client.
    a. Use narcotic analgesia, including patient controlled analgesia (PCA):

    b. Teach client to support chest and abdomen with pillow or hands:

    c. Assess urine output:

    d. Monitor bowel sounds:

22. The primary focus for treatment of nephritis is to heal the glomerular membrane, stop the loss of protein, and break the cycle of edema. Identify four pertinent nursing plans and interventions to achieve these goals.

Plan	Intervention(s)
a.	
b.	
c.	
d.	

KEEPING DRUG SKILLS SHARP

23. Decreased renal function in a diabetic patient requires a _____ in the level of insulin administered.

24. Common analgesics found to cause renal damage as nephrotoxins include: (Select all that apply.)
    1. opioids.
    2. acetaminophen.
    3. phenacetin.
    4. NSAIDs.

25. Clients with hypertension are often prescribed diuretics as part of the medical treatment regimen. Explain how diuretics, which help lower blood pressure, can also cause renal damage.

26. Identify two reasons to make modifications for older clients who are prescribed antibiotics for pyelonephritis.

    a.

    b.

27. The inflammatory condition that results in interstitial nephritis or "tubulointerstitial disease" can be caused by use of: (Select all that apply.)
    1. NSAIDs.
    2. hydrochlorothiazide.
    3. Captopril.
    4. cephalosporins.
    5. acetaminophen.
    6. sodium bicarbonate.
    7. aspirin.
    8. sulfonamide.

28. Commonly used antibiotics for acute pyelonephritis include _____ or
    _____.

29. Management of glomerulonephritis may include plasmapheresis in conjunction with either _____ or _____.

30. Antihypertensive drugs in the _____ class are superior for maintaining blood pressure plus reducing the progression of renal disease.

31. A clot in the renal vein could be treated with _____.

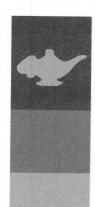

C H A P T E R **36**

Management of Clients with Renal Failure

CHAPTER OBJECTIVES

36.1   Define *uremia, uremic syndrome,* and *renal failure*.
36.2   Distinguish acute renal failure from chronic renal failure related to causes and risk factors.
36.3   Identify prerenal, intrarenal, and postrenal causes of acute renal failure.
36.4   Relate pathophysiology and clinical manifestations of clients with acute and chronic renal failure.
36.5   Distinguish renal excretion in nonoliguric and oliguric renal failure.
36.6   Describe the desired outcomes of medical and nursing management for the client with acute and chronic renal failure.
36.7   Identify self-care activities for the acute renal failure client to prevent further kidney damage.
36.8   Identify treatment modifications and rationale for the older client.
36.9   Describe body system changes for the client with chronic renal failure.
36.10 Identify goals of dialysis therapy.
36.11 Describe different methods of dialysis including advantages, contraindications, specific nursing care, complications, and related psychosocial problems.
36.12 Describe assessment of a vascular access site for the dialysis client.
36.13 Discuss dietary and fluid status concerns for the dialysis client.
36.14 Describe the desired outcomes of the surgical management of the renal transplant client.
36.15 Discuss indications, contraindications, and complications for a renal transplant.
36.16 Identify self-care issues for the renal transplant client.

UNDERSTANDING PATHOPHYSIOLOGY

1.   Common manifestations of acute renal failure (ARF) include: (Select all that apply.)
     1.   abrupt loss of kidney function.
     2.   hematuria.
     3.   elevation in serum creatinine and urea nitrogen levels.
     4.   a decrease in urine production below normal 400ml/24 hrs.

2.   List the three main classifications of ARF and give examples of each:
     a.

     b.

     c.

3.   True or False

     _____   Once renal failure has begun, the ability to reverse the mechanism will depend on the level of destruction of the basement membrane.

     _____   The client diagnosed with diabetes mellitus is protected from renal failure due to high blood glucose levels.

     _____   Hypertension is a major cause of chronic renal failure (CRF).

_____   *Oliguria* refers to a urine output which exceeds 1500 ml/day in a normal healthy client.

_____   Unless treated properly, the client with ARF will develop CRF and require dialysis in the future.

_____   CRF causes more degenerative changes throughout the body than does ARF.

_____   Uremia means "urine in the blood."

_____   Uremic syndrome is a set of manifestations from the loss of renal function.

_____   Renal failure is the loss of renal function.

4.   Compare and contrast the two types of acute renal failure:

	Nonoliguric Renal Failure	Oliguric Renal Failure
Urine output		
Urine		
Clinical signs		
Prognosis		

5. Causes of CRF include all of the following *except*:
   1. diabetes insipidus.
   2. hypertension.
   3. chronic glomerulonephritis.
   4. acute renal failure.
   5. polycystic kidney disease.
   6. obstruction.
   7. repeated episodes of pyelonephritis.
   8. nephrotoxins.

6. Differentiate between ultrafiltration and diffusion.

7. Identify the cause of dialysis disequilibrium syndrome.

APPLYING SKILLS

8. Monitoring the client with ARF includes review of lab data. Discuss the implication for these abnormal lab values.
   a. Increasing BUN level:

   b. Low RBC, Hct, Hgb:

   c. Low platelets:

9. CRF affects every system in the body. For each of the identified areas, give examples of manifestations.
   Hematologic changes:

   Immunologic changes:

Musculoskeletal changes:

Changes in medication metabolism:

Psychosocial changes:

10. Clients who do not respond to conservative treatment for ARF may require dialysis to resolve the problem. Clinical manifestations that require dialysis include: (Select all that apply.)
    1. significant volume overload.
    2. hypovolemia.
    3. progressive uremia (rising BUN and creatinine levels).
    4. altered central nervous system functioning.
    5. pericarditis.

11. Identify the critical nursing assessments that must be performed for a dialysis graft site and explain the implications of the findings.

12. Important self-care activities the nurse should teach the client being discharged after an episode of ARF include: (Select all that apply.)
    1. how to prevent further kidney damage.
    2. follow up with a nephrologist for at least 2 years.
    3. avoiding green leafy vegetables in the diet.
    4. the pathophysiology of renal failure.

13. Compare and contrast the types of dialysis in the chart below.

	Advantages & Disadvantages	Contraindications	Specific Nursing Care
Hemodialysis			
Peritoneal			
Continuous ambulatory peritoneal dialysis			
Continuous cyclic peritoneal dialysis			
Intermittent peritoneal dialysis			
Nightly intermittent peritoneal dialysis			

BEST PRACTICES

14. For each of the following interventions for the treatment of ARF, give the rationale behind the action.
    a. Careful replacement of fluids:

    b. Replacement of other fluid losses:

    c. Cautious use of diuretics to reduce fluid overload:

    d. Electrolyte replacement based on lab data:

    e. Electrocardiograph monitors:

    f. Dietary restrictions:

15. Identify the dietary modifications for the client with ARF. Give a rationale for each action.
    a. High calorie:

    b. Low protein:

    c. Low sodium/magnesium/phosphate/potassium:

    d. TPN:

    e. Adequate/balanced fluids:

16. Identify an appropriate outcome and interventions for a client with the nursing diagnosis Fluid volume excess related to inability of kidneys to produce urine secondary to acute renal failure.
    Outcome:

    Interventions:

17. Identify an appropriate outcome and interventions for a client with the nursing diagnosis Imbalanced nutrition: Less than body requirements related to anorexia and altered metabolic state.
    Outcome:

    Interventions:

18. Constipation is a common problem for the client with CRF. The nurse should advise the client to avoid OTC laxatives because they contain _____ which cannot be excreted when kidneys have failed.

19. List the four basic goals of dialysis therapy.
    a.

    b.

    c.

    d.

20. The nurse should instruct the dialysis patient to avoid salt substitutes because they contain _____ which is not excreted in renal failure.

21. A major goal of kidney transplantation is _____.

22. The nurse counsels the client that the two absolute contraindications to kidney transplant include: (Select all that apply.)
    1. infection.
    2. active malignancy.
    3. hypertension.
    4. COPD.

23. A major cardiovascular complication of kidney transplant is:
    1. hypertension.
    2. stroke.
    3. myocardial infarction.
    4. aneurysm.

24. The nurse tells the client's family that the main reason the death rate after kidney transplantation has dropped is because of _____ _____.

25. One of the main problems with self-care after renal transplantation is _____ _____.

KEEPING DRUG SKILLS SHARP

26. The diuretic _____ is prescribed cautiously for clients with ARF because it can be nephrotoxic and increase risk of further kidney damage.

27. Explain why medications for the older renal client must be adjusted.

28. A client with ARF has a dangerously high laboratory value of potassium. This is a life-threatening situation because of the risk of cardiac arrest. Treatment of the hyperkalemia can include administration of which of the following medications? (Select all that apply.)
    1. Calcium
    2. Insulin
    3. Normal saline
    4. Vitamin C
    5. Kayexalate
    6. Sodium citrate
    7. Sorbitol
    8. Sodium bicarbonate

29. The hormone _____ can be administered either intravenously after hemodialysis or subcutaneously.

CONCEPT MAP EXERCISES

The following questions are based on the concept map *Understanding Chronic Renal Failure and Its Treatment* in your textbook.

30. When the kidneys suffer damage resulting in a decreased glomerular filtration of the blood, what two lab values will be noted initially?

31. What initial clinical manifestations develop when the nephrons of the kidney can no longer concentrate urine?

33. Decreased sodium reabsorption leads to water retention and which common manifestations?

34. A client diagnosed with CRF presents with changes in level of consciousness and pruritus. What is the mechanism for the development of these changes?

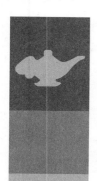

CHAPTER **37**

Assessment of the Reproductive System

CHAPTER OBJECTIVES

37.1   Discuss important lifestyle, health habits, developmental, and other socioeconomic factors to be considered in the assessment of the reproductive system.

37.2   Describe education that should be completed along with assessment.

37.3   Describe the aspects of female and male reproductive assessment including the importance of being nonjudgmental and establishing rapport with the client.

37.4   Describe the health history for the female and male reproductive system including biographic and demographic data.

37.5   Describe a thorough review of clinical manifestations with female and male clients based on their description of current health status.

37.6   List the specific questions to ask the client to elicit information about the clinical manifestations.

37.7   Discuss appropriate questions for the client in the review of systems.

37.8   Identify the aspects of the gynecologic and obstetric history for the female client.

37.9   Identify herbal therapies for female reproductive issues.

37.10   Identify client risk for reproductive system disease based on medical and surgical history.

37.11   Discuss aspects important in the sexual and reproductive history for the male and female client.

37.12   Determine desirable body weight as it impacts reproductive status.

37.13   Discuss social and family history as they relate to the client's clinical manifestations of the reproductive system.

37.14   Identify psychosocial issues for the male client that will decrease sperm count.

37.15   Identify psychosocial issues for the female client such as smoking and use of oral contraceptives that will increase morbidity.

37.16   Perform a physical assessment of the female and male reproductive system assuring caring, comfort, and privacy of the client.

37.17   Identify hernias found on reproductive assessment.

37.18   Describe diagnostic test purposes related to examination of the reproductive system.

37.19   Relate diagnostic testing to specific clinical manifestations and subsequent need to treat the client.

ANATOMY & PHYSIOLOGY REVIEW

1.   Label the structures of the female pelvis.

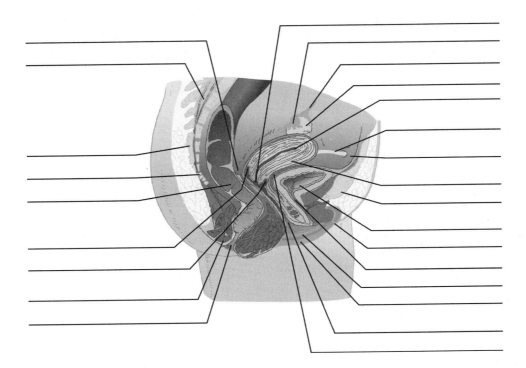

2.   Label the lymph nodes near the female breast.

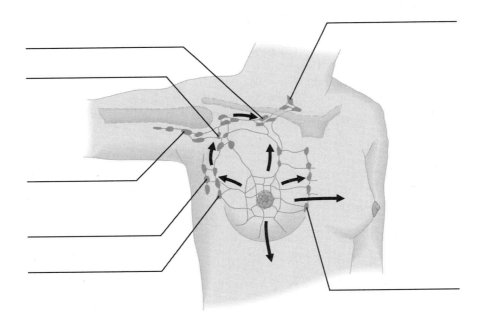

3.   Label the structures of the male pelvis and genitalia.

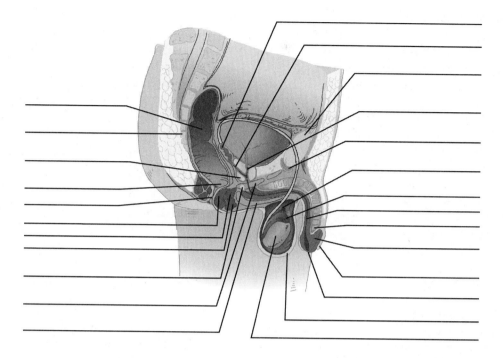

UNDERSTANDING PATHOPHYSIOLOGY

4.   The most serious childhood infectious disease that can affect a woman of childbearing age is:
1.   viral pneumonia.
2.   hepatitis.
3.   endocarditis.
4.   rubella.

5.   The American Cancer Society (ACS) recommends that women who are or have been sexually active and have reached 18 years of age should have annual _____ and
_____.

6.   A mammogram _____
_____ used to detect _____
_____.

7.   Which childhood infection can affect male fertility?
1.   Chicken pox
2.   Measles
3.   Mumps
4.   Hepatitis

8. Match the description or definition to the correct term.

Description/Definition

_____ a. Antigen found in the serum of men with prostate cancer

_____ b. Absence of menstrual flow

_____ c. Excessive uterine bleeding

_____ d. Studies which measure pressure from bladder or urethra, urinary flow, and muscle activity

_____ e. Analysis of sperm for fertility, the effectiveness of a vasectomy, to test DNA, or establish paternity

_____ f. Hypospadias

_____ g. Inguinal hernia

Term

1. Prolapse or protrusion of a loop of intestine through the inguinal wall or canal
2. Prostate-specific antigen (PSA)
3. Malposition of the urinary meatus on the underside of the penile shaft
4. Amenorrhea

5. Urodynamic assessment

6. Semen analysis
7. Menorrhagia

APPLYING SKILLS

9. As part of the reproductive assessment, what information should be included in the data obtained from the client? (Select all that apply.)
   1. Client's lifestyle
   2. Health habits
   3. Self-perceptions
   4. Body image
   5. Developmental stage
   6. Cultural, religious factors
   7. Socioeconomic and educational background

10. The nurse should instruct a client prior to a pelvic examination to: (Select all that apply.)
    1. not douche.
    2. not have sexual intercourse.
    3. take a bath.
    4. not use vaginal products for 2–3 days.

11. The best time to perform a breast exam on a 45-year-old female is:
    1. 7–10 days before menses.
    2. 2–3 days before menses.
    3. 7–10 days after onset of menses.
    4. during menses.

12. If, during a pelvic examination, abnormal cervical or vaginal tissue or a mass is discovered, what other procedures may need to be performed? (Select all that apply.)
    1. Bimanual exam
    2. Colposcopy or biopsy
    3. Lithotripsy
    4. Wet smear

13. An enlargement of the breasts is called _____ _____.

14. The nurse working in an OB/GYN office should discuss health maintenance activities for general health in addition to reproductive health because _____ _____.

15. The _____ is the upper outer quadrant of the breast.

16. The health history for the female reproductive system includes data related to: (Select all that apply.)
    1. genitals.
    2. reproductive system.
    3. breasts.
    4. overall health status.

17. List the common complaints of women seeking gynecologic care.
    a.

    b.

    c.

    d.

    e.

18. List the common complaints of men seeking reproductive care.

    a.

    b.

    c.

    d.

    e.

    f.

BEST PRACTICES

19. During a reproductive assessment of a 40-year-old female, the nurse should also take the opportunity to discuss which of the following health maintenance measures with the client? (Select all that apply.)
    1. Breast self-examinations
    2. Risk factors associated with gynecologic cancer and heart disease
    3. Menstrual hygiene
    4. Lifestyle factors (diet, exercise, sleep, stress)
    5. Protection against sexually transmitted diseases (STDs)

20. A rectal prostate examination should be performed: (Select all that apply.)
    1. in men over the age of 50.
    2. in men over the age of 45 with increased risk.
    3. to detect changes in size or consistency of prostate gland.
    4. to denote tumors or acute or chronic infections.

21. Why is caring and sensitivity so important when conducting a reproductive health history and physical exam? Because: (Select all that apply.)
    1. clients are often humiliated and embarrassed during the exam.
    2. some clients may view reproductive issues as private.
    3. some clients may have guilt feelings and shame about sexuality.
    4. clients may not have adequate information and may feel ignorant.
    5. the genitals may have deep, symbolic meaning for clients.

22. The best way to begin a sexual history is to ask the client _____ _____.

23. The two other body systems that are often assessed at the same time as the reproductive system are the _____ and _____ systems.

24. Explain how weight can be related to reproductive disorders.

25. Why should the physical examination fall at the end of the assessment of the reproductive system?

26. Women are encouraged to begin breast self-exam at age _____.

27. Colposcopy is indicated in all women with _____ _____ _____.

28. True or False

    _____ Laparoscopies can be performed both diagnostically and therapeutically.

    _____ Cervical biopsy is safe to perform on pregnant women.

    _____ The Pap smear screens for common STDs.

    _____ Examination of the male breast is not a routine part of a physical exam.

    _____ Smegma is a cheesy, thick, white, odoriferous substance under the foreskin in uncircumcised males and indicates infection.

    _____ Nodules on the testicles are never normal and are of concern for cancer.

    _____ Testicular biopsy is the best diagnostic test for testicular cancer.

29. What should the nurse do if a male has an erection during a physical examination?

KEEPING DRUG SKILLS SHARP

30. Herbal medications commonly used to treat reproductive disorders include: (Select all that apply.)
    1. saw palmetto.
    2. yohimbe.
    3. St. John's wort.
    4. milk thistle.

31. List the substances that can affect sperm count, contribute to impotence, decrease libido, and encourage risk-taking behavior.
    a.

    b.

    c.

    d.

32. List common drugs that can contribute to sexual function difficulties.
    a.

    b.

    c.

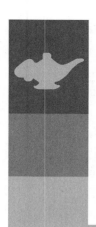

C H A P T E R **38**

Management of Men with Reproductive Disorders

CHAPTER OBJECTIVES

38.1   Identify concerns of men seeking health care for reproductive tract concerns.

38.2   Describe causes and risks for male reproductive disorders.

38.3   Relate the pathophysiology and clinical manifestations of male reproductive disorders.

38.4   Describe desired outcomes of medical, surgical, and nursing management of the male client with reproductive disorders.

38.5   Identify complementary and alternative therapies that improve or impede various male reproductive disorders.

38.6   Identify education for health promotion and self-care activities for male clients with reproductive disorders.

TRENDS AND THEORIES

1. Men are often reluctant to ask for help with prostate or penile problems because _____ _____ _____.

2. Skillful therapeutic interaction with men who have prostate/penile/testicular problems includes:

   a.

   b.

   c.

   d.

3. Partners should be included in discussions about male reproductive disorders because _____ _____ _____.

4. _____% of men in their 50s will have evidence of benign prostatic hypertrophy (BPH).

5. _____ men in the U.S. will be diagnosed with prostate cancer in 2007.

6. Psychosocial demands that infertility places on couples include demands on:

   a.

   b.

   c.

   d.

7. _____ may cause a man with a penis problem to delay seeking treatment for months.

UNDERSTANDING PATHOPHYSIOLOGY

8. The nurse examines a male who has BPH. The nurse explains to the client that BPH is:
    1. hypertrophy of periurethral glands.
    2. hyperplasia of periurethral glands that compresses the normal prostate gland.
    3. dysplasia of prostatic cells that begins in the periphery of posterior gland.
    4. inflammation of prostate glands that compresses the urethra.

9. The cause of testicular cancer is unknown. However, it has been associated with:
    1. prostatitis at an early age.
    2. sexual activity with many partners.
    3. undescended testicles.
    4. cancer of the prostate.

10. Match the following terms with the correct definition or description.

    Terms
    _____ a. Orchitis
    _____ b. Testicular torsion
    _____ c. Epididymitis
    _____ d. Hydrocele
    _____ e. Varicococele
    _____ f. Cryptorchidism
    _____ g. Phimosis
    _____ h. Priapism

    Definition/Description
    1. Acute testicular inflammation caused by a viral infection
    2. Testicle is mobile; spermatic cord twist
    3. Prolonged and painful erection
    4. Penile foreskin constriction
    5. Dilated testicular vein
    6. Undescended testicles
    7. Inflammation of the epididymis
    8. Painless collection of clear, yellow fluid in scrotum

APPLYING SKILLS

11. During a physical assessment, a client with BPH would likely report having which symptoms? (Select all that apply.)
    1. Downward force of stream
    2. Painful urination
    3. Difficulty starting the flow of urine
    4. Pain in lower abdomen

12. Digital rectal examinations are performed on male patients with BPH in order to:
    1. assess prostate size and to differentiate BPH from prostate enlargement.
    2. determine the size of cells.
    3. release a closed stricture above the testes.
    4. allow urine to flow freely.

13. A client with BPH will have which of these symptoms? (Select all that apply.)
    1. Frequency of urination
    2. Urgency, hesitancy
    3. Change in stream of urine
    4. Urinary retention
    5. Nocturia

14. Cancer of the prostate has which of the following diagnostic markers? (Select all that apply.)
    1. Hard nodules, unilateral enlargement of outer prostate
    2. Elevated PSA greater than 10 ng/m, DRE exam positive
    3. Increased acid phosphatase levels
    4. Positive transrectal ultrasound and biopsy

15. The nurse examines a 28-year-old male with a testicular nodule that is highly suspicious for testicular cancer. What laboratory exam would provide further evidence to support this diagnosis?
    1. Elevated testosterone level
    2. Alpha-fetoprotein (AFP), human chorionic gonadotropin (HCG)
    3. Carcinoembryonic antigen (CEA)
    4. Antinuclear antibodies (ANA)

BEST PRACTICES

16. A 65-year-old male is scheduled for a transurethral prostatectomy (TURP). The nurse explains to the client that in this procedure:
    1. a low abdominal incision is made in order to approach the prostate without entering the bladder.
    2. an incision is made into the area between the anus and the prostate.
    3. a transurethral incision of the prostate is made, followed by balloon dilation of the stricture.
    4. a lighted tube is placed in the urethra and excess prostatic tissue is removed.

17. What is a common nursing diagnosis for a client with TURP in the postoperative phase? (Select all that apply.)
    1. Ineffective tissue perfusion related to deep vein thrombosis
    2. Altered comfort related to pain of bladder spasm
    3. Disturbed body image related to disfiguring surgery
    4. Imbalanced nutrition, less than body requirement

18. Discharge teaching for clients with TURP should include:
    1. use enemas to avoid straining.
    2. increase intake of coffee, tea, and sodas.
    3. avoid heaving lifting, heavy climbing, driving, and prolonged sitting.
    4. do not have more than two servings of alcohol per day.

19. The nurse counsels a client that the important psychosocial factors that can combine to cause erectile dysfunction (ED) include: (Select all that apply.)
    1. Performance anxiety
    2. Stress and fatigue
    3. Low self-esteem
    4. Depression
    5. Changes in relationships

20. The nurse describes the two types of penile prostheses to a client considering a penile implant as _____ and _____.

21. A 75 kg client has a closed-irrigation system after an open prostatectomy. The saline is infusing at 200 ml/hour. At the end of the 8-hour shift, the nurse empties the Foley bag of 1700 ml. The most appropriate action by the nurse is to:
    1. document the urine output.
    2. call the physician.
    3. reduce the rate of the irrigation.
    4. reposition the catheter.

22. The nurse teaches a client with infertility that which of the following measures may be helpful? (Select all that apply.)
    1. Take a warm, relaxing bath before intercourse.
    2. Refrain from wearing tight clothing.
    3. Abstain from recreational drugs and alcohol.
    4. Use a commercial scrotal cooling device.

KEEPING DRUG SKILLS SHARP

23. Because they may aggravate the condition, clients with BPH should avoid taking which of these medications? (Select all that apply.)
    1. Antipsychotic medications, antidepressants
    2. Calcium channel blockers
    3. Cold medicines, diet pills
    4. Topical agents for urinary constriction

24. Clients with BPH should be encouraged to drink fluids because concentrated urine acts as an irritant to the _____.

25. True or False

    _____ The use of phototherapeutic agents such as herbs to help control BPH has been increasing.

    _____ The most commonly used herbal agent in treating BPH is saw palmetto.

26. _____ is commonly given to men after an open prostatectomy to maintain blood flow to the corpora cavernosa during the recovery period.

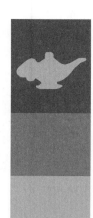

CHAPTER 39

Management of Women with Reproductive Disorders

CHAPTER OBJECTIVES

39.1   Identify cultural influences and reactions to menstrual disorders.

39.2   Identify common menstrual disorders and their manifestations.

39.3   Explain desired outcomes of medical and nursing management of menstrual disorders.

39.4   Describe causes and risk factors of pelvic inflammatory disease, endometrial disorders, uterine and ovarian malignant disorders, urogenital prolapse, polyps, benign uterine and ovarian tumors, and vaginal and vulvar disorders.

39.5   Relate the pathophysiology and clinical manifestations of pelvic inflammatory disease, endometrial disorders, uterine and ovarian malignant disorders, urogenital prolapse, polyps, benign uterine and ovarian tumors, and vaginal and vulvar disorders.

39.6   Describe the desired outcomes of medical, surgical, and nursing management for pelvic inflammatory disease, endometrial disorders, uterine and ovarian malignant disorders, urogenital prolapse, polyps, benign uterine and ovarian tumors, and vaginal and vulvar disorders.

39.7   Explain postoperative care following hysterectomy.

UNDERSTANDING PATHOPHYSIOLOGY

1.   A 35-year-old female complains of irritability, depression, frequent crying spells, migraine headaches, and abdominal bloating—all before her menses. These symptoms are probably related to:

1.   taking medications for extreme psychosis.

2.   iron and vitamin deficiency.

3.   PMS syndrome relating to hormonal imbalance.

4.   excessive retention of thyroid stimulating hormone (TSH).

2. Match the following terms with the correct description.

Term

_____ a. Cystocele

_____ b. Vaginal prolapse

_____ c. Rectocele

_____ d. Vaginitis

_____ e. Toxic shock syndrome

_____ f. Vaginal fistulae

_____ g. Vulvitis

Description

1. Descent of urinary bladder
2. Inflammation of the vulva
3. Protrusion of vaginal wall musculature
4. Inflammation of the vagina
5. Abnormal tube-like passage from the vagina to bladder
6. Toxins of *Staphylococcus aureus*
7. Descent of the bowel/protrusion of posterior wall of vagina

3. A 45-year-old female has just had a hysterectomy and is anxious about experiencing severe symptoms of menopause. The nurse can respond appropriately by saying:
   1. "Only older women have this problem."
   2. "Menopausal symptoms occur when the ovaries are removed."
   3. "You must wait until symptoms are severe to have treatment."
   4. "Symptoms from this surgery only start when you are 55 years and older."

4. More than 50% of women with history of pelvic inflammatory disease (PID) have difficulty becoming pregnant after an infection of PID due to:
   1. fallopian tube enlargement, which allows the harboring of more bacteria.
   2. cervical canal stretched by past infections.
   3. scarring by inflammatory process and subsequent closing and scarring of fallopian tubes.
   4. ruptured fallopian tubes unable to hold eggs.

5. A total hysterectomy is the removal of the _____ and the _____.

6. Total hysterectomy with bilateral salpingo-oophorectomy is a total hysterectomy along with the removal of the _____ and the _____.

APPLYING SKILLS

7. The clinical symptoms of PID that a patient would present with are: (Select all that apply.)
   1. malaise, fever, chills.
   2. nausea and vomiting.
   3. acute sharp severe pain on both sides of abdomen.
   4. heavy, purulent vaginal discharge.

8. What is the most serious long-term complication that can result from endometriosis?
   1. Infertility
   2. Cancer of the uterus
   3. Prolapsed uterus
   4. Cervical cancer

9. List clinical manifestations of vasomotor instability associated with menopause.
   a.

   b.

   c.

   d.

10. When a Foley catheter is discontinued after a hysterectomy, the nurse should report which of the following to the physician? (Select all that apply.)
    1. Voiding frequently in small amounts
    2. Inability to void
    3. Bladder distention
    4. Hematuria

BEST PRACTICES

11. A 26-year-old female has been complaining of persistent dysmenorrhea for the past 6 months. In providing patient education, the nurse should: (Select all that apply.)
    1. encourage exercise, including swimming.
    2. tell her to decrease sodium and increase calcium and vitamin D.
    3. discuss oral contraceptives to relieve menstrual discomfort.
    4. encourage use of narcotics for extreme pain.

12. What are the priority nursing actions for a client who has just had a vaginal hysterectomy?
    1. Assist with tub and shower bath.
    2. Provide a high carbohydrate diet.
    3. Teach client exercises to strengthen chest and stomach.
    4. Observe client for decreased urine output.

13. The primary diagnostic tool for cervical cancer is:
    1. gram stain and culture.
    2. Pap smear.
    3. cervical ovulation.
    4. C-reactive protein.

14. During evaluation of the client with cervical cancer, the nurse would expect the client to have which of the following assessment findings? (Select all that apply.)
    1. Vaginal discharge
    2. Metrorrhagia and bleeding
    3. Painful intercourse
    4. Pressure in bladder and bowel
    5. Abdominal pain

15. When providing care for a client being treated at home for PID, the nurse should instruct the client to:
    1. continue to take medications for blood pressure elevations.
    2. avoid sexual contact with partner, no douching.
    3. ambulate at least 3–4 times per day.
    4. resume vaginal cleansing.

16. To promote drainage and comfort, a client with PID should: (Select all that apply.)
    1. maintain semi-Fowler's position to promote downward drainage.
    2. take a sitz bath or apply heat to lower back and abdomen.
    3. maintain reverse Trendelenburg position for comfort.
    4. only take pain medication every 8 hours.

17. A 26-year-old female is admitted for a workup for PID. This condition is also associated with: (Select all that apply.)
    1. bacterial vaginal infections (untreated).
    2. sexually transmitted diseases.
    3. lack of condom use with high incidence of passing bacteria between partners.
    4. recent viral infections of the lung.

18. While preparing discharge instructions for the client after an abdominal hysterectomy, the client asks when she can return to work. The nurse should respond:
    1. "It's possible to return to normal activities within 4–6 weeks."
    2. "When the abdomen incision has healed in about 3–4 months."
    3. "In 2 weeks if you have no pain."
    4. "Following your next visit to the doctor's office."

19. A 55-year-old female client diagnosed with cancer of the uterus is to receive radioactive implants. Where would you place the client on the clinical unit?
    1. While radioactive implants are in place, the client can be placed in a ward
    2. A private room with adjoining bathrooms
    3. Far away from the nurses' station
    4. Private room with radiation precautions

KEEPING DRUG SKILLS SHARP

20. A client scheduled for discharge after an abdominal hysterectomy with removal of ovaries and fallopian tubes wants information regarding hormone replacement therapy. What hormone will be most likely prescribed by the physician?
    1. Thyroxin
    2. Estrogen
    3. Testosterone
    4. Lactin

21. A woman with endometriosis wants to have children. Drug therapy for her will probably include which of the following?
    1. Estrogen
    2. Motrin
    3. Acetaminophen
    4. Progestin

THEORIES AND TRENDS

22. Culturally competent nurses understand the influence of culture on attitudes towards menstruation and sexuality. List five culturally based or religious-based influences.

   a.

   b.

   c.

   d.

   e.

UNDERSTANDING TERMINOLOGY

23. Match the following menstrual disorders with their description.

Menstrual Disorder	Description
_____ a. Primary amenorrhea	1. Vaginal spotting or bleeding between menses
_____ b. Secondary amenorrhea	2. Not yet starting menstruation in a girl 16 years or older
_____ c. PMS	3. Cyclical combination of emotional and physical manifestations that occur before menses
_____ d. Dysmenorrhea	4. Absence of menses in a woman who previously had been menstruating
_____ e. Metrorrhagia	5. Excessive vaginal bleeding at normal cyclical intervals
_____ f. Menorrhagia	6. Painful periods

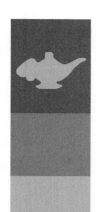

CHAPTER 40

Management of Clients with Breast Disorders

CHAPTER OBJECTIVES

40.1 Describe the nurse's role in increasing public awareness of early detection of breast cancer.

40.2 Identify facts indicating success of treatment in the beginning decline of breast cancer new cases and deaths.

40.3 Relate the impact of ethnicity and psychosocial and socioeconomic factors on breast cancer incidence relative to risk for the disease.

40.4 Discuss ovarian and hormone function as well as hormone replacement therapy (HRT) related to etiology and risk for breast cancer.

40.5 Relate other factors including family history, diet, environment, health promotion, and health maintenance activities to the occurrence of breast cancer.

40.6 Describe the role of the nurse in assisting clients to assess risk of breast cancer in a reasonable manner and according to American Cancer Society guidelines.

40.7 Describe breast self-exam (BSE) as a method of health maintenance for breast cancer detection.

40.8 Identify the pathophysiology and clinical manifestations of various malignant breast tumors.

40.9 Identify the types and purpose of each diagnostic method for breast cancer.

40.10 Describe the TNM staging system as it relates to the extent of breast cancer disease and prognosis.

40.11 Describe the medical and surgical treatment strategies for primary, local recurrence, and metastatic breast cancer.

40.12 Describe the preoperative and postoperative nursing management for the breast cancer client and the breast cancer reconstruction client including education for self-care.

40.13 Discuss the coping and body image issues that are likely for the breast cancer client.

40.14 Describe the appropriate nursing assessment and management of the breast cancer client receiving radiation and chemotherapy including nutrition and treatment compliance.

40.15 Discuss types and uses of radiation, chemotherapy, and hormone therapy effective for breast cancer treatment.

40.16 Describe the incidence of breast cancer in men including treatment.

40.17 Discuss breast surgeries for benign disease.

UNDERSTANDING PATHOPHYSIOLOGY

1. The most important single risk factor for breast cancer is _____.

2. The overall risk of breast cancer is greatest in women:
   1. over 60 years of age.
   2. who do not have breast changes.
   3. who have BRCA$_1$/BRCA$_2$ genes.
   4. who have tumor suppressor.

3. While examining a female client, the nurse becomes alarmed when she palpates:
   1. a painful reddened mass in the upper outer quadrant of breast.
   2. a 3 cm movable mass in the axillary region.
   3. a large, tender, movable mass in upper area of breast.
   4. a hard, painless, immobile, nontender lesion in an irregularly shaped mass in the upper outer quadrant.

4. True or False

_____ African-American women are more at risk of dying from breast cancer than Caucasian women.

_____ Having Medicaid significantly improves the chances of survival.

_____ Asian women born in this country have the same risk of breast cancer as do Caucasian women.

_____ Early menarche and late menopause increases the risk of breast cancer.

_____ Hormone replacement therapy (HRT) carries the same risk for breast cancer whether it is used long-term or short-term.

APPLYING SKILLS

5. The most accurate diagnostic test used for assisting in the diagnosis of breast cancer is:
   1. fine needle aspiration.
   2. closed biopsy.
   3. mammography.
   4. steriotactic core biopsy.

6. During the postoperative period for a client who has had breast surgery, possible complications include: (Select all that apply.)
   1. lymphedema, infection.
   2. hematoma.
   3. cellulitis.
   4. seroma.

7. During the early postoperative period following a mastectomy, the nurse would encourage the client to:
   1. perform active elbow flexion and extension exercises on the affected side.
   2. perform full range of motion exercises.
   3. adduct the affected arm daily.
   4. keep affected arm straight and aligned for 24–48 hours.

8. What organization will be able to assist the mastectomy client who has had radiation and surgery with body image concerns?
   1. American Cancer Society
   2. Reach to Recovery
   3. National Cancer Foundation
   4. Society of American Mastectomy Society

9. Match these terms with the correct definition or description.

	Term		**Definition/Description**
_____	a. Tissue expanders	1.	Done to achieve symmetry, delayed for several months following breast reconstruction
_____	b. Transverse rectus abdominal muscle flap	2.	"Tummy tuck"
_____	c. Latissimus dorsi muscle flap	3.	Deflated saline envelope inserted under chest muscle that expands over 6–8 weeks
_____	d. Gluteal muscle free flaps	4.	Large, fan-shaped muscle beneath the scapula that is used when inadequate skin is available at mastectomy site
_____	e. Nipple areola reconstruction	5.	Breast construction involves use of gluteus muscle

BEST PRACTICES

10. Lifestyle changes that can to help reduce the potential risk for breast cancer include: (Select all that apply.)
    1. decreasing alcohol consumption.
    2. decreasing fat intake to 20% of dietary calories.
    3. exercising regularly.
    4. ingesting large quantities of niacin.

11. The National Cancer Advisory Board (NCAB) recommends to the National Cancer Institute (NCI) that women between 40–49 years of age:
    1. have mammograms every 5 years.
    2. have screening mammograms every 1–2 years if they are at average risk for breast cancer.
    3. only do manual breast self-exams monthly.
    4. have diagnostic mammograms every 2–4 years.

12. Fine needle aspiration determines whether a solid lump is a _____ _____.

13. Stereotactic needle guided biopsy is used mainly to identify _____ _____.

14. A _____ is an en bloc removal of the breast, axillary lymph nodes, and overlying skin, with the muscles left intact.

KEEPING DRUG SKILLS SHARP

15. Additional treatments for clients who have breast cancer may include: (Select all that apply.)
    1. chemotherapy.
    2. radiation therapy.
    3. hormone therapy.
    4. DNA screening.

16. True or False

    _____   Tamoxifen is an agent commonly used in clients who have breast tumors with receptors for estrogen.

17. Radiation therapy used to treat micrometastatic disease following a mastectomy:
    1. enables the healing process to progress faster.
    2. successfully reduces the risk of local recurrence and distant metastasis.
    3. promotes skin grafts to become less infected.
    4. enhances the chemotherapy to be given in a shorter period of time.

18. Radiation therapy for breast cancer can be administered through which of these methods? (Select all that apply.)
    1. External beams
    2. Brachytherapy
    3. Iridium implants
    4. Intravenous via large bore needles

19. Skin care teaching for the client receiving radiation therapy includes: (Select all that apply.)
    1. wash the area with mild soap and water daily.
    2. do not apply lotion or powder to the radiation field.
    3. a soft clean gauze pad can be used between skinfolds to prevent skin breakdown.
    4. wearing a pressure garment will help prevent skin irritation.

20. Assessments the nurse should make on a client receiving radiation therapy include: (Select all that apply.)
    1. skin changes.
    2. fatigue.
    3. dry throat.
    4. GI complaints.

21. A client on chemotherapy has the nursing diagnosis Risk for imbalanced nutrition, less than body requirements due to nausea and vomiting after her treatments. Nursing interventions could include: (Select all that apply.)
    1. encourage the client to eat lightly or only take liquids for 3 days after chemotherapy.
    2. use germ-fighting commercial mouthwashes to prevent oral infections.
    3. have the client suck on ice if she has mouth soreness.
    4. take antiemetic medications on a schedule, not on an as-needed basis.

22. Common assessment findings in men with breast cancer are:
    1. a suspicious lump seen on an incidental chest x-ray.
    2. nipple discharge or retraction.
    3. a small, localized lesion.
    4. estrogen receptor negative histology.

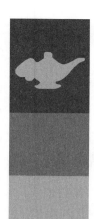

CHAPTER 41

Management of Clients with Sexually Transmitted Infections

CHAPTER OBJECTIVES

41.1   Define terms related to sexually transmitted infections (STIs).
41.2   Identify the social significance of STIs.
41.3   Identify characteristics of specific STIs.
41.4   Examine current treatment guidelines of the CDC website.
41.5   Identify causes of and risk factors for STIs.
41.6   Relate pathophysiology to the specific disease condition and clinical manifestations.
41.7   Describe medical and nursing management of the client with an STI including assessment and interventions directed toward specific outcomes.
41.8   Relate diagnostic testing for STIs to clinical manifestations.
41.9   Identify specific drug therapy for various STIs.
41.10   Describe education necessary for the client with an STI in the adolescent and older populations.
41.11   Describe a therapeutic relationship with the client who has an STI including therapeutic communication and supportive intervention.
41.12   Describe an appropriate method of sexual history taking.
41.13   Identify community-based practices that affect those at risk for STIs.
41.14   Discuss right-to-know issues related to STIs and partners.

UNDERSTANDING TERMINOLOGY

1. Compare and contrast the terms *venereal disease* and *sexually transmitted infection*.

2. Define *sexarchy*.

UNDERSTANDING PATHOPHYSIOLOGY

3. Which of the following diseases are most commonly referred to as STIs? (Select all that apply.)
   1. Chlamydia
   2. Gonorrhea
   3. Syphilis
   4. Genital herpes
   5. Genital warts

4. A _____ is a highly contagious infection caused by *Haemophilus ducreyi*.

5. Lymphogranuloma is caused by strains of _____.

6. Individuals at high risk for acquiring STIs include: (Select all that apply.)
   1. IV drug users.
   2. people involved in high-risk sexual activity.
   3. adolescents who have unprotected sex.
   4. chronic renal failure patients.

7. The organism that causes Chlamydia is:
   1. genital herpes.
   2. *Chlamydia trachomatis*.
   3. human papillomavirus.
   4. *Neisseria gonorrhoeae*.

8. A female client who presents with a heavy, yellow-green, purulent vaginal discharge probably has:
   1. vaginitis.
   2. Chlamydia.
   3. syphilis.
   4. gonorrhea.

9. The principal clinical manifestation of primary syphilis is:
   1. enlarged lymph node.
   2. warts on the genitals.
   3. genital chancre sores.
   4. vaginal and rectal bleeding.

10. Women with genital warts have an increased risk for:
    1. carcinoma of the cervix.
    2. sterility.
    3. fibroid tumors.
    4. Candida yeast infections.

APPLYING SKILLS

11. Male clients who present with mucopurulent discharge should have which initial exam done to confirm a preliminary diagnosis of Chlamydia?
    1. DFA (direct fluorescent antibody)
    2. Urine culture
    3. GC culture and gram stain for gonorrhea
    4. Clinical examination of the pelvic area

12. The most common complication of gonorrhea in women is:
    1. salpingitis that can progress to pelvic inflammatory disease (PID).
    2. reversible PID.
    3. meningitis.
    4. urethral enlargement.

13. Which laboratory studies can confirm a diagnosis of syphilis in its primary stages? (Select all that apply.)
    1. DFM (dark field microscopy)
    2. Culture and sensitivity of urethra
    3. Serologic test for syphilis
    4. Fluorescent treponemal antibody absorption test (FTA-ABS)

14. A young woman is newly diagnosed with genital herpes lesion type 2. Which clinical manifestations would she present with? (Select all that apply.)
    1. Small vesicles with erythematous borders on genital regions
    2. Burning sensation at site of inoculation
    3. Anuria
    4. Leukorrhea

BEST PRACTICES

15. A 16-year-old adolescent comes to the clinic for treatment of an STI and is concerned about her boyfriend. The nurse should provide which of the following information to the adolescent when she is being discharged from the clinic?
    1. All sexual partners need to evaluated and treated.
    2. You can return in 1 month for follow-up and see if he needs it.
    3. He will need to be treated only if he is having symptoms.
    4. His treatment will only start after you have completed the course of medications.

16. The most effective mechanical barriers to STIs are:
    1. oral contraceptives.
    2. IUDs (intrauterine devices).
    3. rhythm methods.
    4. latex condoms.

KEEPING DRUG SKILLS SHARP

17. The treatments of choice for Chlamydial infections include: (Select all that apply.)
    1. gentamycin three times a day for 7 days.
    2. doxycycline (Vibramycin) for 7 days orally.
    3. azithromycin (Zithromax) in one dose.
    4. penicillin G in two doses IM.

18. The current recommended treatment regimen for uncomplicated gonorrhea is:
    1. amoxicillin.
    2. a single dose of IM rocephin (Ceftriaxone) or Cefixin.
    3. tetracycline three times a day for 7 days.
    4. gentamycin IM.

19. The recommended treatment for an acute primary infection of genital herpes is: (Select all that apply.)
    1. streptomycin in two doses.
    2. penicillin G topical.
    3. zovirax (Acyclovir) for 7–10 days.
    4. famciclovir.

TRENDS

20. Go to the CDC website (http://www.cdc.gov/std/treatment/2006/toc.htm) and explore the section on Clinical Prevention Guidance. Write down the three most important things you learn.

DEMONSTRATE AGE-RELATED COMPETENCIES

21. What special challenges does the nurse need to overcome in order to educate teens about STIs? (Select all that apply.)
    1. Different understanding of the phrase "long-term relationship."
    2. Concrete thinking typical of that age group.
    3. Lower perceived risk, especially with their "main partner."
    4. Difficult to access this population.

22. List some alternative sites where STI education could be provided for teens.

23. What is a major barrier to assessing for STIs in the older population?

USING ASSESSMENT SKILLS

24. How can a nurse best take a sexual history from a client? (Select all that apply.)
    1. Use a tool specific for sexual history taking.
    2. Ask questions in a sensitive, nonjudgmental manner.
    3. Have the client fill out a questionnaire.
    4. Become comfortable with terminology and your own values.

ETHICS DISCUSSION

25. Discuss with a partner right-to-know guidelines regarding exposure to STIs. Are there any ethical conflicts? Are there pros and cons to requiring a client with an STI to provide names of his/her contacts to public health authorities for tracking and case management?

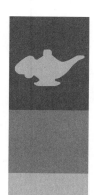

CHAPTER 42

Assessment of the Endocrine and Metabolic Systems

CHAPTER OBJECTIVES

42.1 Describe the aspects of endocrine and metabolic disorders assessment related to presenting manifestations.

42.2 Discuss the components of the health history.

42.3 Identify the clinical manifestations often associated with endocrine and metabolic dysfunction.

42.4 List the specific questions to ask the client to elicit information about the clinical manifestations.

42.5 Discuss appropriate questions for the client in the review of systems related to clinical manifestations.

42.6 Identify client potential for endocrine and metabolic problems based on medical and surgical history.

42.7 Discuss food or medication allergies such as iodine.

42.8 Discuss interactions of medications and alternative therapies.

42.9 Describe the use of medications such as hormones or herbal therapy.

42.10 Identify dietary habits concerning any foods that cause clinical manifestations.

42.11 Describe social and family history that contributes to a diagnosis of endocrine or metabolic problems.

42.12 Perform a physical assessment on the entire body to assess for endocrine and metabolic interferences.

42.13 Describe diagnostic testing including the appropriate use for each test regarding possible endocrine or metabolic disorders.

ANATOMY & PHYSIOLOGY REVIEW

1. Label the diagram below with the name of each endocrine gland.

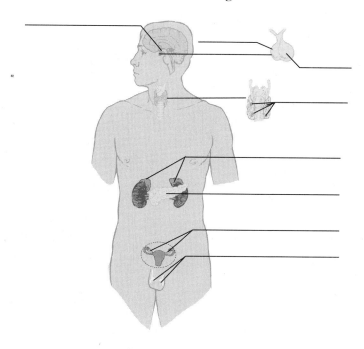

UNDERSTANDING PATHOPHYSIOLOGY

2. True or False

   _____ A client's sexual history is not important in a workup for endocrine or metabolic disorders.

   _____ Exposure to mercury and lead can lead
   to liver damage.

   _____ Serum cortisol is measured in clients
   suspected of having hyperfunctioning
   or hypofunctioning adrenal glands.

3. Match the terms with the correct definition or description of clinical manifestations.

   Term

   _____ a. Gynecomastia
   _____ b. Pancreatic disorder
   _____ c. Hyperthyroidism
   _____ d. Hypothyroidism
   _____ e. Biliary tract disorders
   _____ f. Gallbladder disorders
   _____ g. Acromegaly
   _____ h. Hypopituitarism
   _____ i. ADH suppression
   _____ j. Steatorrhea
   _____ k. Hepatocellular disease
   _____ l. Hyperparathyroidism

   Definition/Description

   1. History of childhood head trauma
   2. Fatty, foul-smelling stools
   3. Dehydration
   4. Dark-colored, tarry stools
   5. Calcium stone formation
   6. Dark yellow, tea-colored urine
   7. Right upper quadrant pain
   8. Enlarging hands, feet, or head
   9. Dry, brittle, thinning hair
   10. Elevation of body temperature/exophthalmos
   11. Pain radiating to back
   12. Breast enlargement in males

APPLYING SKILLS

4. In evaluating a client with metabolic and endocrine disorders, which of the following areas
   should be explored? (Select all that apply.)
   1. Health history
   2. Physical examination
   3. Diagnostic tests
   4. Family and social history

5. Family history is important when questioning
   clients with endocrine and metabolic disorders
   because: (Select all that apply.)
   1. history of previous disorders increases risk
      for development.
   2. a number of disorders are inherited and tend
      to run in families.
   3. family members are not prone to inherit
      these disorders.
   4. most psychosocial concerns are limited.

6. When examining a client for hepatic or biliary
   pain, on which areas of the abdomen should the
   nurse concentrate? (Select all that apply.)
   1. Right lower quadrant
   2. Mid-abdomen
   3. Lower back portion
   4. Right upper quadrant

7. Ultrasound exams are particularly valuable for
   diagnosing conditions of the:
   a.

   b.

   c.

BEST PRACTICES

8. True or False

   _____ Assessment of clients with metabolic
   or endocrine problems focuses on the
   manifestations of hormone excess or
   deficiency, or on metabolic dysfunction.

   _____ Visceral pain can be described as dull,
   aching, burning, cramping, or colicky.

   _____ Referred pain is pain that has a specific
   cause it can be referred to.

   _____ Fatty food intolerance can indicate pancreatic or biliary tract disease.

   _____ It is not important to assess skin when
   investigating a possible endocrine or
   metabolic problem.

9. _____ is a diagnostic procedure used to remove a sample of living tissue for analysis.

10. _____ is the extraction of fluid accumulated in the peritoneum.

11. A client has altered mental status and has begun having seizures. Disorders the nurse might suspect include:
    1. hepatic encephalopathy.
    2. diabetes.
    3. hyperparathyroidism.
    4. Hashimoto's disease.

12. A client with an endocrine disorder might present with: (Select all that apply.)
    1. decreased libido.
    2. irregular menstrual cycle.
    3. impotence or infertility.
    4. emotional lability.

13. A nurse assessing a client with suspected endocrine or metabolic disorder needs to complete a thorough history and physical because _____
    _____
    _____.

14. Radiation may cause problems with _____
    _____.

15. List procedures that can increase the client's risk of acquiring hepatitis virus.
    a.

    b.

    c.

    d.

    e.

    f.

16. A history of alcohol abuse can accompany _____ or _____ disorders.

17. The nurse should inspect the skin for:
    a.

    b.

    c.

    d.

    e.

18. The nurse should inspect the nails for:
    a.

    b.

    c.

    d.

    e.

19. Tests of the endocrine pancreas include measuring the _____.

20. Serum cholesterol may be elevated in _____.

KEEPING DRUG SKILLS SHARP

21. Many drugs and chemicals are hepatotoxic, including: (Select all that apply.)
    1. alcohol.
    2. gold compounds.
    3. anabolic steroids.
    4. halothane.

22. True or False

    _____ Allergy to iodine or fish would not be a contraindication for a contrast dye study.

    _____ Infusion of IV saline can decrease the plasma level of aldosterone.

    _____ Anabolic steroids can affect endocrine and metabolic function.

    _____ A client who stops taking corticosteroids abruptly is at risk of developing Hashimoto's thyroiditis.

    _____ Black tea has antihypertensive effects.

    _____ Milk thistle may be used by clients who have liver disorders.

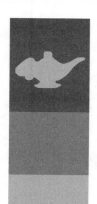

C H A P T E R **43**

Management of Clients with Thyroid and Parathyroid Disorders

CHAPTER OBJECTIVES

43.1   Describe normal and abnormal states of thyroid and parathyroid function.

43.2   Identify etiology and risk factors for thyroid and parathyroid disorders.

43.3   Relate the pathophysiology, clinical manifestations, and laboratory diagnostics to thyroid and parathyroid disorders.

43.4   Distinguish clinical manifestations of hypothyroidism and hyperthyroidism.

43.5   Describe desired outcomes of medical and surgical management for clients with thyroid and parathyroid disorders.

43.6   Relate the need for specific medications or cautionary measures about medications to thyroid and parathyroid disorders.

43.7   Identify nursing assessments, diagnoses, outcomes, and interventions for clients with thyroid and parathyroid disorders.

43.8   Describe education that promotes self-care for clients with thyroid and parathyroid disorders.

43.9   Distinguish differences in treatment of hypothyroidism and older adults.

43.10   Describe the emergent nature of complications of thyroid and parathyroid disorders.

UNDERSTANDING PATHOPHYSIOLOGY

1. A normal functioning thyroid gland is referred to as _____.

2. Enlargement of the thyroid gland may be due to: (Select all that apply.)
   1. lack of iodine.
   2. inflammation.
   3. benign tumors.
   4. malignant tumors.

3. Which of the following may cause primary hypothyroidism? (Select all that apply.)
   1. Antithyroid drugs
   2. Surgery and treatment with radioactive agents for hyperthyroidism
   3. Hashimoto's disease
   4. Defective hormone synthesis

4. The physiologic process of exophthalmos in hyperthyroidism is due to:
   1. accumulation of fluid in the fat pads and muscles that lie behind the eyeballs.
   2. increased venous pressure.
   3. retro-orbital dryness.
   4. excessive tearing from the duct.

5. What is likely to happen if a client has a diet lacking sufficient iodine or if production of thyroid hormone is suppressed?
   1. The thyroid decreases in size.
   2. The thyroid enlarges to compensate for hormonal deficiency.
   3. The gland uses more T_3.
   4. Positive feedback occurs.

6. Hypothyroidism results in a deficiency of thyroid hormones, causing: (Select all that apply.)
   1. slowed body metabolism.
   2. decreased heat production.
   3. decreased oxygen consumption.
   4. increased appetite.

7. Hypothyroidism is also known as _____ _____.

8. The thyroid gland needs iodine in order to:
   1. synthesize and secrete thyroid hormones.
   2. enable the adrenal gland to operate.
   3. break down HCl.
   4. absorb trace elements in the system.

9. The reduction in thyroid hormones causes an increase in: (Select all that apply.)
   1. ammonia levels.
   2. triglyceride levels.
   3. serum cholesterol.
   4. arteriosclerosis and coronary heart disease.

10. Hyperthyroidism is also known _____ _____.

11. Hyperthyroidism may be due to: (Select all that apply.)
   1. excessive stimulation of the adrenal gland.
   2. excessive levels of circulating thyroid hormone (TH).
   3. increased regulatory control.
   4. decreased metabolism.

APPLYING SKILLS

12. Laboratory values indicative of hypothyroidism in a client being admitted to the hospital would include: (Select all that apply.)
   1. decreased TH level.
   2. increased thyroid-stimulating hormone (TSH) level.
   3. normal CBC.
   4. decreased aspartate transaminase (AST).

13. Signs and symptoms most identifiable in a patient with hypothyroidism would include: (Select all that apply.)
   1. sensitivity to cold.
   2. sensitivity to heat.
   3. dry skin or hair.
   4. weight gain.
   5. irregular menses.

14. Myxedema coma can be brought on by stressors from surgery or infections. When identifying common characteristics, the nurse would see certain clinical manifestations, including: (Select all that apply.)
   1. decreased metabolic rate.
   2. hypoventilation.
   3. respiratory distress.
   4. hypothermia, hypotension.

15. In identifying thyrotoxicosis, the nurse will assess which of the following in the client? (Select all that apply.)
   1. Tachycardia
   2. Increased appetite, sweating
   3. Diarrhea
   4. Agitation and tremors

16. Laboratory values indicative of hyperthyroidism include: (Select all that apply.)
   1. increased TH levels.
   2. decreased cholesterol.
   3. normal hemoglobin and hematocrit.
   4. elevated antiglobulin test (AGT).

17. In assessing a patient with thyroid storm (thyrotoxicosis), the nurse will look for: (Select all that apply.)
   1. increased fever.
   2. severe tachycardia.
   3. delirium.
   4. dehydration.
   5. extreme irritability.

18. The client having a thyroidectomy is at risk for which of the following complications? (Select all that apply.)
   1. Thyroid storm
   2. Tetany
   3. Respiratory obstruction
   4. Laryngeal edema
   5. Vocal cord injury

19. The major clinical and diagnostic manifestations of thyroid cancer are: (Select all that apply.)
   1. a hard, irregular, painless nodule.
   2. a "cold" nodule which does not take up radioactive iodine.
   3. greater than 10 cm mass.
   4. enlargement of the vocal area.

20. Hypercalcemia produces gastrointestinal symptoms such as: (Select all that apply.)
   1. nausea.
   2. thirst.
   3. anorexia.
   4. constipation.
   5. abdominal pain, ileus.

21. Lab values indicative of hypoparathyroidism include:
   1. decreased calcium.
   2. increased calcium.
   3. decreased TSH.
   4. increased sodium.

22. Manifestations of hyperparathyroidism are seen in which body systems?

23. Why are thyroid and parathyroid disorders so often overlooked in older adults?

24. Manifestations of hypoparathyroidism are mainly related to _____.

BEST PRACTICES

25. To prevent negative nitrogen balance and weight loss, the hyperthyroid client must follow a: (Select all that apply.)
    1. high-calorie diet.
    2. high-protein diet.
    3. 1200-calorie diet.
    4. diet consisting only of meat intake for 48 hours.

26. Total thyroidectomy is performed to remove _____.

27. Subtotal thyroidectomy is performed to correct _____.

28. Immediate postoperative care for a thyroidectomy client includes: (Select all that apply.)
    1. maintaining patent airway.
    2. minimizing strain on the suture line.
    3. relieving sore throat and tracheal irritation.
    4. relieving complications.

29. Which of the following are appropriate nursing diagnoses for the client with hypoparathyroidism? (Select all that apply.)
    1. Risk for injury
    2. Knowledge deficit
    3. Risk for ineffective therapeutic regimen management
    4. Constipation

30. What are two appropriate outcomes for the client with hyperparathyroidism and the nursing diagnosis Impaired urinary elimination?
    a.

    b.

KEEPING DRUG SKILLS SHARP

31. Endemic goiter can be prevented by the ingestion of:
    1. fruits.
    2. potassium-sparing diuretic.
    3. iodized salts.
    4. synthetic salt supplements.

32. Administration of low-dose levothyroxine (Synthroid) helps improve: (Select all that apply.)
    1. cardiac function.
    2. lipid profile.
    3. liver toxicity.
    4. respiratory adjuncts.

33. The major medications used to control hyperthyroidism are: (Select all that apply.)
    1. iodide replacements.
    2. propylthiouracil.
    3. methimazole (Tapazole).
    4. Meganin.

34. The most serious toxic effect of propylthiouracil is:
    1. agranulocytosis.
    2. decreased RBCs.
    3. lymphedema.
    4. liver toxicity.

35. Iodine therapy is prescribed for which of the following reasons? (Select all that apply.)
    1. Decrease vascularity of the thyroid gland
    2. Treat thyroid storm
    3. Prevent release of TH
    4. Increase amount of TH stored in the thyroid gland

36. The iodine medication of choice is _____ _____.

37. The administration of I-131 will have which of the following effects on clients with hyperthyroidism? (Select all that apply.)
    1. The thyroid gland will pick up radioactive iodine.
    2. Cells concentrating I-131 will make T_4 and are destroyed by local irradiation.
    3. TH secretion will diminish.
    4. Oversecretion of gland will occur.

38. _____ is a major complication of I-131 administration.

39. Drugs given to treat a thyroid storm include: (Select all that apply.)
    1. sodium iodine.
    2. glucocorticoids.
    3. beta blockers.
    4. propylthiouracil.

40. What medication will be given to a client who is experiencing tetany after removal of a parathyroid gland?
    1. Calcium chloride (IM)
    2. Synthroid
    3. Lasix
    4. Calcium gluconate (IV)

41. Which medication is used along with calcium supplements in hypoparathyroidism?

    _____

42. Pharmacologic management of hypercalcemia seen with hyperparathyroidism includes: (Select all that apply.)
    1. normal saline.
    2. furosemide (Lasix).
    3. gallium nitrate (Ganite).
    4. thiazide diuretics.
    5. glucocorticoids.

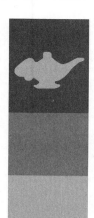

CHAPTER 44

Management of Clients with Adrenal and Pituitary Disorders

CHAPTER OBJECTIVES

44.1 Compare and contrast adrenocortical disorders of hyper- or hypofunction of the adrenal cortex.

44.2 Relate hypofunction of the adrenal gland to primary or secondary disorders.

44.3 Describe the causes and risk factors for adrenal insufficiency, hypocortisolism, hyperaldosteronism, pheochromocytoma, pituitary disorders, and gonadal disorders.

44.4 Relate the pathophysiology to clinical manifestations and diagnostic testing.

44.5 Describe the urgency of treatment for Addisonian crisis.

44.6 Describe the desired outcomes of medical and nursing management of Addisonian crisis.

44.7 Describe the desired outcomes for medical, surgical, and nursing management of adrenalectomy clients and hypophysectomy clients.

UNDERSTANDING PATHOPHYSIOLOGY

1. Risk factors for primary adrenal insufficiency include: (Select all that apply.)
   1. a history of endocrine disorders.
   2. taking glucocorticoids for 3 weeks and suddenly stopping.
   3. taking glucocorticoids more than every other day.
   4. adrenalectomy and tuberculosis.

2. _____ is the most common cause of adrenal insufficiency.

3. Which of the following would be consistent with primary adrenal insufficiency? (Select all that apply.)
   1. Decreasing cortisol production rate
   2. Increasing plasma adrenocorticotropic hormone (ACTH)
   3. Decreasing sodium concentration
   4. Cachexia

4. Addisonian crisis or acute adrenal insufficiency may be brought on by: (Select all that apply.)
   1. pregnancy.
   2. surgery.
   3. infections.
   4. emotional upsets.

5. Cushing's syndrome is caused by: (Select all that apply.)
   1. overactivity of the adrenal gland.
   2. hypersecretion of the glucocorticoids.
   3. decreased circulating adrenal cortisol.
   4. diabetes insipidus.

6. _____ is hypersecretion of aldosterone resulting from an adrenal lesion.

7. _____ results from a variety of conditions that cause overproduction of aldosterone.

8. _____ is oversecretion of one or more of the hormones by the pituitary gland.

9. _____ is deficiency of one or more of the hormones produced by the anterior lobe of the pituitary.

10. A client with pheochromocytoma has an excessive amount of:
    1. renin.
    2. aldosterone.
    3. catecholamines.
    4. glucocortisol.

11. True or False

    _____ The diagnosis of Addison's disease depends on blood and urine hormonal assays.

    _____ Manifestations of hypopituitarism do not appear until at least 75% of the gland has been destroyed.

APPLYING SKILLS

12. Assessments the nurse would expect to find in a client with hypopituitarism include: (Select all that apply.)
    1. short stature.
    2. sexual and reproductive disorders.
    3. hyperthyroidism.
    4. secondary adrenocortical insufficiency.

13. A client with adrenal crisis will experience which of the following clinical manifestations? (Select all that apply.)
    1. Pain
    2. Hypoglycemia
    3. Decreased fluid volume
    4. Edema

14. A client with Addison's disease will exhibit which of these clinical manifestations?
    1. Weight gain
    2. Hunger
    3. Lethargy
    4. Muscle spasm

15. What findings should be normal with a client with Addison's disease?
    1. Blood glucose
    2. Serum sodium
    3. Serum potassium
    4. White blood cell count

16. A newly admitted 45-year-old male client reports a 20 lb. weight gain and states, "My face and the middle section of my body are round and fat." The nurse also notes that his legs and arms are thin. Based on this assessment and the information the client has provided, what other clinical sign should the nurse look for in order to make a tentative diagnosis of Cushing's syndrome?
    1. Bruises on the skin
    2. Hypotension
    3. Muscle hypertrophy of the extremities
    4. Excessive hair on the head

17. The primary feature of pheochromocytoma's effect on blood pressure is:
    1. systolic hypertension.
    2. diastolic hypertension.
    3. hypertension resistant to drug management.
    4. muffled systolic sounds.

18. Secondary hyperaldosteronism is caused by continuous secretion of aldosterone because of high levels of _____. This is caused by high _____.

19. The major etiology of secondary hyperaldosteronism is _____ from several different causes.

20. List the syndromes associated with hyperpituitarism.

BEST PRACTICES

21. Which assessment by the nurse would alert him/her to a potentially severe complication following transfrontal hypophysectomy? (Select all that apply.)
    1. Urine output of more than 200 ml/hour
    2. Blood pressure 10 mm Hg above baseline
    3. Blood glucose reading of 88
    4. Urine specific gravity <1.005

22. A nursing priority for a client with Addisonian crisis is to:
    1. promote anxiety.
    2. treat infections.
    3. prevent hypotension.
    4. control hypertension.

23. Nursing management of patients with Addison's disease includes: (Select all that apply.)
    1. monitoring vital signs.
    2. monitoring for exposure to colds and infections.
    3. assessing physical vitality and emotional status.
    4. avoiding stress.

24. Clients with Cushing's disease need to modify their diets by increasing their protein intake and:
    1. restricting sodium.
    2. restricting potassium.
    3. reducing fat by 20%.
    4. increasing calorie consumption.

KEEPING DRUG SKILLS SHARP

25. When a client with Addison's disease develops hypoglycemia, it should be corrected with: (Select all that apply.)
    1. IV D_5W infusion.
    2. IV D_5W push bolus.
    3. D_5NS 500 ml.
    4. normal saline 1000 ml.

26. Excessive use of glucocorticoids may lead to _____.

27. Prior to surgery for an adrenalectomy, the physician will order cortisol preparations IM or IV to be given to the client. The nurse knows that this preparation is given because:
    1. cortisol protects against the development of acute adrenal insufficiency.
    2. insulin per sliding scale will help regulate glucose uptake.
    3. antibiotics during surgery will need to be given.
    4. hormones will be readily decreased.

28. True or False

    _____ Kayexalate may be administered orally or as an enema, in combination with sorbitol, to release sodium ions in exchange for potassium ions.

UNDERSTANDING AGE-RELATED DIFFERENCES

29. A prepubescent boy diagnosed with hypogonadotropic hypogonadism would display which features? (Select all that apply.)
    1. Eunuchoid body type
    2. Small testes
    3. Lack of virilization
    4. Early coronary artery disease

30. Which age-related considerations are appropriate to a discussion of adrenal disorders? (Select all that apply.)
    1. Adrenal disorders are not common in older adults.
    2. Symptoms are often attributed to age-related illnesses.
    3. Increased age is a risk factor for hypopituitarism.
    4. Older adults might have more problems with the side effects of steroids.

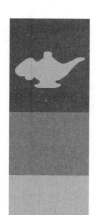

Management of Clients with Diabetes Mellitus

CHAPTER OBJECTIVES

45.1   Explain the significance of diabetes mellitus as a significant public health problem in the early 21st century.

45.2   Classify diabetic states.

45.3   Describe the etiology and risk factors for the different classifications of diabetes.

45.4   Relate the pathophysiology and clinical manifestations of diabetes.

45.5   Differentiate the pathophysiology of type 1 and type 2 diabetes.

45.6   Describe diagnostic testing necessary to conclusive diagnosis of diabetes.

45.7   Describe additional laboratory testing for diabetes.

45.8   Explain self-monitoring of blood glucose.

45.9   Describe the desired outcomes of medical management of diabetes mellitus including the various insulin therapies.

45.10   Describe the desired outcomes of nursing management of the client with diabetes.

45.11   Adapt diabetes management to the older client.

45.12   Describe surgical management, including pancreas transplants and islet cell transplants, and the desired outcomes.

45.13   Describe nursing management and self-care education for the surgical client.

45.14   Identify complications of diabetes.

45.15   Describe the urgent nature of treatment for hyperglycemia and diabetic ketoacidosis.

45.16   Differentiate diabetic ketoacidosis and hyperglycemic, hyperosmolar, nonketotic syndrome (HHNK).

45.17   Describe hypoglycemia as a complication of diabetes, along with medical management.

45.18   Discuss the Somogyi effect and the dawn phenomenon and their impact on diabetes management.

45.19   Discuss the chronic macrovascular and microvascular complications of diabetes, along with interventions to manage these complications.

45.20   Discuss the management of a diabetic client undergoing surgery.

THEORIES AND TRENDS

1.   _21_ million people in the U.S. have diabetes, which is _7_ % of the population.

2.   _6 million_ people have undiagnosed diabetes.

3.   Diabetes is a significant public health problem because it is the _6th_ leading cause of death and the total estimated cost of diabetes in the U.S. is _$132 billion_.

4.   _Islet cell_ transplant is a new treatment under investigation for type 1 diabetes.

UNDERSTANDING PATHOPHYSIOLOGY

5.   Type 2 diabetes is the result of a progressive _insulin deficiency_ along with _insulin resistance_ and is commonly associated with _obesity_.

Copyright 2009 by Elsevier, Inc. All rights reserved.

195

6. Diabetes mellitus is a chronic systemic disease resulting from: (Select all that apply.)
   1. deficiency of insulin.
   2. absent alpha cells distribution.
   3. decreased ability of the body to use insulin.
   4. abnormal glucose metabolism involving the spleen and muscle.

7. Type 1 diabetes mellitus is characterized by: (Select all that apply.)
   1. destruction of pancreatic beta cells.
   2. absolute insulin deficiency.
   3. backup of liver and spleen distribution.
   4. abnormal cellular metabolism by the delta cells.

8. The most common form of diabetes mellitus is _type 2_.

9. Gestational diabetes mellitus is discovered during:
   1. labor and delivery.
   2. pregnancy. \book says pregnancy
   3. delivery.
   4. a routine eye exam.

10. Type 1 diabetes is also referred to as _IDDM_.

11. Populations at greatest risk for developing diabetes mellitus are: (Select all that apply.)
    1. Native Americans.
    2. Hispanics.
    3. African-Americans.
    4. Asians.

12. Glucose in the urine is commonly referred to as _glycosuria_.

13. Fat metabolism causes breakdown products called _Ketones_.

14. One major action of insulin is to:
    1. increase hepatic production of glucose.
    2. inhibit glucose storage as glycogen.
    3. promote breakdown of fat and glycogen.
    4. promote glucose uptake in skeletal muscle and adipose tissue.

15. Insulin increases:
    1. storage of glycogen and fatty acids.
    2. protein breakdown.
    3. breakdown of fats.
    4. blood glucose levels.

16. The _HbA1C_ lab test measures the average blood glucose level over the last 3 months.

17. All diabetics should test their urine for _Ketones_ when they are sick, under stress, or when their blood glucose levels are high.

18. Urine _glucose_ testing is not considered reliable.

19. Diabetics should have annual urine testing for _microalbuminuria / proteinuria_, which is an early sign of renal damage from diabetes.

20. The key to keeping glucose levels under control by using immediate feedback is _self-monitoring glucose (SMBG)_.

APPLYING SKILLS

21. Clients who would *not* need an oral glucose tolerance test would have a fasting glucose level of:
    1. between 140 and 200 mg/dl.
    2. above 110 mg/dl.
    3. between 60 and 100 mg/dl.
    4. above 120 mg/dl.

22. The classic clinical manifestations in clients with diabetes are: (Select all that apply.)
    1. polyuria.
    2. polydipsia.
    3. polyphagia.
    4. postload glucose.

23. A diagnosis of diabetes is made when a client's fasting blood glucose level is greater than:
    1. 126 mg/dl.
    2. 150 mg/dl.
    3. 160 mg/dl.
    4. 200 mg/dl

24. The best time to obtain a postprandial glucose level is _2 hrs. p a meal_.

25. The presence of protein in the urine (microalbuminuria) is an early sign of:
    1. liver toxicity.
    2. hepatic overload.
    3. kidney disease.
    4. peripheral liver destruction.

26. The polydipsia and polyuria related to diabetes are caused primarily by:
    1. the release of ketones from cells during fat metabolism.
    2. fluid shifts resulting from osmotic effects of hyperglycemia.
    3. damage to the kidneys from exposure to high levels of glucose.
    4. changes in RBCs resulting from attachment of excessive glucose to hemoglobin.

27. The primary difference between HHNK and keto-acidosis is that in HHNK there is:
    1. greater production of lactic acid.
    2. greater production of ketones.
    3. lesser production of lactic acid.
    4. no production of ketones.

28. Diabetic ketoacidosis and hyperglycemic hyper-osmolar nonketotic (HHNK) coma are alike in that:
    1. both occur most often in insulin-dependent (type 1) diabetes.
    2. both may be caused by an infection or some other stress.
    3. metabolic acidosis is a prominent feature of both.
    4. serum glucose levels are usually greater that 800 mg/dl.

29. Factors that could cause hypoglycemia in a diabetic client are:
    1. decreased dose of insulin, too much exercise, eating too much carbohydrates.
    2. excessive dose of insulin, stress, injecting into an area of hypertropic lipodystrophy.
    3. excessive dose of insulin, too much exercise, eating too little.
    4. excessive dose of insulin, too little exercise, illness.

30. Which of the following would suggest to a nurse that a diabetic client is suffering from hypoglycemia?
    1. Cold clammy skin, weakness, headache
    2. Drowsiness, nausea, vomiting, soft eyeballs
    3. Fruity smell to breath, warm dry skin
    4. Intense thirst, abdominal pain

31. Which of these lab data would support the inference that a diabetic client is experiencing severe ketoacidosis?
    1. Decreased pH, decreased Hct, decreased serum CO_2
    2. Decreased pH, increased Hct, decreased serum CO_2
    3. Increased pH, increased Hct, decreased serum CO_2
    4. Increased pH, increased Hct, increased serum CO_2

32. List the times when clients need to increase the frequency with which they perform self-monitoring of blood glucose (SMBG).

    - starting new diabetic agent
    - starting a medication that effects B glucose
    - when sick / stressed
    - when you think sugars are too high / too low
    - lose / gain weight
    - Δ in medical plan, diet plan, activity regimen

33. What is the goal of nursing education for the diabetic client?

    Help client become responsible for & competent to , make informed decisions r/t diabetic care.

34. True or False
    ___T___ Clients with type 1 diabetes may benefit from pancreas transplant.
    ___T___ Clients with type 2 diabetes do not benefit from pancreas transplant.
    ___F___ The client's own pancreas is removed and the new pancreas supplies both exocrine and endocrine functions.
    ___F___ The goal of a pancreas transplant is to decrease the frequency of insulin injections.
    ___F___ A rapid rise in blood glucose after pancreas transplant indicates rejection.

REVIEWING YOUR KNOWLEDGE

35. Matching. Match the description on the left with the condition on the right. Answers may be used more than once.

Description

_1_ a. Occurs rarely

_1_ b. Results from excessive evening insulin dosage

_2_ c. Early morning hyperglycemia without nocturnal hypoglycemia

_2_ d. Use of Ultralente insulin may alleviate the problem

_1_ e. Decreasing suppertime intermediate acting insulin can help

_2_ f. Seen in both type 1 and type 2 diabetics

Condition

1. Somogyi effect
2. Dawn phenomenon

36. List the macrovascular and microvascular complications of diabetes. Which is the most common reason for hospitalization of the diabetic client?

MAC — coronary artery disease
CVA, HTN, PVD, Infections

MIC — Retinopathy, nephropathy, neuropathy

37. The most characteristic lipid abnormality in diabetes mellitus is ___↑ triglycerides___.

38. List health promotion and health maintenance activities for the diabetic client with macrovascular disease.

HP: managing obesity & maintaining ideal body weight, exercising, not smoking, achieving normal blood lipid levels,
HM: prompt recognition + tx, of hyperglycemia, aggressive management of HTN, Screening of risk clients

39. ___urinary tract___ are the most common type of infection in diabetics.

40. List the three types of diabetic retinopathy.

nonproliferative
preproliferative
proliferative.

KEEPING DRUG SKILLS SHARP

41. The main purpose of giving insulin to a client with type 1 diabetes is to:
    1. improve the functioning of the pancreas.
    2. replace the insulin not being produced by the pancreas.
    3. decrease the functioning of the pancreas.
    4. supplement the production of insulin by the pancreas.

42. Which drug would the nurse anticipate administering to a diabetic client with gastroparesis?
    1. cimetadine (Tagamet)
    2. metoclopramide (Reglan)
    3. famotidine (Pepcid)
    4. dicyclomine (Bentyl)

43. After an injection of Humalog insulin, the client should eat breakfast:
    1. immediately.
    2. in 10–15 minutes.
    3. in 30 minutes or so.
    4. whenever he/she can.

DEMONSTRATE AGE-RELATED COMPETENCIES

44. The nurse caring for an older diabetic client understands that the aging process affects the client because: (Select all that apply.)
    1. changes due to aging can affect blood glucose levels.
    2. the amount of circulating glucose regulating hormones decreases.
    3. peripheral insulin receptor sites become more sensitive.
    4. impairments in mental status may affect self-care ability.
    5. changes in liver and kidney function may exacerbate hypoglycemia.

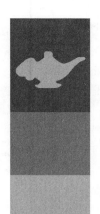

CHAPTER 46

Management of Clients with Exocrine Pancreatic and Biliary Disorders

CHAPTER OBJECTIVES

46.1 Examine disorders of the exocrine pancreas and biliary tract, including causes, risk factors, and pathophysiology.

46.2 Relate clinical manifestations to possible pancreatic or biliary tract diagnoses.

46.3 Describe possible critical care clinical situations related to pancreatic clinical manifestations.

46.4 Describe priorities of medical management outcomes including pain management, fluid volume corrections, and nutrition.

46.5 Describe priorities of nursing management outcomes including pain management, comfort, volume, and nutrition management.

46.6 Describe potential surgical management of specific diagnoses including postoperative management.

46.7 Discuss client education needed for appropriate self-care.

46.8 Relate diagnostic testing to clinical manifestations and treatment.

UNDERSTANDING PATHOPHYSIOLOGY

1. Clients with pancreatic disorders may have problems with _digestion_ and _utilization of glucose_.

2. True or False
   _T_ In the United States, alcohol abuse is the number-one cause of acute pancreatitis.
   _T_ Inflammation of the gallbladder may be acute or chronic.

3. Biliary pancreatitis occurs when: (Select all that apply.)
   (1.) edema or an obstruction blocks the ampulla of Vater.
   (2.) there is reflux of bile into pancreatic ducts.
   (3.) there is direct injury to the acinar cells.
   4. there is blockage of spleen vats.

4. List seven risk factors for pancreatitis.
   a. _Cholecystitis_
   b. _Cholelithiasis_
   c. _Hyperlipidemia_
   d. _Hypercalcemia_
   e. _Pancreatic Tumor_
   f. _Pancreatic ischemia_
   g. _Certain meds + alcohol abuse._

5. A cholecystectomy is the _removal of the gallbladder_.

6. _jaundice_ appears only when common duct obstruction is present.

7. List three types of gallstones and provide a brief description of each.
   a. _Cholesterol - most common; ↑ c age; prevalent in women; stones smooth + whitish/yellow-tan._
   b. _pigment - present in 30% of people c cholelithiasis in U.S. stones are black or calcium bilirubinate_
   c. _mixed - combo of pigment + cholesterol stones w/ either c some other substance; Ca carbonate, phosphates, bile salts, + palmitate are the other constituents._

8. Clinical signs of acute pancreatitis are a result of ___autodigestion___ of the pancreas.

APPLYING SKILLS

9. Turner's sign is ___bluish discoloration of the (L) flank.___

10. Cullen's sign is ___bluish discoloration of the periumbilical area.___

11. A client admitted to the clinic with a confirmed case of pancreatitis will show elevation of which of the following in the lab results? (Select all that apply.)
    1. Amylase
    2. Glucose
    3. Potassium
    4. Trypsin

12. Signs of shock in clients with acute pancreatitis can result from: (Select all that apply.)
    1. hypovolemia.
    2. vasodilating effect of kinin enzymes.
    3. development of congestive heart failure.
    4. increase of tubular necrosis.

13. What symptoms would the nurse expect to see in a client with acute pancreatitis? (Select all that apply.)
    1. Diarrhea
    2. Jaundice
    3. Abdominal pain
    4. Abdominal distention

14. What conditions would be consistent with acute pancreatitis?
    1. Leukopenia
    2. Thrombocytopenia
    3. Hyperkalemia
    4. Hyperglycemia

15. What complication must the nurse watch for in a client with acute pancreatitis? (Select all that apply.)
    1. Altered fluid volume
    2. Duodenal ulcer
    3. Cirrhosis
    4. Respiratory problems

16. The most specific and characteristic manifestation of cholelithiasis is ___pain or biliary colic___

17. Assessment of the client with cholelithiasis becomes important because the manifestations are similar to and need to be distinguished from ___coronary heart disease___.

BEST PRACTICES

18. The overall management of a client with acute pancreatitis requires: (Select all that apply.)
    1. managing the pain.
    2. correcting hypovolemia.
    3. restoring electrolyte balance.
    4. elevating the hemoglobin margins.

19. Dietary instructions for a client with pancreatitis being discharged from a clinic should include: (Select all that apply.)
    1. eating frequent meals high in protein.
    2. following a low-fat diet.
    3. ensuring moderate to high carbohydrate intake.
    4. avoiding alcohol.

20. The nurse must evaluate the client with pancreatitis for the development of:
    1. diabetes mellitus.
    2. hepatitis.
    3. cholelithiasis.
    4. irritable bowel syndrome.

21. Complications associated with cholecystectomy include: (Select all that apply.)
    1. hemorrhage.
    2. pneumonia.
    3. thrombophlebitis.
    4. urinary retention and ileus.

22. True or False
    ___F___ Nonsurgical intervention for the cholelithiasis client is the most common intervention in the U.S. to treat gallstones.

    ___T___ Assessment following the cholecystectomy includes monitoring breath and bowel sounds, vital signs, hemorrhage, and respiratory problems.

    ___T___ After laparoscopic cholecystectomy, referred pain to the shoulder is a common occurrence of pain.

KEEPING DRUG SKILLS SHARP

23. _____*Morphine*_____ has been contraindicated in patients with pancreatitis because it causes spasms of the sphincter of Oddi. Current evidence suggests that it may be a viable alternative for pain management.

24. When extreme hyperglycemia is present in clients with acute pancreatitis, which of the following medications will be ordered?
    1. Oral agents
    2. Insulin
    3. Narcotic
    4. Muscle relaxants

25. In the treatment of acute pancreatitis, _____*Calcium gluconate*_____ must be administered intravenously if there is evidence of hypocalcemia with tetany.

26. Pancreatic enzyme replacements should be taken:
    1. three times per day.
    2. with each meal.
    3. in the morning and at bedtime.
    4. every 4 hours.

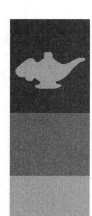

CHAPTER 47

Management of Clients with Hepatic Disorders

CHAPTER OBJECTIVES

47.1 Explain the importance of the liver to normal physiologic processes.
47.2 Relate jaundice as a symptom of liver disease.
47.3 Relate etiology and clinical manifestations of jaundice.
47.4 Describe the desired outcomes of medical, surgical, and nursing management of the client with jaundice with a focus on skin integrity.
47.5 Describe the different forms of hepatitis, causative agents, transmission, and laboratory tests.
47.6 Explain the pathophysiology of hepatitis along with the clinical manifestations.
47.7 Describe the desired outcomes of medical and nursing management for hepatitis.
47.8 Describe complications of hepatitis.
47.9 Relate the use of interferon therapy to types of hepatitis.
47.10 Compare and contrast the different forms of cirrhosis along with the etiology and risk factors.
47.11 Relate the pathophysiology and clinical manifestations of cirrhosis.
47.12 Describe the desired outcomes of medical and nursing management for the client with cirrhosis.
47.13 Relate laboratory data for the client with cirrhosis to subsequent nursing interventions.
47.14 Describe portal hypertension, ascites, and hepatic encephalopathy as complications of cirrhosis, including their related pathophysiology, clinical manifestations, and medical, surgical, and nursing management.
47.15 Identify specific problems such as hemorrhage related to portal hypertension.
47.16 Discuss liver neoplasms that may be benign, malignant, primary, or metastatic.
47.17 Relate diagnostic studies to specific pathophysiologic conditions.
47.18 Discuss liver transplant as a treatment to prolong life in clients with liver disease.

UNDERSTANDING PATHOPHYSIOLOGY

1. Jaundice is caused by:
   1. excessive accumulation of bile pigments in the blood.
   2. large amounts of ketones.
   3. intake of cellular hepatic cells.
   4. breakdown of carbohydrates in the cells.

2. Obstructive jaundice can also be caused by: (Select all that apply.)
   1. stones.
   2. hepatic cellular damage.
   3. intake of excessive ketones.
   4. distribution of cellular wastes.

3. Hepatitis is an inflammation of the liver caused by which of the following? (Select all that apply.)
   1. Viruses
   2. Toxins
   3. Chemicals
   4. Drugs

4. Portal vein hypertension develops in severe cirrhosis due to: (Select all that apply.)
   1. a retrograde increase in pressure resistance.
   2. ascites due to osmotic or hydrostatic shifts.
   3. incomplete clearing of protein metabolic wastes.
   4. increase in ammonia levels.

5. Match the type of hepatitis with the correct description or definition. (More than one answer may apply.)

2,5,9   a.   Hepatitis A

2,3,6,8   b.   Hepatitis B

__2__   c.   Hepatitis C

__1__   d.   Hepatitis D

__10__   e.   Hepatitis E

__7__   f.   Toxic hepatitis

1. Always found with hepatitis B
2. Also known as infectious hepatitis
3. Spread by carriers
4. Spread by blood
5. Primary prevention by careful handwashing
6. Primary prevention by active immunity
7. Caused by benzene and chloroform
8. Health care workers at risk
9. Spread by contaminated shellfish, water, and milk
10. Contracted through travel in high incidence areas

APPLYING SKILLS

6. An extremely dangerous complication of portal hypertension is ___hemorrhage___ .

7. Clinical manifestations of alcoholic hepatitis include: (Select all that apply.)
   1. anorexia.
   2. nausea.
   3. abdominal pain, jaundice.
   4. spleen enlargement.

8. Complications of cirrhosis of the liver include: (Select all that apply.)
   1. ascites.
   2. bleeding esophageal varices.
   3. hepatic encephalopathy.
   4. renal failure.

BEST PRACTICES

9. Clients who have cirrhosis of the liver have high ammonia levels. If ammonia levels rise, the diet should be restricted in:
   1. protein.
   2. carbohydrates.
   3. fats.
   4. calcium.

10. The most appropriate candidates for a liver transplant are those: (Select all that apply.)
    1. with severe liver disease with no alternative medical/surgical treatment.
    2. with end-stage liver disease.
    3. experiencing life-threatening complications.
    4. experiencing neurologic effects of liver damage.

11. Clinical care of the hepatic client includes: (Select all that apply.)
    1. preventing nausea by decreasing fatty food intake.
    2. minimizing transmission to family members.
    3. managing fatigue.
    4. administer bile acid sequestrants.

12. Ascites as a complication of cirrhosis is managed by which of the following interventions? (Select all that apply.)
    1. Fluid restriction
    2. Administer albumin and diuretics
    3. Percussion of abdomen for dull sounds
    4. Monitor vital signs after paracentesis

KEEPING DRUG SKILLS SHARP

13. Clinicians administer very few medications to clients with hepatitis because of hepatotoxicity. Medications that should be avoided include: (Select all that apply.)
    1. aspirin.
    2. acetaminophen.
    3. various sedatives.
    4. chlorpromazine.

14. Clients with cirrhosis of the liver who are receiving thiazide diuretics should maintain a diet high in:
    1. potassium.
    2. sodium.
    3. calcium.
    4. protein.

15. Medications may be given to clients with cirrhosis of the liver to improve clotting factors. The medication that will be ordered is:
    1. heparin.
    2. vitamin K.
    3. calcium gluconate.
    4. dextran.

16. When a client has a rupture of esophageal varices, the physician will routinely order:
    1. vasopressin.
    2. Pitocin.
    3. oxytocin.
    4. Benadryl.

17. The purpose of administering vasopressin IV is to: (Select all that apply.)
    1. achieve temporary lowering of portal pressure.
    2. reduce portal venous blood flow.
    3. constrict afferent arterioles.
    4. maintain liver functions.

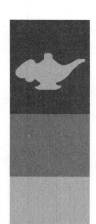

C H A P T E R **48**

Assessment of the Integumentary System

CHAPTER OBJECTIVES

48.1   Describe skin assessment including a health history, chief complaint, and clinical manifestations.
48.2   Examine the client using the systems review.
48.3   Relate past medical and surgical history to the current clinical manifestations.
48.4   Describe allergic reactions that may contribute to the current skin condition.
48.5   Describe potential interactions of medications and herbal drug therapy.
48.6   Examine dietary choices for potential contributions to skin disorders.
48.7   Describe social and family history that may contribute to skin disorders such as sun exposure, hair loss, skin cancer, or diabetes.
48.8   Discuss important aspects of the physical examination.
48.9   Relate culture and ethnicity to predisposition or lack of to certain skin disorders.
48.10   Identify specific primary and secondary skin lesions.
48.11   Relate diagnostic testing to clinical manifestations and subsequent treatment.

ANATOMY & PHYSIOLOGY REVIEW

1.   Label the specific parts of the three layers of the skin.

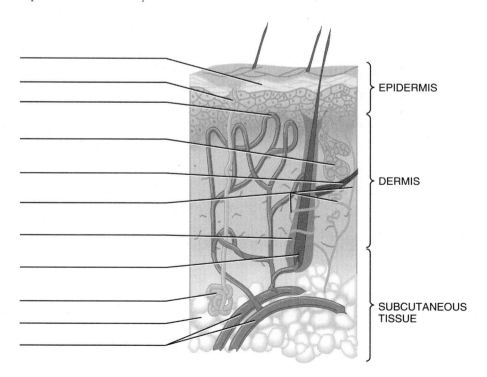

UNDERSTANDING PATHOPHYSIOLOGY

2. The clinical manifestation that most often brings a client to the health care provider is _____ _____.

3. Differentiate between allergy and irritation.

4. List the dermatologic conditions that are genetically transmitted.
   a.

   b.

   c.

   d.

5. The skin disease that may be passed on to family members because of close and frequent exposure is _____ _____.

6. Excess body hair is known as _____ _____.

7. Nails indicate _____ _____ and _____ _____ status.

8. Pallor in the nail bed may be indicative of _____.

9. Differentiate between a callus and a corn.

10. Differentiate between linear and satellite patterns.

11. True or False
    _____   A bulla is a secondary lesion.
    _____   An excoriation is a primary lesion.
    _____   Inflammation often goes unrecognized in Caucasians.
    _____   Skin turgor increases with age.
    _____   Food allergies can cause atopic dermatitis or urticaria.

12. Identify the ABCDs of melanoma.
    A.

    B.

    C.

    D.

APPLYING SKILLS

13. Explain why it is important to ask clients about previous trauma or surgical interventions.

14. Explain the rationale for assessing occupational history in a client who presents with a skin disorder.

15. Match each dermatologic term with the appropriate description.

	Dermatologic Term		**Description**
_____	a. Circumscribed	1.	Thickened, scaly skin
_____	b. Nummular	2.	Areas of decreased pigment
_____	c. Dermatome	3.	Unusual thinning
_____	d. Erythema	4.	Loss of patches of hair
_____	e. Ichthyosis	5.	The redness of inflammation
_____	f. Alopecia	6.	Limited to a certain area by sharply defined borders
_____	g. Primary lesion	7.	Circular lesion about the size of a large coin
_____	h. Secondary lesion	8.	Area of skin supplied by a single dorsal nerve root
_____	i. Rubor	9.	The first lesion to appear on the skin
_____	j. Hypopigmentation	10.	A primary lesion that has changed
_____	k. Atrophy	11.	Redness

16. Explain the rationale for conducting a dermatologic assessment in a well-lit, private room with moderate temperature and neutral, white, or cream-colored walls.

17. Identify the body area where it is easiest to detect the following:
    a. Pallor:

    b. Cyanosis:

    c. Jaundice:

    d. Jaundice in dark-skinned clients:

18. Skin temperature should be assessed using the _____.

19. Identify the order used to assess and describe lesions.

20. In order to assess the contour and consistency of lesions, the nurse would need to _____ _____ the lesions.

21. True or False

    _____ The location of lesions is described in reference to anatomic landmarks.

22. Label each assessment finding of the nails.

About 160°

_____   _____

_____   _____

_____

BEST PRACTICES

23. Explain when a skin culture would be indicated.

24. Explain the purpose of a patch test.

25. Identify contraindications to a patch test.

26. Explain the rationale for instructing clients to avoid taking aspirin for 48 hours prior to a biopsy.

27. Explain the postprocedure care following a biopsy.

KEEPING DRUG SKILLS SHARP

28. The most common type of allergic drug reaction is _____.

29. Describe the type of reaction that may occur when taking a photosensitizing drug.

30. Match each type of reaction to the medication.

Type of Reaction		Medication
_____	a. Maculopapular without blistering	1. Prednisone
_____	b. Sunburn-like rash	2. Penicillin
_____	c. Eczematous rash	3. Tetracycline
_____	d. Acne breakout	4. Diphenhydramine hydrochloride

31. _____ is a complementary/alternative treatment used for relief of eczema, psoriasis, and to increase wound healing.

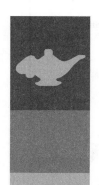

CHAPTER **49**

Management of Clients with Integumentary Disorders

CHAPTER OBJECTIVES

49.1 Describe the magnitude and impact of skin diseases on clients.

49.2 Define terms related to common skin disorders, pressure ulcers, precancerous skin changes, skin cancer, and bullous and infectious disorders.

49.3 Identify causes and risk factors of common skin disorders, pressure ulcers, precancerous skin changes, skin cancer, and bullous and infectious disorders.

49.4 Relate the pathophysiology and clinical manifestations of common skin disorders, pressure ulcers, precancerous and cancerous skin conditions, and bullous and infectious disorders.

49.5 Describe the desired outcomes of medical and nursing management for common skin disorders and medical, surgical, and nursing management for pressure ulcers, precancerous and cancerous skin conditions, and bullous and infectious disorders.

49.6 Identify the purpose of the numerous cosmetic and/or restorative, reconstructive, or traumatic injury plastic surgical procedures.

UNDERSTANDING PATHOPHYSIOLOGY

1. Match each example of eczema or dermatitis with the correct description.

	Eczema or Dermatitis		Description
_____	a. Atopic dermatitis	1.	Eruptions from allergy to poison ivy, sumac, or oak or a proven allergen
_____	b. Seborrheic dermatitis	2.	Eruption from direct contact with irritating substances, which can be almost anything including cosmetics, chemicals, dyes, or detergents
_____	c. Irritant dermatitis	3.	Characteristic distribution of eczema in person with a family history of asthma, hay fever, or eczema
_____	d. Allergic contact dermatitis	4.	Eruption resulting from peripheral venous disorders
_____	e. Nummular eczema	5.	Yellowish-pink scaling of the scalp, face, and trunk
_____	f. Stasis dermatitis	6.	Appearance of coin-shaped, oozing, crusting patches

2. The major clinical manifestation of atopic dermatitis that causes the greatest morbidity is _____ _____.

3. The most common cause of intertrigo is contamination with _____ _____.

4. The length of time it takes for normal skin cells to grow, move to the surface, and slough off is _____; however, in psoriasis this cycle speeds up and takes only _____.

5. List the most common sites for psoriasis eruptions.
   a.

   b.

   c.

   d.

   e.

6. Acne rosacea occurs most often between the ages of _____ and _____. _____ are affected more frequently than _____.

7. Differentiate first-degree from second-degree sunburn.

8. List the three most common types of skin cancer.
   a.

   b.

   c.

9. The greatest risk for skin cancer would be found in a client who:
   1. never burns and always tans.
   2. burns once or twice and then tans.
   3. always burns.

10. List the five risk factors for malignant melanoma.
    a.

    b.

    c.

    d.

    e.

11. List the four changes in a skin lesion that are suspicious of malignant melanoma.
    a.

    b.

    c.

    d.

12. Survival for clients with malignant melanoma is directly related to the _____ _____ of tumor invasion.

13. The malignant disease involving the T helper cells is _____.

14. The two major complications of herpes zoster are _____ and _____ _____.

15. The two types of plastic surgery are _____ and _____.

16. The most common cause of free flap failure is _____.

17. True or False
    _____ Pruritus is a skin disease.
    _____ Xerotic skin lacks moisture in the top layer of the skin and is common in the younger population.
    _____ Stasis dermatitis results from venous insufficiency.
    _____ Changes in physical and emotional health can precede flares of psoriasis.
    _____ Skin tears are most common in older adults due to thinning of the epidermis.

_____ It is believed that pressure ulcers are a specific indicator of malnutrition.

_____ Actinic keratosis is the most common epithelial precancerous lesion caused by sun exposure.

_____ Basal cell carcinoma almost always metastasizes.

_____ Unlike other skin cancers, squamous cell carcinoma occurs frequently in dark-skinned clients.

_____ Malignant melanoma is the deadliest form of skin cancer.

_____ Pemphigus vulgaris is an autoimmune disease caused by circulating immunoglobulin G autoantibodies.

_____ A person who has never had chickenpox cannot get it from someone who has herpes zoster.

_____ Paronychia is an infection under the nail.

_____ Onychomycosis is a fungal infection of the nail.

APPLYING SKILLS

18. Explain why a quantitative culture versus a swab culture is used to diagnose an ulcer infection.

19. A score below _____ on the Braden Scale indicates a client is at high risk for pressure ulcer development.

20. An assessment finding that may indicate that the rhinoplasty client is experiencing excessive bleeding is _____.

21. True or False

_____ For a client with a nursing diagnosis of Impaired skin integrity related to pressure ulcer, an appropriate outcome statement is "Stage IV ulcer will heal to Stage III."

BEST PRACTICES

22. Explain how the care of pruritus is altered for the older client.

23. Match each type of ulcer care with the appropriate description.

Type of Ulcer Care (Debridement)	Description
_____ a. Mechanical debridement	1. Use of synthetic dressings to cover an ulcer, allowing enzymes in the wound bed to digest the devitalized tissues
_____ b. Biodebridement	2. Use of wet-to-dry dressings, hydrotherapy, and high-pressure wound irrigation to soften and remove devitalized tissues
_____ c. Sharp debridement	3. Use of topical debriding agents to dissolve the collagen anchors that hold the necrotic slough tissue to the wound bed
_____ d. Autolytic debridement	4. Debridement is carried out at the bedside using a scalpel and forceps to remove loose necrotic tissue
_____ e. Enzymatic debridement	5. Use of sterile larvae (maggots), which secrete enzymes that digest wound tissue
_____ f. Conservative sharp debridement	6. Use of a scalpel to excise devitalized thick, adherent eschar; this is completed in the operating room

24. Explain the benefit of cool tap water soaks for the treatment of superficial, partial-thickness sunburn.

25. An appropriate nursing intervention for a client with an altered body image is to:
    1. be sensitive to the client's feelings and needs.
    2. reassure the client that plastic surgery will change everything.
    3. empathize with the client and tell them you know exactly how he or she feels.
    4. ignore client statements about his or her feelings.

26. Match each facial resurfacing procedure with the appropriate description.

Procedure

_____ a.   Skin peel

_____ b.   Laser resurfacing

_____ c.   Dermabrasion

_____ d.   Dermal fillers

_____ e.   Botulinum injection

Description

1. Products are used to fill in small wrinkles or depressed blemishes in the skin.
2. Substance is injected to temporarily improve the appearance of moderate to severe frown lines between eyebrows.
3. Various products are used to lift superficial layers of skin and remove fine wrinkles from the skin.
4. Treatment creates a shallow burn injury to the skin.
5. Process of sanding the surface layers of skin on cheeks and forehead with an electric rotating brush to smooth out pitting and surface blemishes.

27. The primary nursing responsibility for a client with a flap is to _____ _____ _____.

28. The most important emergency measure for a client who has sustained a traumatic amputation is to _____ _____.

29. True or False

    _____ Ultraviolet light is used to cause desquamation.

    _____ Cryotherapy is common, painless therapy for the treatment of multiple lesions of actinic keratosis.

    _____ Because of the risk of tumor spread during biopsy, clients who have malignant melanoma removed in a two-stage process (biopsy first followed by tumor removal in a separate procedure) have poorer outcomes than clients who have the procedure done in one step.

    _____ A rhytidectomy is a procedure that restores youthful appearance and removes all of the wrinkles of the face.

    _____ Clients can expect to see immediate results following liposuction.

    _____ A client with intermaxillary wires should avoid alcoholic and carbonated beverages.

KEEPING DRUG SKILLS SHARP

30. List the factors that influence the absorption, penetration, and permeation of topically applied preparations.
    a.

    b.

    c.

    d.

    e.

    f.

31. Which of the following medications draw moisture into the cell structure of the stratum corneum? (Select all that apply.)
    1. Menthol
    2. Urea
    3. Camphor
    4. Lactic acid

32. Identify the two topical immunomodulators (TIMs) that are approved for the treatment of atopic dermatitis.
    a.

    b.

33. The most important thing to consider when using a short course of topical steroid therapy is to _____.

34. A client with psoriasis is being treated with methotrexate. What laboratory value should be monitored before and during treatment?
    1. Lipids
    2. Blood glucose
    3. Creatinine
    4. CBC

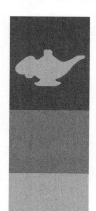

CHAPTER 50

Management of Clients with Burn Injury

CHAPTER OBJECTIVES

50.1 Define *burns* and *burn injury*.
50.2 Describe the impact of burn injury in the United States each year.
50.3 Identify the mechanism of injury for different types of burns.
50.4 Explain the pathophysiology of burn injury to the body systems.
50.5 Relate the clinical manifestations to the pathophysiologic mechanisms.
50.6 Describe the desired outcomes of medical and nursing management of the resuscitative, acute, and rehabilitation phases of burn care.
50.7 Identify multiple priority nursing diagnoses and interventions during the phases of burn care.
50.8 Describe the outcomes of surgical intervention during he acute phase of burn care.
50.9 Discuss the psychosocial issues related to body image following major burn injury.

UNDERSTANDING PATHOPHYSIOLOGY

1. Match each statement on the left with the answer on the right. Not all answers will be used.

_____	a.	Sunburn is an example of a _____ burn.
_____	b.	There are over _____ million burns/year.
_____	c.	Contact with current over _____ volts is potentially dangerous.
_____	d.	_____ probably causes most deaths in structure fires.
_____	e.	This fails, leading to edema.
_____	f.	This is important in considering radiation burns.

1. 60
2. Sodium-potassium pump
3. Shielding
4. 1 million
5. Smoke inhalation
6. 40
7. 700,000
8. Radiation burn
9. Chemical burn
10. Free radicals

2. List the three protective measures the body loses due to destruction of the skin in burn injury.
    a.

    b.

    c.

3.   Match each type of burn injury with the appropriate definition.

Type of Burn Injury

_____   a.   Partial-thickness

_____   b.   Full-thickness

_____   c.   First-degree

_____   d.   Second-degree
_____   e.   Third-degree
_____   f.   Fourth-degree

Definition

1.   Characterized by damage throughout the dermis and skin appears dry and may be black, brown, white, or ivory
2.   Involves skin, fat, muscle, and sometimes bone and skin appears charred or may be completely burned away
3.   Involves injury to the epidermis and portions of the dermis
4.   Damage throughout the dermis
5.   Superficial, painful, and skin appears red
6.   Skin appears wet or blistered and is extremely painful

4.   The clinical manifestations of CO poisoning do not usually occur until COHb levels reach _____.

5.   Basal metabolic rates of the burn client are _____.

6.   The two complications that inhibit the return of optimal physical functioning are _____ _____ and _____ _____.

7.   True or False

_____   Seventy-five percent of all burn injuries result from the actions of the victim.

_____   Scalding liquids are the leading cause of burn injury.

_____   Ignition from cigarettes is the nation's largest single cause of all fire deaths.

_____   Immune function is increased in burn injury.

_____   Donor sites for skin grafts can only be used one time.

APPLYING SKILLS

8.   Differentiate between the causes of thermal, chemical, electrical, and radiation burns.

9.   A 197 lb. client's urine output is less than 0.5 ml/kg/hour after a burn injury. Calculate the urinary output that would be considered minimally adequate.

10.   Following a major burn injury, the nurse would expect the bowel sound to be:
      1.   hypoactive.
      2.   hyperactive.
      3.   absent.

11.   Following a burn injury to the upper airway, the client is at risk for upper airway obstruction. Typically, the nurse would be vigilant of this complication between _____ and _____ hours.

12.   When assessing a client for possible smoke exposure, the nurse would note:
      1.   complaints of dizziness.
      2.   soot in the nares.
      3.   pallor.
      4.   inflamed nares.

13.   An assessment finding consistent with decreased cardiac output in the first 24 hours after burn injury is:
      1.   increased urine output.
      2.   bounding peripheral pulse.
      3.   normal capillary refill.
      4.   decreased blood pressure.

14. Differentiate between background and procedural pain experienced by burn victims.

15. Pulmonary assessment is performed every _____ to _____ hours during the first 24 hours after injury.

16. List the nursing assessments that are performed to determine adequacy of circulation in a client with a nursing diagnosis of Ineffective tissue perfusion.

    a.

    b.

    c.

    d.

    e.

17. Using the Curreri formula, calculate the energy requirements for a 146 lb. female with 36% TBSA burn.

18. Using the consensus formula for fluid resuscitation, calculate the fluid requirements for the first 24 hours for a 212 lb. man with a 45% TBSA burn.

19. A 33-year-old male has large, thick-walled blisters over deep red, wet, and shiny tissue over all his upper extremities and half of his face. He has four irregular-shaped red burns on his chest that each appears to be the size of his hand. Compute the TBSA burned.

20. Sheet autografts are used in areas of the body that are _____.

21. Meshed autografts are used in areas of the body that are _____ or on _____, _____ wounds.

22. Matching. Match the type of graft on the left with its description on the right.

Type of Graft		**Description**
_____ a. Allograft		1. Pig skin
_____ b. Xenograft		2. Nylon fabric
_____ c. Biobrane		3. Human cadaver skin

BEST PRACTICES

23. A nursing intervention that can be initiated to decrease facial edema and facilitate lung expansion is to _____ _____.

24. A client is at risk for acute tubular necrosis secondary to myoglobin and hemoglobin released from damaged muscles. The goal is maintain a urinary output of _____ to _____ ml/hr.

25. Explain why it is important to debride burn wounds of loose, nonviable tissue.

26. The single most important measure to prevent infection is _____ _____ _____.

27. A nursing consideration for a client using 0.5% silver nitrate for wound care is to:
    1. store the antimicrobial agent in a warm environment.
    2. assess adequacy of pain management.
    3. check serum electrolytes daily.
    4. assess for hypersensitivity.

28. List the measures used to prevent wound contracture.
    a.

    b.

    c.

    d.

29. The therapeutic position that should be used when the burn injury involves the hip is _____ _____.

30. An intervention that will help the client feel some control over his or her situation would be to:
    1. provide passive ROM.
    2. provide dressing changes at a time the client specifies.
    3. allow the client to assist with wound care.
    4. apply splints and pressure garments before visitors arrive.

31. Meals provided during the acute phase of treatment should be high in _____ and _____.

32. Explain why wound debridement for burn injury clients is scheduled at the end of the day.

33. True or False
    _____ A static splint exercises the affected joint.

34. A client is in the acute phase of burn care. Place the following nursing diagnoses in priority order.
    _____ Pain
    _____ Ineffective airway clearance
    _____ Impaired physical mobility
    _____ Hypothermia
    _____ Disabled family coping
    _____ Impaired gas exchange
    _____ Imbalanced nutrition
    _____ Risk for stress ulceration (Collaborative problem)
    _____ Risk for infection
    _____ Disturbed personal identity
    _____ Anxiety

35. During the rehabilitation phase, which nursing diagnosis would take priority?
    1. Impaired airway clearance
    2. Disturbed personal identity
    3. Hypothermia
    4. Impaired physical mobility

36. Interventions for hypothermia during the acute phase of burn care include: (Select all that apply.)
    1. limit hydrotherapy session to 30 minutes or less.
    2. use warmed IV fluids.
    3. expose limited areas of the body during dressing changes.
    4. wear cotton gowns.
    5. use heating lamps.

37. A day pass for a therapeutic outing might help meet the outcomes listed for which nursing diagnosis/diagnoses? (Select all that apply.)
    1. Impaired physical mobility
    2. Disturbed personal identity
    3. Disabled family coping
    4. Anxiety

38. Describe psychological responses to burn injury that are common in each phase.

KEEPING DRUG SKILLS SHARP

39. The drug of choice in treating pain in the client with a moderate or major burn is IV _____ _____.

40. If NSAIDs are used in the treatment of mild to moderate pain, measures need to be initiated to prevent _____.

41. True or False

    _____ Analgesic medications are given so that the client receives the benefit of the drug's peak effect immediately following dressing changes.

    _____ Silver sulfadiazine is rarely used anymore for wound care.

    _____ Proton pump inhibitors can be used during the acute phase of burn care.

    _____ Anxiolytics are contraindicated for the burned client with inhalation injury because of the risk of respiratory depression.

    _____ Fentanyl is an acceptable alternative to morphine for pain control.

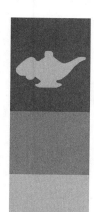

CHAPTER 51

Assessment of the Vascular System

CHAPTER OBJECTIVES

51.1 Describe the aspects of vascular system assessment related to presenting manifestations.
51.2 Identify risk factors for the development of vascular disease when assessing the client.
51.3 Discuss the components of the health history.
51.4 Distinguish arterial and venous disorders related to the client's chief complaint and clinical manifestations.
51.5 Identify the clinical manifestations often associated with vascular disorders.
51.6 Discuss appropriate questions for the client in the review of systems related to clinical manifestations.
51.7 Identify client potential for vascular disorders based on medical and surgical history.
51.8 Discuss food or medication allergies such as iodine.
51.9 Discuss interactions of medications and alternative therapies.
51.10 Identify dietary habits concerning any food and fluid intake and body weight.
51.11 Describe social and family history that contributes to a diagnosis of vascular disorders.
51.12 Perform a physical assessment of the entire body to assess for vascular disorders.
51.13 Compare bilateral vital signs, color, and temperature measurements that would indicate vascular disease.
51.14 Describe diagnostic testing including the appropriate use for each test regarding possible vascular disorders.

ANATOMY & PHYSIOLOGY REVIEW

1. Label the structures of each type of blood vessel.

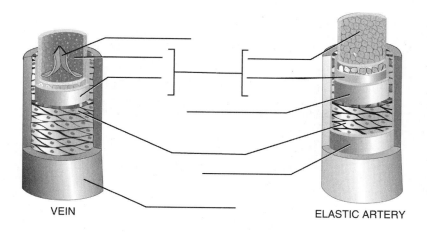
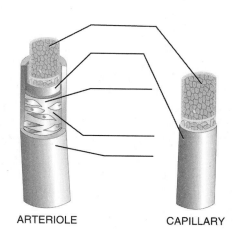

VEIN   ELASTIC ARTERY   ARTERIOLE   CAPILLARY

UNDERSTANDING PATHOPHYSIOLOGY

2. List the two classic characteristics for intermittent claudication.
   a.

   b.

3. Factors that may predispose a client to venous disorders include: (Select all that apply.)
   1. positive family history of venous disorders.
   2. occupation requiring high levels of physical activity.
   3. multiple pregnancies.
   4. obesity.

4. _____ is discoloration of the skin from chronic venous disorders.

5. True or False
   _____ Dependent cyanosis is caused by venous pooling in the extremities.
   _____ Dependent rubor is caused by venous disorders affecting circulation.

APPLYING SKILLS

6. Assessment of the vascular system includes biographic and demographic data. Identify the rationale for obtaining this information in relation to the vascular system.
   Age:

   Occupation:

7. When completing a medical history on a client, the nurse should inquire about *current* health status and the presence of any clinical manifestations to establish a _____ to aid in diagnosis and treatment.

8. True or False
   _____ Clients with arterial insufficiency will have shiny, hairless skin and thick, ridged toenails.
   _____ Edema is not usually present in clients with pure arterial insufficiency.

9. When assessing temperature in extremities, the nurse should compare one extremity with the
   _____ limb.

10. _____ is performed on a client with vascular problems to assess for blood flow in the arm prior to performing a stick for ABGs.

11. _____ studies for deep vein thrombosis (DVT) are more accurate than the test for Homans' sign.

12. The nurse assessing a client for risk factors for vascular disorders would inquire about: (Select all that apply.)
    1. diabetes.
    2. hypertension.
    3. family history of vascular problems.
    4. work situation.
    5. activity level.

13. Which allergy, if present, could pose a problem for the client undergoing diagnostic testing for vascular disorders and why?
    1. Gentamycin
    2. Iodine
    3. Aspirin products
    4. Furosemide

14. Match the disease condition on the right to the herbal remedy used on the left. Disorders may be used more than once or not at all. Herbs may be used for more than one disorder.

Disease Condition
_____ 1. Garlic
_____ 2. Horse chestnut
_____ 3. Valerian
_____ 4. Ginkgo
_____ 5. Onion

Herbal Remedy
a. Hypertension
b. Antispasmodic
c. Varicose veins
d. Phlebitis

15. _____ measures venous blood volume changes in the extremities.

16. The treadmill test can provide information on the severity of _____ and the extent to which it affects the client's _____.

BEST PRACTICES

17. A male client has come to the clinic complaining of impotence. The nurse would assess for problems related to which structure?
    1. Aorta
    2. Heart
    3. Subclavian artery
    4. Peripheral veins
    5. Lymphatics

18. Changes in skin color are best demonstrated by:
    1. using a standardized chart.
    2. comparing with the contralateral limb.
    3. referencing a table with skin-tone references.
    4. checking appearance with a family member.

19. Important aspects of the social history related to vascular disorders that the nurse should include in a complete examination are: (Select all that apply.)
    1. use of nicotine.
    2. occupation.
    3. activity and rest.
    4. sleep habits.

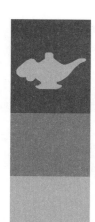

C H A P T E R **52**

Management of Clients with Hypertensive Disorders

CHAPTER OBJECTIVES

52.1 Discuss the trends related to the care of the hypertensive client.
52.2 Describe the cause, epidemiology, and modifiable and nonmodifiable risk factors of hypertensive disease.
52.3 Relate the pathophysiology and clinical manifestations of primary and secondary hypertension.
52.4 Describe the desired outcomes of medical and nursing management of hypertension.
52.5 Explain the modification in treatment regimen for older clients.
52.6 Describe the urgent nature of hypertensive crisis along with the need for blood pressure reduction.
52.7 Describe public health goals for community screening and self-care initiatives.
52.8 Define *syncope* and its relationship to postural hypotension.

TRENDS AND THEORIES

1. Despite the advances made in detection and treatment of hypertension, there is a trend of *increasing* mortality rates for heart disease and strokes among all of the following *except*:
   1. older adults.
   2. Asian-Americans.
   3. African-Americans.
   4. lower socioeconomic groups.

2. Arterial hypertension affects more than _____ people in the United States.

3. _____% of people with hypertension have their blood pressures controlled to their target level.

4. The two major factors that contribute to a decline in improved client outcomes are _____ _____ and _____ _____.

UNDERSTANDING PATHOPHYSIOLOGY

5. The most common complication of untreated hypertension is _____ _____.

6. The elevation in blood pressure in hypertension is caused by persistent and progressive _____ _____ _____.

7. Compare and contrast between primary and secondary hypertension.

Type	Characteristics
Primary (essential)	
Secondary	

8. List the steps in the renin-angiotensin-aldosterone system to control blood pressure.
   a.

   b.

   c.

   d.

   e.

9. The increase in _____ seen in Cushing's disease causes increases in sodium retention and angiotensin II levels, resulting in increased blood pressure.

10. Untreated hypertension causes damage to which of the following "target organs"? (Select all that apply.)
    1. Brain
    2. Liver
    3. Eyes
    4. Kidneys

11. All medications given to treat hypertension have the potential to cause _____ _____; some more than others.

12. In a hypertensive crisis, the major problem is not so much the elevation of blood pressure as it is _____.

APPLYING SKILLS

13. The diagnosis of hypertension is made when the average of two or more separate blood readings is _____ or higher for the systolic blood pressure and _____ or higher for the diastolic blood pressure.

14. List the factors that should be used to evaluate whether a treatment regimen for controlling hypertension is effective.
    a.

    b.

    c.

15. True or False

    _____ When completing a physical assessment, the nurse notes a client to be overweight with increased fat around the midriff, waist, and abdomen. This body shape has been shown to be associated with the development of hypertension.

    _____ Clients should have blood pressure readings taken immediately upon arrival at the clinic to reflect normal pressures at home.

    _____ Clients who report complaints of persistent headaches, fatigue, dizziness, blurred vision, or epistaxis may have undiagnosed hypertension.

    _____ If a blood pressure reading is classified as "prehypertension" category, measures should be taken to address modifiable risk factors immediately.

    _____ Visible changes to the blood vessels of the eye can be seen resulting from untreated hypertension.

16. Essential nursing care of the client experiencing a hypertensive emergency include: (Select all that apply.)
    1. reducing arterial pressure no more than 25% in the first moments to hours.
    2. monitoring blood pressure frequently, as often as every 5–15 minutes.
    3. prevent target organ ischemia by preventing rapid falls in blood pressure.
    4. liberal use of sublingual nifedipine for rapid control of blood pressure.

BEST PRACTICES

17. For each *modifiable* risk factor for hypertension, discuss what lifestyle changes the nurse should advise the client to take to reduce blood pressure.

Risk Factor	Action
Stress	
Obesity	
Nutrients	
Substance abuse	

18. State the critical nursing action that should be implemented prior to taking a blood pressure reading in a client.

19. List the two key aspects to dietary intervention in clients with hypertension.
    a.

    b.

20. In planning treatment regimens, the nurse recognizes that _____ usually improves when the client understands the reasons for treatment and consequences of inadequate interventions.

21. List the nursing interventions that can be implemented to prevent injury from syncope.
    a.

    b.

22. List five revised goals of the National Public Health Plan to address hypertension.

23. Describe the importance of community blood pressure screening events.

24. List an appropriate outcome and three interventions with rationale for the nursing diagnosis Risk for noncompliance.

KEEPING DRUG SKILLS SHARP

25. List the first line choices for drug therapy to treat hypertension.
    a.

    b.

26. It would be appropriate to evaluate reducing the number and amounts of antihypertensive medications for a client if the client's blood pressure has been controlled effectively for _____ _____.

27. A client newly diagnosed with hypertension is concerned about "remembering all the information" related to medications and monitoring her blood pressure at home. The nurse develops the diagnosis of Risk for ineffective management of therapeutic regimen related to lack of knowledge. Identify outcomes to meet the learning needs of this client.

28. Explain the phrase "start low and go slow" in relation to medication for older clients with hypertension.

CONCEPT MAP EXERCISES

The following questions are based on the Concept Map *Understanding Hypertension and Its Treatment* in the textbook.

29. Combination therapy is often used to control hypertension, including ACE inhibitors and diuretics. How do ACE inhibitors affect elevated blood pressure?

30. A 67-year-old client with hypertension has been prescribed a new medication, which is a calcium channel blocker. She doesn't understand how a "calcium" drug helps with blood pressure. How would the nurse explain the effect of this medication in treating her hypertension?

31. Increased pressure detected by the baroreceptors in the carotid arteries causes what clinical manifestation?

32. When is secondary prevention of hypertension instituted?

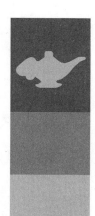

CHAPTER 53

Management of Clients with Vascular Disorders

CHAPTER OBJECTIVES

53.1 Define *peripheral arterial disorders*.
53.2 Identify the cause and risk factors for arterial, venous, and lymphatic disorders.
53.3 Relate the pathophysiology and clinical manifestations for arterial, venous, and lymphatic disorders.
53.4 Identify diagnostic testing for arterial, venous, and lymphatic disorders.
53.5 Describe desired outcomes of the medical, surgical, and nursing management of the client with arterial, venous, and lymphatic disorders.
53.6 Identify modifications of treatment necessary for the older client.
53.7 Identify postoperative complications of surgical intervention for arterial bypass surgery.
53.8 Identify self-care activities following arterial surgery.

UNDERSTANDING PATHOPHYSIOLOGY

1. Peripheral arterial occlusive diseases are caused primarily by _____ _____.

2. List the primary risk factors for the development of atherosclerosis.
    a.

    b.

    c.

3. Differentiate between primary and secondary lymphedema.

4. Physical manifestations of peripheral vascular disease (PVD) include: (Select all that apply.)
    1. lack of pulses in brachial artery.
    2. pallor of legs.
    3. thick, brittle nails.
    4. hairy shins.
    5. poorly healing ulcers.
    6. mottling color.
    7. paralysis.
    8. lack of pulse in dorsalis pedis artery.

5. The most successful grafting material used today for bypass surgery is _____ _____.

6. The major indication for the "open" or guillotine type of amputation over a "flap" amputation is _____.

7. List the classic manifestations of acute ischemia caused by peripheral thrombus or embolism (the 6 P's).

a.

b.

c.

d.

e.

f.

8. List the risk factors for development of an aneurysm.

a.

b.

9. Ruptures occur most often in abdominal aortic aneurysms larger than _____.

10. Color changes to the hands are a classic manifestation of a Raynaud's vasospasm. Describe the physiologic reason for each of the stages of the spasm.

Stage	Physiologic Changes
Pallor (white) color in hands	
Cyanotic (blue) color in hands	
Rubor (red) color in hands	

11. List the three conditions of Virchow's triad for the development of venous thrombosis and their etiologies.

a.

b.

c.

12. True or False

_____ A dissecting aneurysm is not a true aneurysm.

_____ The classic sign for an abdominal aortic aneurysm is colicky pain.

_____ A client can feel a pulsating mass in the abdomen, with or without pain, from an abdominal aneurysm.

_____ Abdominal aortic aneurysms (AAA) are the most common type of aneurysm.

_____ If the aneurysm is smaller than 4–5 cm and asymptomatic, it is safe to surgically correct it.

_____ Repair of AAA requires an incision from the xiphoid process to the symphysis pubis.

_____ If a client has cardiac disease, he or she will undergo a coronary artery bypass before repairing an aneurysm.

_____ The spinal cord can become ischemic, resulting in paraplegia, if an AAA ruptures.

_____ The client who undergoes AAA repair faces the greatest risk of cardiac and pulmonary complication during the 4 hours of surgery under anesthesia.

_____ A client's sexual functioning will be greatly improved after correction of an AAA due to increased blood flow.

APPLYING SKILLS

13. List the three characteristics of intermittent claudication.

    a.

    b.

    c.

14. Mr. Thomas, a 78-year-old construction worker, has had PVD for a number of years. He now tells the nurse that his sleep is being interrupted by pain in his legs that requires him to get up and walk around. He states that the pain used to occur when walking but now it hurts when he is stationary. State the clinical significance of "pain at rest" for the client with intermittent claudication.

15. When evaluating vascular disorders, a _____ can determine the quality of blood flow of the vessels.

16. List four anatomical areas where pulses should be assessed in a client with a possible peripheral vascular disorder.

    a.

    b.

    c.

    d.

17. A nurse assesses a postoperative client who has undergone a bypass grafting of a lower extremity. Manifestations that would indicate a clot blocking blood flow include that the limb has become: (Select all that apply.)

    1. cool.
    2. pale in appearance.
    3. painful.
    4. pulseless.

18. List the critical nursing assessments that should be performed in the *preoperative* time period for a client who will undergo a bypass grafting for an extremity with PVD.

    a.

    b.

    c.

19. A change in urine color from yellow to brown in a client who underwent arterial bypass surgery indicates a critical postoperative complication of

    _____

    _____

    _____.

20. True or False

    _____ Tachypnea is the most frequent manifestation of a pulmonary embolism.

BEST PRACTICES

21. For each medical management goal, identify specific client teaching areas for the nurse to discuss.

Goal	Specific Teaching Area
a. Reduce risk	
b. Promote arterial flow	
c. Save the limb of clients with intermittent claudication	

22. A nursing intervention for a client with arterial insufficiency would be to place the client in _____ position to aid blood flow through gravity.

23. Identify the priority nursing action for the client with a nursing diagnosis of Risk for impaired skin integrity related to decreased peripheral circulation.

24. When planning an exercise program for a client with vascular disorders, the nurse should exclude clients who have: (Select all that apply.)
    1. leg ulcers.
    2. gangrene.
    3. cellulitis.
    4. deep vein thrombosis (DVT).

25. When teaching a client about phantom sensations, the nurse would explain that: (Select all that apply.)
    1. the sensations are often felt immediately after surgery but gradually decrease over the next 2 days.
    2. the client may feel warmth, cold, itching, or pain, which is caused by intact peripheral nerves above the amputation site.
    3. most phantom pain occurs in clients who had pain prior to amputation.
    4. phantom sensations are unusual and may indicate a complication from the amputation surgery.

26. To prevent edema at the stump postoperatively, the nurse would elevate the stump only for the first _____ and then place it flat.

27. Compare and contrast the types of nursing care required for a client who has undergone a traumatic amputation and for a client who has undergone a planned amputation.
    Traumatic:

    Planned:

28. List the activity restrictions the nurse should instruct a client who has undergone AAA repair to follow as part of discharge teaching.
    a.

    b.

    c.

    d.

29. True or False

     _____ Clients at risk for DVT should not position pillows under the knee for comfort.

     _____ Clinical manifestations of DVT include bilateral swelling of the legs.

     _____ Homans' sign is not considered an accurate test for DVT anymore.

     _____ Venous duplex scanning is the primary diagnostic test for DVT.

     _____ Elastic wraps applied to the legs of clients with venous stasis should be rewrapped once a day to assess the skin.

     _____ Nurses do not need to document the lack of manifestations of pulmonary embolism in clients with DVT if they are stable.

30. List modifications in the nursing care plan for the older adult who is being treated for an arterial problem.

31. List common possible complications following arterial bypass surgery.
    a.

    b.

    c.

KEEPING DRUG SKILLS SHARP

32. Compare and contrast common medications used for anticoagulant therapy.

Medication	Indication	Route	Nursing Considerations
Coumadin			
Heparin			
Low-molecular–weight heparin (LMWH)			

33. The calcium antagonist _____ _____ is the first choice for decreasing the frequency, duration, and intensity of vasospastic attacks.

34. True or False

_____ Anticoagulant agents do not break up or dissolve clots; they prevent new clots from forming.

_____ Heparin therapy requires monitoring of a client's partial thromboplastin time (PTT) levels but low-molecular–weight heparin does not.

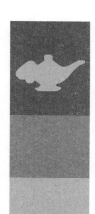

CHAPTER 54

Assessment of the Cardiac System

CHAPTER OBJECTIVES

54.1   Describe the effect of cardiovascular disease (CVD) in the U.S. and the world.
54.2   Describe the health history presenting with manifestations of CVD.
54.3   Determine appropriate questions to elicit the chief complaint from the client.
54.4   Identify clinical manifestations of CVD.
54.5   Distinguish types of syncope and dyspnea.
54.6   Identify risk factors for CVD.
54.7   Describe primary and secondary prevention to modify known risk factors of CVD.
54.8   Relate surgical history and allergies to CVD manifestations.
54.9   Determine interactions between prescription medications and herbal medicines.
54.10 Determine dietary habits that become risk factors for CVD.
54.11 Examine social and family history issues that impact DVD.
54.12 Describe important aspects of the physical examination including neck vein and carotid artery assessment.
54.13 Distinguish normal and abnormal heart sounds.
54.14 Relate abdominal assessment to cardiac competence.
54.15 Describe important aspects of extremity assessment to CVD.
54.16 Relate the need for specific diagnostic testing to clinical manifestations.
54.17 Describe nursing responsibilities for diagnostic testing.

ANATOMY & PHYSIOLOGY REVIEW

1. Label the structures of the heart and trace the flow of blood through the heart systemic circulation.

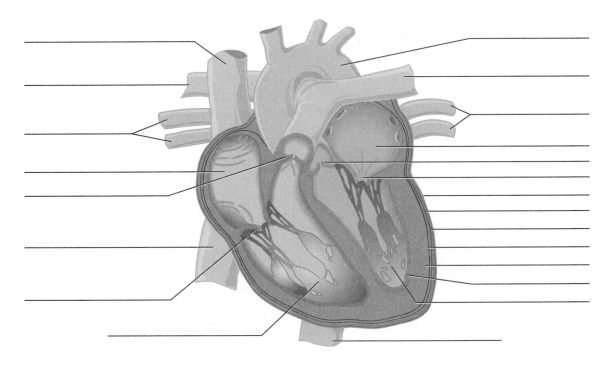

TRENDS AND THEORIES

2. Cardiovascular disease is the #_____ cause of death in the United States and in 2003 accounted for _____% of all deaths in the United States.

3. The total cost of cardiovascular disease in the United States is _____.

4. A major problem for society is that cardiovascular disease affects _____

   _____.

5. Demographic data is important to assess because

   _____

   _____.

UNDERSTANDING PATHOPHYSIOLOGY

6. True or False

   _____ Chest pain is one of the most important manifestations of cardiac disease.

_____ There are greater CVD risk factors among African-American and Mexican-American women than among white women of comparable socioeconomic status.

_____ Murmurs are heard as a consequence of turbulent blood flow through the heart and large vessels.

7. Clients who smoke increase their risk for

   _____ and

   _____.

8. Nicotine, a major ingredient in cigarettes, causes: (Select all that apply.)
   1. peripheral vasoconstriction.
   2. increasing resistance to left ventricular emptying.
   3. increased myocardial workload.
   4. no reduction in cardiac output.

9. The most common causes of fatigue include: (Select all that apply.)
   1. anemia.
   2. anxiety.
   3. chronic diseases.
   4. depression.
   5. thyroid dysfunction.

10. The cardiac cycle is composed of: (Select all that apply.)
    1. the first heart sound (S_1).
    2. the second heart sound (S_2).
    3. rhythm direct forces.
    4. cardiac noding.

APPLYING SKILLS

11. When taking the past medical history of a client at risk for cardiovascular disease, the nurse should include questions about:

    a.

    b.

    c.

    d.

    e.

    f.

    g.

    h.

12. When evaluating chest pain, it is important to assess: (Select all that apply.)
    1. timing.
    2. quality.
    3. quantity.
    4. location.
    5. any precipitating or aggravating factors.

13. True or False

    _____ Tachycardia (rapid heartbeat) can occur as a result of increased force of myocardial contraction caused by the ingestion of caffeine or emotional stress.

    _____ Exertional dyspnea is the most common form of cardiac-related dyspnea.

    _____ Syncope is a transient loss of consciousness related to inadequate cerebral perfusion.

    _____ Clubbing of the fingernails is seen in clients with significant cardiopulmonary disease.

    _____ Elevated serum cholesterol levels are associated with coronary artery disease.

    _____ Neck vein distention can be used to estimate central venous pressure (CVP).

    _____ Crackles frequently signal left ventricular failure and usually occur just after the onset of an S_3 gallop.

    _____ Orthopnea is the need to sit up to breathe easily.

    _____ Paroxysmal nocturnal dyspnea (PND) is a sudden sensation of not being able to breathe, which wakes the client from sleep.

14. Compare and contrast heart sounds.

Characteristic	S$_1$	S$_2$	Gallop	Friction Rub	Murmur
Physiology					
Heard best					
Sounds like					

15. List three things to assess in the abdomen of a client during a head-to-toe assessment related to cardiovascular disease.

a.

b.

c.

16. List five things to assess in the extremities of a client during a head-to-toe assessment related to cardiovascular disease.

a.

b.

c.

d.

e.

17. Describe the significance of the following laboratory studies as they relate to cardiovascular disease.
    a. Hematocrit:

    b. WBC:

    c. Myoglobin:

    d. CK-MB:

    e. Troponin:

    f. PT/PTT:

    g. LDL:

    h. HDL:

    i. Sodium:

    j. Potassium:

    k. BUN/creatinine:

    l. Glucose:

18. List five things that should be assessed as part of social and family history as it pertains to cardiovascular disease.
    a.

    b.

    c.

    d.

    e.

BEST PRACTICES

19. The American Heart Association recommends that health care providers routinely assess a client's general risk of CVD beginning at age _____.

20. Describe primary and secondary risk factor modification for the modifiable risk factors and the metabolic risk factors.

	Modifiable Risk Factors	Metabolic Risk Factors
Primary prevention		
Secondary prevention		

21. Auscultation of the precordium yields valuable information about: (Select all that apply.)
    1. normal or abnormal heart rate and rhythm.
    2. ventricular filling.
    3. blood flow across heart valves.
    4. constant flux of arteries.

22. The most common diagnostic procedures used to diagnose CVD are: (Select all that apply.)
    1. laboratory tests.
    2. ECG.
    3. radiographic studies.
    4. hemodynamic studies.

23. Clients with chronic conditions such as cardiovascular disorders should be vaccinated against _____.

KEEPING DRUG SKILLS SHARP

24. Oral contraceptives increase the incidence of _____.

25. Numerous medications can affect the cardiovascular system, including: (Select all that apply.)
    1. antihypertensives.
    2. diuretics.
    3. cardiotonic drugs.
    4. bronchodilators.

26. Tricyclic antidepressants and other psychotropic medications can cause _____ _____.

27. List seven herbs known to have antidysrhythmic action.
    a.

    b.

    c.

    d.

    e.

    f.

    g.

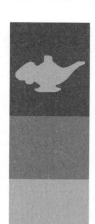

CHAPTER **55**

Management of Clients with Structural Cardiac Disorders

CHAPTER OBJECTIVES

55.1   Describe disorders of the heart that impair the efficiency of the heart as a pump.
55.2   Define the various structural cardiac disorders.
55.3   Describe the causes and risk factors for structural cardiac disorders.
55.4   Relate the pathophysiology and clinical manifestations of structural cardiac disorders.
55.5   Describe the desired outcomes of medical, surgical, and nursing management of structural cardiac disorders.
55.6   Identify diagnostic testing for clients with structural cardiac disorders.
55.7   Differentiate types of cardiomyopathy.
55.8   Identify self-care for clients with cardiomyopathy.
55.9   Discuss valve reconstruction for structural cardiac disorders.
55.10 Discuss cardiac transplant for the client with end-stage structural cardiac disorders.
55.11 Identify infectious disorders, such as rheumatic fever, infective endocarditis, myocarditis, or chronic constrictive pericarditis, that may alter the structural integrity of the heart.

TRENDS AND THEORIES

1. In 2001, _____ hearts were transplanted in the United States.

2. The biggest obstacle to heart transplantation is _____.

3. For people on the heart transplant list, the mortality rate is _____.

4. Heart transplantation clients who die after the procedure usually do so _____ _____.

5. Heart transplantation is considered a standard therapy for _____.

UNDERSTANDING PATHOPHYSIOLOGY

6. Factors that can lead to the development of acquired valvular disease include: (Select all that apply.)
   1. myocardial ischemia.
   2. rheumatic fever.
   3. infectious endocarditis.
   4. connective tissue disorders.

7. The most common preventable cause of mitral stenosis is _____ _____.

8. Inflammation of the endocardium resulting from acute rheumatic fever or infectious endocarditis is caused by: (Select all that apply.)
   1. inflammation causing the valve leaflets and chordae tendinae to become fibrous.
   2. shortening of chordae tendinae, which narrows the outflow tract.
   3. abnormal respiratory reserve remains.
   4. rhythm disturbances.

9. Mitral valve prolapse occurs when:
   1. anterior and posterior cusps of the mitral valve billow upward into the atrium during systolic contraction.
   2. unable to detect current conduction of atrial valve.
   3. posterior centers of the heart relax and cause stress.
   4. upward flow of cardiac strain produces exertional dyspnea.

10. Myocardial oxygen consumption is higher in aortic stenosis due to:
    1. hypertrophy of the right ventricle.
    2. hypertrophy of the left ventricle.
    3. enlarged ventricular tissue.
    4. venous congestion.

11. Risk factors known to contribute to development of rheumatic fever include: (Select all that apply.)
    1. poor hygiene.
    2. crowding.
    3. poverty.
    4. chronic infections.

12. Aortic regurgitation is most often a result of which of these infectious disorders? (Select all that apply.)
    1. Rheumatic fever
    2. Syphilis
    3. Infective endocarditis
    4. Mild pneumonia

13 _____ is a syndrome resulting from inflammation of the pericardial and visceral pericardium.

14. Match the type of cardiomyopathy on the left with its description on the right. More than one descriptor may be used for each type of cardiomyopathy.

Cardiomyopathy

_____ a. Hypertrophic
_____ b. Restrictive

_____ c. Dilated

Description

1. The most common form, seen in 60% of cases
2. Most people with the idiopathic form of this type of cardiomyopathy die within 5 years after onset of manifestations
3. Hydralazine and nitrates have improved outcomes
4. May be genetically transmitted or caused by hypertension
5. The most common manifestation is dyspnea
6. The client with this is at risk for endocarditis
7. The least common type
8. Must be differentiated from pericarditis
9. These clients are often refractory to antidysrhythmics

APPLYING SKILLS

15. Most clients with structural cardiac problems will present with a classic _____.

16. The organism responsible for rheumatic fever is:
    1. *Staphylococcus aureus*.
    2. group A beta-hemolytic streptococci (GAS).
    3. nongroup streptococci.
    4. *Candida albicans*.

17. Rheumatic fever directly impacts which areas of the body? (Select all that apply.)
    1. Layers of the heart
    2. Joints
    3. Subcutaneous tissue
    4. Central nervous system
    5. Skin

18. True or False

    _____ Atrial fibrillation is a common finding in clients with mitral stenosis.

    _____ Biologic, or tissue, valves are more durable than other types.

_____ Mechanical heart valves are prone to emboli.

_____ An indication for valve replacement is progressive impairment of cardiac function despite medical therapy.

_____ If a heart valve is not pliable enough for reconstruction, a heart transplant is the client's only surgical option.

_____ A commissurotomy is used to repair the leaflets of a valve which have become fused at the base.

_____ Mild leaking is common with valvuloplasty.

19. Complications of rheumatic fever include: (Select all that apply.)
    1. valvular disorders.
    2. cardiomegaly.
    3. heart failure.
    4. venous congestion.

20. The inflamed myocardium of the heart in rheumatic fever has areas of necrosis called _____
    _____.

21. The nurse needs to obtain which of the following to assist in confirming a diagnosis of rheumatic fever?
    1. Urine culture
    2. Blood culture
    3. Throat culture
    4. Immunoassay of stool

22. Additional diagnostic tests that will be ordered for a client with rheumatic fever include: (Select all that apply.)
    1. CBC with WBC elevation.
    2. erythrocyte sedimentation rate (ESR).
    3. C-reactive protein.
    4. ECG.

23. Clinical signs that a client with cardiac tamponade will present with include: (Select all that apply.)
    1. hypotension and muffled heart sounds.
    2. tachycardia and dyspnea.
    3. jugular venous distention.
    4. cyanosis of lips and nails.

24. Clinical manifestations of tricuspid stenosis include: (Select all that apply.)
    1. dyspnea and fatigue.
    2. pulsations in the neck.
    3. peripheral edema.
    4. weight loss.

BEST PRACTICES

25. The primary focus of nursing management of valvular heart disease includes: (Select all that apply.)
    1. helping the client maintain a normal cardiac output.
    2. preventing manifestations of heart failure.
    3. avoiding venous congestion.
    4. preserving tissue perfusion.

26. Most clients treated in the hospital for rheumatic fever are put on the bed rest because it: (Select all that apply.)
    1. reduces myocardial oxygen demands.
    2. reduces cardiac effort.
    3. helps inflammation around the heart to subside.
    4. aids in promoting rest.

27. When teaching a client being discharged from the hospital with rheumatic fever, it is important to stress avoidance of exposure to streptococcal infections. To do this, the nurse would encourage the client to: (Select all that apply.)
    1. avoid people who have upper respiratory infections.
    2. avoid people who have had a recent strep infection.
    3. notify physician if any symptoms of sore throat or pharyngitis develop.
    4. guard against infections for the rest of his or her life to avoid development of heart disease.

28. The emergency intervention of choice for treating cardiac tamponade is _____
    _____.

29. Self-care measures the nurse should teach the client being dismissed with dilated cardiomyopathy include:
    1. sticking to the prescribed exercise regimen.
    2. avoiding alcoholic beverages.
    3. limiting daytime napping to 30 minutes.
    4. maintaining weight by eating foods that are appealing.

30. A client with restrictive cardiomyopathy is being discharged on digoxin. Specific instructions for this client include:
    1. taking the medication as prescribed.
    2. counting the pulse before administering the medication.
    3. being especially vigilant for toxic effects of digoxin.
    4. keeping follow-up appointments as directed.

KEEPING DRUG SKILLS SHARP

31. The drug of choice for treatment of rheumatic fever is:
    1. oral penicillin.
    2. oral diuretics.
    3. beta blockers.
    4. angiotensin-releasing agents.

32. Clients with rheumatic fever will be given prophylactic antibiotics for an extended period of time post-treatment. How long would the nurse tell a client he would be taking oral penicillin?
    1. 10 years or more
    2. Up to 5 years after the initial attack
    3. No more than 1 year
    4. Up to 6 months

33. Digitalis is useful for slowing the ventricular heart rate in clients with _____ _____.

34. _____ are helpful in reducing the risk of embolus.

35. Which of the following medications bring about significant hemodynamic changes in clients with chronic mitral regurgitation? (Select all that apply.)
    1. Angiotensin-converting enzymes
    2. Nitrates
    3. Digitalis
    4. Sulfonamides

36. _____ has been given to prevent transient ischemic attacks.

37. Prophylactic antibiotics may be given on an individual basis for invasive medical or dental procedures in order to prevent _____ _____ in persons who have rheumatic heart disorders.

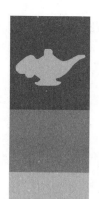

CHAPTER **56**

Management of Clients with Functional Cardiac Disorders

CHAPTER OBJECTIVES

56.1 Identify the significance of atherosclerosis to coronary heart disease (CHD).
56.2 Relate CHD to the development of heart failure.
56.3 Describe the etiology and risk factors for CHD and heart failure.
56.4 Explain risk factors that can be modified versus those that are nonmodifiable or contributing.
56.5 Relate the pathophysiology and clinical manifestations of CHD and heart failure.
56.6 Describe the desired outcomes of medical, surgical, and nursing management of the CHD and heart failure client.
56.7 Describe specific pre- and post-care nursing management of the coronary artery bypass graft (CABG) client.
56.8 Identify complications of CABG surgery.
56.9 Identify specific manifestations of left and right heart failure.
56.10 Discuss diagnostic findings that assist to determine the cause of heart failure.
56.11 Differentiate management of the client with decompensated heart failure from the client with chronic heart failure.

TRENDS AND THEORIES

1. True or False

_____ Heart disease is the number-one killer of both men and women.

_____ Death rates for both CHD and for heart failure (HF) have been decreasing since the 1990s.

_____ Women entering the workforce may have increased rates of CHD.

_____ CHD is the major causative factor for HF.

_____ Exercise and low-fat, low-cholesterol diets increase the amount of HDL in the blood.

_____ Heart failure is a physiologic state in which the heart cannot pump enough blood to meet the metabolic needs of the body.

_____ In chronic heart failure, the increased workload of the heart and the extreme work of breathing increases the metabolic demands of the body.

_____ Dependent edema is one of the early signs of right ventricular failure.

UNDERSTANDING PATHOPHYSIOLOGY

2. True or False

_____ In CHD, atherosclerosis develops in the coronary arteries, causing them to become narrowed or blocked.

3. List six modifiable risk factors for CHD.
   a.

   b.

   c.

   d.

   e.

   f.

4. When compared to the white population, the risk of CHD is greatest among which of the following groups? (Select all that apply.)
   1. Mexican-Americans
   2. American Indians
   3. Native Hawaiians
   4. Asians

5. The incidence of CHD markedly increases among women after _____.

6. Atherosclerosis primarily affects the _____ _____ of the _____ and normally takes years to develop.

7. _____ is the presence of more than one artery supplying blood to a muscle.

8. List some causes of heart failure.
   a. Conditions that increase preload:

   b. Conditions that increase afterload:

   c. Conditions that precipitate heart failure:

9. Compare and contrast the manifestations of right-sided heart failure and left-sided heart failure in the box below.

Right-Sided Heart Failure	Left-Sided Heart Failure

APPLYING SKILLS

10. True or False

    _____ Elevated serum cholesterol levels increase as blood cholesterol levels increase.

    _____ High levels of HDL seem to protect against the development of CHD.

11. Diagnostic studies used to determine underlying causes and degrees of heart failure include: (Select all that apply.)
    1. B-type natriuretic peptide (BNP).
    2. echocardiogram.
    3. chest x-ray.
    4. ECG.

BEST PRACTICES

12. True or False

    _____ The primary goals that guide the medical management of a client with CHD are reducing and controlling risk factors and restoring blood supply to the myocardium.

    _____ Coronary artery bypass graft surgery involves the bypass of a blockage in one or more of the coronary arteries using the saphenous veins, mammary artery, or radial artery.

13. Postoperative complications that are more prevalent in the older client who has had a CABG include: (Select all that apply.)
    1. dysrhythmias related to aged sinoatrial node cells.
    2. drug toxicity associated with impaired hepatic and renal function.
    3. multiple drug interactions.
    4. decreased physical stamina.

14. Prior to discharge, the nurse will instruct the family of a client who has had a CABG regarding: (Select all that apply.)
    1. medication actions and side effects.
    2. dietary restrictions.
    3. physical activity restrictions.
    4. incisional care.

15. Other terms used to denote heart failure include: (Select all that apply.)
    1. cardiac decompensation.
    2. cardiac insufficiency.

    3. ventricular failure.
    4. heart pump syndrome.

16. The nursing care of the client with decompensated heart failure includes which nursing diagnoses?
    a.

    b.

    c.

    d.

    e.

    f.

    g.

17. Write an outcome for the nursing diagnosis Decreased cardiac output appropriate for the client in decompensated heart failure.

18. List some interventions that would assist the client to meet the outcome written in #17 above.

19. Describe the teaching a client needs prior to having a CABG.

20. A client had a CABG and has the nursing diagnosis Risk for hemorrhage. Appropriate interventions include: (Select all that apply.)
    1. monitoring mediastinal chest tubes hourly for drainage.
    2. keep chest tubes positioned correctly without kinking tubing.
    3. monitor for manifestations of cardiac tamponade.
    4. monitor for manifestations of pulmonary edema.

KEEPING DRUG SKILLS SHARP

21. Which of the following are true regarding glycoprotein IIb/IIIa receptor antagonists? (Select all that apply.)
    1. Prevent platelet aggregation in the acute coronary syndromes
    2. When combined with aspirin, decrease the incidence of recurrent cardiac events
    3. Help to smooth the lining of the heart
    4. Decrease the need for heparin

22. Beta-adrenergic antagonists are used to inhibit the effects of the _____ _____.

23. Diuretics are given to clients to: (Select all that apply.)
    1. reduce circulating blood volume.
    2. diminish preload.
    3. lessen systemic and pulmonary congestion.
    4. relieve systemic threshold.

24. True or False
    _____   Hypokalemia can potentiate digitalis toxicity and cause myocardial weakness and cardiac dysrhythmias.

25. Digoxin exerts which of the following effects? (Select all that apply.)
    1. Improves cardiac output; enhances kidney perfusion
    2. Creates a mild diuresis of sodium and water
    3. Helps in treating heart failure
    4. Helps control ventricular response in atrial fibrillation

26. What drug has both beneficial hemodynamic effects and can reduce anxiety?

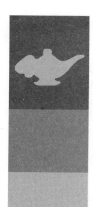

CHAPTER **57**

Management of Clients with Dysrhythmias

CHAPTER OBJECTIVES

57.1 Define *normal sinus rhythm*.
57.2 Define *dysrhythmia*.
57.3 Identify the three major causes of dysrhythmias.
57.4 Relate the pathophysiology and clinical manifestations of dysrhythmias.
57.5 Identify diagnostic assessments and outcome management for dysrhythmias.
57.6 Identify characteristics of the specific dysrhythmias and the treatment of each dysrhythmia.
57.7 Describe desired outcomes of medical, surgical, and nursing management of non–life-threatening and life-threatening dysrhythmias.
57.8 Identify self-care activities for the client with potential for dysrhythmia.

UNDERSTANDING PATHOPHYSIOLOGY

1. The conduction and rhythm system of the heart is susceptible to damage by heart disease as a result of: (Select all that apply.)
   1. ischemia of the heart tissue.
   2. decreased coronary artery blood flow.
   3. too much calcium in the chambers.
   4. inability of the vessels to return the blood.

2. Abnormal rhythms are referred to as: (Select all that apply.)
   1. dysrhythmias.
   2. arrhythmias.
   3. abnormal sounds.
   4. irregular tones.

3. A heart rhythm that begins in the sinoatrial (SA) node is referred to as:
   1. normal sinus rhythm.
   2. normal conduction.
   3. atrial sinus pattern.
   4. ectopic rhythm.

4. The most serious complication of a dysrhythmia is _____.

5. Dysrhythmias result from disturbances in: (Select all that apply.)
   1. automaticity.
   2. conduction.
   3. reentry of pulses.
   4. endocardial swings.

6. Automaticity is used to describe:
   1. alterations in the normal heart rates produced by various pacemaker cells in the myocardium.
   2. impulses driven from sinus activity.
   3. aberrant sounds that collect in the sinus nodes.
   4. abnormal gateway keeping of sounds from the ventricles.

7. Latent pacemaker cells can also fire at increased rates beyond their inherent rate. When rates exceed these values, the rhythm is _____ _____.

8. _____ is the activation of muscle for a second time by the same impulse.

9. A _____ _____ is a conduction delay that occurs between the sinus node and atrial muscle.

251

APPLYING SKILLS

10. The nurse will evaluate clients for dysrhythmias based on which of the following clinical observations? (Select all that apply.)
    1. Heart rate below 50 or above 140 beats per minute
    2. An extremely irregular heart rhythm or pulse
    3. A first heart sound that varies in intensity
    4. Sudden appearance of heart failure, shock, and angina
    5. Slow, regular heart rate that does not change with activity or medications

11. Sinus tachycardia has which of the following clinical characteristics? (Select all that apply.)
    1. Regular rhythm at a rate of 100–180 beats per minute
    2. Normal P wave and QRS complex
    3. Occurs in response to an increase in sympathetic stimulation
    4. Occurs in response to a decreased vagal stimulation

12. _____ is a delay in passage of the impulse from the atria to the ventricles.

13. Which of the following characteristics describe ventricular tachycardia? (Select all that apply.)
    1. A life-threatening dysrhythmia
    2. Occurs when irritable ectopic focus in ventricles takes over
    3. Occurs in significant cardiac disease
    4. Mild cases treated with aspirin

14. Which identifying features of ventricular tachycardia are evident on the ECG monitor? (Select all that apply.)
    1. Rapidly occurring series of PVCs (three or more)
    2. P waves are absent
    3. Ventricular rate ranges between 100–220 beats per minute
    4. QRS complex is wide and bizarre

15. A client with ventricular tachycardia will be experiencing which of the following clinical manifestations? (Select all that apply.)
    1. Cerebral ischemia
    2. Myocardial ischemia
    3. Feels like impending death
    4. Feeling faint, weak, and dizzy

16. Ventricular fibrillation is a life-threatening dysrhythmia characterized by: (Select all that apply.)
    1. extreme, rapid, erratic impulse formation and conduction.
    2. abrupt cessation of effective cardiac output.
    3. bizarre fibrillatory wave patterns on ECG.
    4. impossible-to-identify P waves, QRS complexes, or T waves.

17. Ventricular fibrillation can be either _____ or _____ _____.

18. Clients with sinus bradycardia must be evaluated for: (Select all that apply.)
    1. hypotension.
    2. light-headedness.
    3. syncope.
    4. fatigue.

19. Sinus dysrhythmia is characterized by: (Select all that apply.)
    1. changes in the automaticity of the SA node.
    2. firing at varying speeds.
    3. heart rate between 60–100 beats per minute.
    4. abnormal ECG.

20. A dysrhythmia arising in an ectopic pacemaker or the site of a rapid reentry circuit in the atria is called _____ or _____.

21. An atrial flutter appears on the ECG with which of these identifying characteristics? (Select all that apply.)
    1. Inverted P waves
    2. Picket fences or sawtooth pattern
    3. Rate generally around 220–350 beats per minute
    4. No noted changes in the QRS complex

22. Patients with atrial flutter may experience which of the following clinical signs and symptoms? (Select all that apply.)
    1. Palpitations
    2. Chest pains
    3. Lightheadedness and dizziness
    4. Hypertension

23. Atrial fibrillation can best be described as: (Select all that apply.)
    1. rapid, chaotic atrial depolarization from a reentry disorder.
    2. impulses between 400–700 beats per minute.
    3. extremely slow response and reactivity.
    4. mechanical depolarization.

24. Atrial fibrillation has which of these identifying characteristics on an ECG?
    1. Erratic or no identifiable P waves and an underlying irregular ventricular rhythm
    2. Identifiable QRS complex
    3. P–P ratio is normal
    4. T wave high

25. Causes of atrial fibrillation include: (Select all that apply.)
    1. sick sinus syndromes.
    2. hypoxia.
    3. increased atrial pressure.
    4. pericarditis.

26. Cardioversion is used to treat: (Select all that apply.)
    1. SVT.
    2. atrial fibrillation.
    3. atrial flutter.
    4. ventricular tachycardia in an unstable client.

Using the information in Box 57-1 of the textbook, interpret the following ECG tracings.

27.

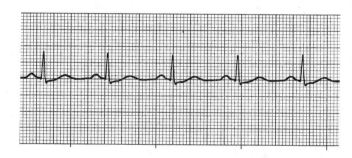

28.

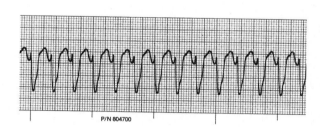

29.

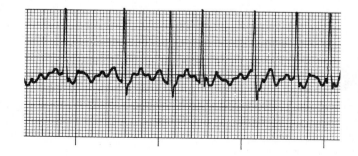

30.

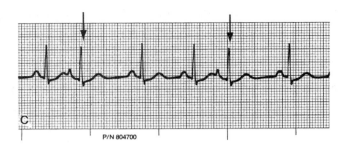

31.

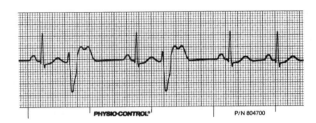

32.

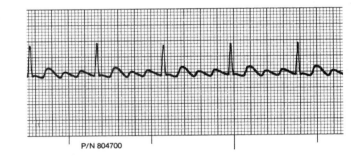

33.

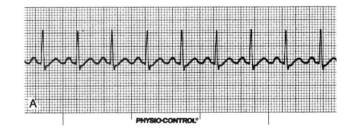

34.

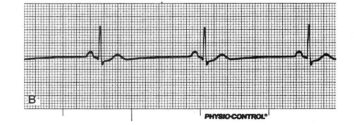

35. The nurse could teach a client with the potential to develop a dysrhythmia to do which of the following? (Select all that apply.)
    1. Take medications as ordered.
    2. Keep routine follow-up appointments.
    3. Wear a MedicAlert bracelet.
    4. Avoid things known to trigger the dysrhythmia.

KEEPING DRUG SKILLS SHARP

36. Medications used in the treatment of atrial flutter in combination with cardioversion include: (Select all that apply.)
    1. digitalis.
    2. quinidine.
    3. verapamil.
    4. Inderal and procainamide.

37. If the client has been taking digitalis preparations, a current therapeutic drug level must be obtained prior to cardioversion because:
    1. digitalis toxicity may predispose the client to ventricular dysrhythmias during cardioversion.
    2. abnormal heart rhythms will be noted.
    3. cardiac cycle will be slowed.
    4. QRS complexes will not be identifiable on the ECG.

38. Which medications might be used to treat sinus tachycardia? (Select all that apply.)
    1. Beta blockers
    2. Calcium channel blockers
    3. Digitalis
    4. Lidocaine

39. If symptomatic, the nurse would administer which medication to the client with sinus bradycardia?
    1. Lidocaine
    2. Adenosine
    3. Atropine
    4. Sotalol

40. A client in atrial fibrillation would receive which drug in addition to antidysrhythmic medications?
    _____

41. The nurse would prepare to administer which drug to the client who has frequent PVCs that cause symptoms? (Select all that apply.)
    1. Amiodarone
    2. Lidocaine
    3. Atenolol
    4. Atropine
    5. Verapamil

42. What is the drug of choice for Torsades de Pointes? _____

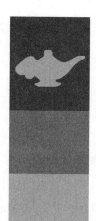

CHAPTER **58**

Management of Clients with Myocardial Infarction

CHAPTER OBJECTIVES

58.1   Describe the magnitude of coronary heart disease (CHD) in the United States.
58.2   Relate CHD to chest pain, angina, and myocardial infarction (STEMI).
58.3   Identify the causes and risk factors for angina and STEMI.
58.4   Relate the pathophysiology of angina and STEMI to the clinical manifestations.
58.5   Differentiate the patterns of angina.
58.6   Identify the diagnostic evaluation for angina and STEMI.
58.7   Describe the desired outcomes of medical and nursing management of the client with angina and other forms of CHD.
58.8   Identify the importance of the acronyms A, B, C, D, E and MONA in the treatment of CHD.
58.9   Describe the self-care necessary for prevention of further attacks of CHD.
58.10 Describe the potential for complications following STEMI and myocardial infarction.
58.11 Discuss the rehabilitation phase of treatment for STEMI.

TRENDS AND THEORIES

1. _____ Americans will have a new or recurrent acute coronary syndrome this year.

2. Acute coronary syndromes are responsible for more than _____ deaths annually.

3. Angina pectoris is a common manifestation of heart disease and affects _____ Americans.

4. The client who leads a hectic life and needs to slow down to prevent further anginal attacks can explore which options?
    a.
    b.
    c.
    d.
    e.
    f.

5. Complications of STEMI include:
    a.
    b.
    c.
    d.
    e.
    f.
    g.
    h.
    i.

UNDERSTANDING PATHOPHYSIOLOGY

6. Angina pectoris is associated with _____ _____.

7. Myocardial ischemia develops when: (Select all that apply.)
    1. blood supply through the coronary vessels is not adequate.
    2. oxygen content of the blood is not adequate to meet body demands.
    3. walls of the vessels are too thin.
    4. venous congestion exists.

8. _____ is paroxysmal chest pain or discomfort triggered by a predictable degree of exertion or emotion.

9. _____ is paroxysmal chest pain triggered by an unpredictable degree of exertion or emotion, which may occur at night.

10. _____ is chest discomfort similar to classic angina but of longer duration, and that may occur while the client is at rest.

11. The most common site of a myocardial infarction (MI) is the _____.

APPLYING SKILLS

12. Clients with angina are likely to have which of the following symptoms? (Select all that apply.)
    1. Pain as retrosternal or slightly to the left of the sternum
    2. Burning, pressing pain
    3. Pain usually lasting 5 minutes
    4. Dyspnea, pallor, sweating

13. The most common laboratory tests and noninvasive tests of clients suspected of having angina are: (Select all that apply.)
    1. resting ECG.
    2. chest x-ray.
    3. fasting glucose.
    4. fasting lipid profile.

14. The major clinical manifestation in a client who is experiencing an MI is _____ _____.

15. Symptoms that clients with MI are likely to describe upon admission to the hospital include: (Select all that apply.)
    1. pain radiating to the neck, jaw and shoulder, back, or left arm.
    2. some epigastric indigestion.
    3. nausea and dizziness.
    4. unexplained anxiety and weakness.

16. When blood flow to the heart is decreased, ischemia and necrosis of the heart muscle occur, causing which of the following ECG changes? (Select all that apply.)
    1. Altered Q waves
    2. ST segment changes
    3. T waves changes on a 12-lead ECG
    4. QRS changes

17. What laboratory findings would indicate that a client has just suffered an MI? (Select all that apply.)
    1. Elevated levels of serum creatine kinase–MB
    2. Cardiac troponin T elevated
    3. Cardiac troponin I elevated
    4. Ldh, AST, ESR are elevated

18. True or False

    _____ A client is at the highest risk of sudden death during the first 24 hours after an MI.

    _____ Rehabilitation programs begin with admission.

    _____ Using a bedside commode is recommended for the first 24 hours.

    _____ Early mobilization activities following STEMI should not exceed 1–2 metabolic equivalent tests (METs).

    _____ Stage II rehabilitation programs should include increased exercise as well as discussions about sexual activity.

    _____ Stage IV rehabilitation is supervised in the community.

19. The most common cause of death after an MI is _____.

BEST PRACTICES

20. When educating a client about weight reduction, it is important to explain that: (Select all that apply.)
    1. weight reduction can reduce blood pressure.
    2. weight reduction can reduce cholesterol.
    3. weight reduction can decrease risk for diabetes mellitus.
    4. eating high-calorie foods is important.

21. Nursing actions performed when a client is admitted to the emergency room with suspected MI include administering:

   M.

   O.

   N.

   A.

22. Describe the components of the ABCDE mnemonic for CHD.

   A.

   B.

   C.

   D.

   E.

23. Dietary self-care for the client with angina includes which of the following? (Select all that apply.)
   1. Eat small low-fat meals.
   2. Abstain from gas-forming foods.
   3. Rest after eating.
   4. Increase fiber.
   5. Decrease alcohol to 2–3 drinks a day.

KEEPING DRUG SKILLS SHARP

24. When treating angina, the physician will most likely prescribe:
   1. nitroglycerin.
   2. aspirin.
   3. heparin.
   4. lovenox.

25. Several different types of medications are used to treat acute angina pectoris, including: (Select all that apply.)
   1. vasodilators.
   2. beta-adrenergic blockers.
   3. calcium channel blockers.
   4. vitamins and minerals.

26. Sublingual nitroglycerin is given to clients to: (Select all that apply.)
   1. reduce pain.
   2. dilate coronary arteries.
   3. restore coronary blood flow.
   4. increase upper levels of cytokines.

27. When at home, clients who experience chest pain or suspect they are having an MI should: (Select all that apply.)
   1. ingest aspirin.
   2. resume usual activity for 30 minutes to see if pain goes away.
   3. go to bed and wait until the pain subsides.
   4. ingest large quantities of glucose.

28. Not all clients are suitable candidates for thrombolytic therapy. Which clients have absolute contraindications? Clients: (Select all that apply.)
   1. with a prior intracranial hemorrhage.
   2. with known malignant neoplasm.
   3. who are currently pregnant.
   4. who are taking anticoagulants.

29. List the steps the client should take if angina occurs while he or she is at home.

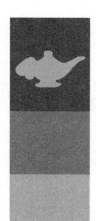

CHAPTER **59**

Assessment of the Respiratory System

CHAPTER OBJECTIVES

59.1   Describe the health history of a client presenting with manifestations of respiratory disorders.
59.2   Determine appropriate questions to elicit the chief complaint from the client.
59.3   Identify clinical manifestations of respiratory disease.
59.4   Distinguish cardiac and noncardiac chest pain.
59.5   Relate medical history to common clinical manifestations and other symptoms of respiratory disorders.
59.6   Relate new client problems to a chronic respiratory condition.
59.7   Relate surgical history and allergies to respiratory manifestations and treatment for the manifestations.
59.8   Determine interactions between prescription medications and herbal medicines.
59.9   Determine increased dietary needs for clients with respiratory disease.
59.10   Relate social history such as living and working conditions, hobbies, travel, or smoking that impact respiratory disorders.
59.11   Relate family history of respiratory diseases or smoking that impacts respiratory manifestations.
59.12   Describe important aspects of the physical examination including assessing for the presence of hypoxia, tachycardia, and weight loss.
59.13   Distinguish normal and abnormal lung sounds.
59.14   Locate appropriate anatomical sites for lung sounds.
59.15   Relate the need for specific diagnostic testing to clinical manifestations.
59.16   Describe nursing responsibilities for diagnostic testing.

UNDERSTANDING PATHOPHYSIOLOGY

1. Common clinical manifestations of the respiratory system include: (Select all that apply.)
   1. cardiac chest pain.
   2. dyspnea.
   3. cough.
   4. clear sputum.
   5. wheezing.
   6. stridor.

2. When clients discuss important information about the clinical manifestations related to respiratory illnesses, nurses often follow the mnemonic OLDCARTS. Which of the following is *not* a question included in this type of assessment?
   1. Onset
   2. Location
   3. Previous illnesses
   4. Characteristics
   5. Factors that make it worse
   6. Factors that make it better

3. Compare and contrast noncardiac and cardiac chest pain.

4. Sputum production with a cough is not normal. Findings about sputum that might characterize this abnormality include: (Select all that apply.)
    1. yellow, green, rusty sputum.
    2. frothy, thick mucus.
    3. clear sputum.
    4. less than 3 ounces per day.

5. True or False

    _____   *Hemoptysis* refers to blood expectorated from the mouth that appears bright red in color.

    _____   Wheezing may or may not be audible.

    _____   Aspiration can produce stridor but is usually not life-threatening.

    _____   Nosebleeds, hay fever, and referred ear pain are examples of nose and sinus complaints of the respiratory system.

APPLYING SKILLS

6. Breathlessness can be quantified by the _____ and the intensity of dyspnea can be rated by the _____ _____.

7. Client complaints of a foul taste in the mouth, unpleasant breath odor, and nasal obstruction may indicate _____.

8. The nurse inquires whether the client has had any changes in voice character, hoarseness, difficulty swallowing, or sleep-related disorders, such as snoring. These changes are associated with _____.

9. Compare and contrast factors of a client's psychosocial history.

Factor	Area to Be Assessed
Occupation	
Geographic location	
Environment	
Habits	
Exercise	
Nutrition	

10. The nurse notes that her client complained of not being able to smell as well lately. This assessment could be associated with _____, _____, _____, or_____ _____.

11. When examining the thorax by inspection, palpation, percussion, and auscultation, the nurse should _____ _____.

12. The nurse is assessing for tactile fremitus on the posterior chest wall. The nurse does this assessment by asking the client to _____ _____ and then _____ _____.

13. True or False

    _____   Upon percussion of the chest wall, a resonant sound is heard. This is a normal finding.

_____ Hyperresonant sounds are normally heard in adults with good air exchange.

_____ If the nurse percusses an area and hears a flat note, the area is solid tissue such as bone.

_____ Tympanic notes can be heard when percussing over the stomach.

_____ Percussion is done over the entire chest wall, including ribs and sternum, to check for abnormalities.

14. Provide a description of adventitious breath sounds along with a clinical example.
    a. Fine crackles:

    b. Pleural friction rub:

    c. High-pitched wheeze:

15. When assessing the client's medication use for respiratory problems, the nurse notes that most of the client's medications are _____ through a _____ _____.

16. A client is resting in bed. Upon assessment, the nurse notes a pulse oximetry reading of 80%. The nurse determines that the client is _____ and requires further evaluation and action of oxygen status.

BEST PRACTICES

17. Based on pulmonary function tests, the client with obstructive lung disease will have a decreased _____ and forced _____ with increased _____, _____, and _____.

18. In arterial blood gas analysis, the _____ reflects the effectiveness of alveolar ventilation.

19. A client will undergo a ventilation-perfusion lung scan for pulmonary emboli because it is _____ than pulmonary angiography.

20. A 23-year-old male college student has been ordered to have a chest x-ray for a suspected respiratory infection. It is likely that the x-ray was ordered because _____ _____.

21. Thoracentesis and lung biopsy may be performed if the health care provider suspects _____ _____ or _____ conditions.

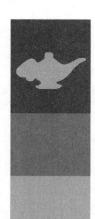

C H A P T E R **60**

Management of Clients with Upper Airway Disorders

CHAPTER OBJECTIVES

60.1 Identify the major impact of upper airway disorders on clients.
60.2 Differentiate upper airway disorders from lower airway disorders.
60.3 Define *tracheotomy* and *tracheostomy*.
60.4 Identify tracheostomy as a method of airway control.
60.5 Differentiate tracheostomy tubes and purposes.
60.6 Describe problems with tracheostomy tubes and cuffs.
60.7 Discuss tracheostomy tube weaning and removal.
60.8 Describe postoperative nursing assessment, diagnosis, and outcomes for tracheostomy.
60.9 Identify neoplastic, hemorrhagic, inflammatory, and obstructive disorders of the upper airway.
60.10 Describe causes and risk factors for neoplastic, hemorrhagic, inflammatory, and obstructive disorders of the upper airway.
60.11 Relate the pathophysiology and clinical manifestations of neoplastic, hemorrhagic, inflammatory, and obstructive disorders of the upper airway.
60.12 Describe the diagnostic findings of neoplastic, hemorrhagic, inflammatory, and obstructive disorders of the upper airway.
60.13 Describe the desired outcomes of medical, surgical, and nursing management for clients with neoplastic, hemorrhagic, inflammatory, and obstructive disorders of the upper airway.
60.14 Discuss surgery of the larynx and neck dissection including pre- and postoperative care.

UNDERSTANDING PATHOPHYSIOLOGY

1. A client has a nursing diagnosis of Risk for impaired gas exchange. List the three factors that affect removal of carbon dioxide.
   a.

   b.

   c.

2. The primary etiologic agent in laryngeal cancer is
   _____.

3. Risk factors for laryngeal cancer include: (Select all that apply.)
   1. history of smoking.
   2. exposure to asbestos.
   3. chronic pharyngitis.
   4. concurrent alcohol and smoking use.

4. Factors that contribute to altered nutrition in clients with laryngeal tumors include: (Select all that apply.)
   1. dysphagia.
   2. altered sense of taste.
   3. weight loss.
   4. loss of appetite.

5. The client with a laryngectomy will remain on tube feedings until _____ has subsided, _____ has occurred, and the client can _____.

6. All of the following are clinical manifestations suggestive of sinusitis *except*:
   1. fever and chills.
   2. pain in the lower teeth.
   3. headaches.
   4. purulent nasal discharge.

7. The most common infection organism in pharyngitis is _____.

8. All of the following are clinical manifestations of pharyngitis *except*:
   1. sore throat.
   2. difficulty swallowing.
   3. malaise.
   4. otalgia.
   5. fever.

9. Rhinitis medicamentosa is caused by abuse or overuse of _____ or _____.

10. Hoarseness in clients with GERD is caused from the chemical irritation by _____ _____ on the vocal cords.

11. When only one vocal cord is paralyzed, the primary clinical manifestation is _____ _____.

12. True or False

   _____ Once the stoma of a permanent tracheostomy is healed, most clients do not need a tube.

   _____ Subcutaneous emphysema is a serious condition that requires treatment immediately.

   _____ It is harmless for others to smoke in a room with a client who has a tracheostomy.

   _____ It is safe to use room deodorizers in a room with a client who has a tracheostomy.

   _____ Cancer of the larynx most often occurs in women.

   _____ Metastasis is uncommon in subglottic tumors.

   _____ Voice quality is maintained in clients that have supraglottic laryngectomy.

   _____ The sense of smell is lost with total laryngectomy.

   _____ Blood-tinged sputum is not expected in tracheal secretions in the immediate postoperative period following laryngectomy.

   _____ Viral and bacterial pharyngitis is contagious by droplet spread.

   _____ Laryngitis may be the result of GERD.

   _____ Abnormal voice may be the result of vocal abuse.

   _____ Laryngeal injury most often results from trauma during a motor vehicle accident.

APPLYING CONCEPTS

13. Which of the following clients are not good candidates for a single-cannula tracheostomy tube? (Select all that apply.)
    1. Client with excessive secretions
    2. Client who has difficult clearing secretions
    3. Client with a thick neck
    4. Client with an altered airway

14. The client's biggest concern about weaning is:
    1. the experience of pain.
    2. fear of not being able to breathe.
    3. inability to manage secretions on his or her own.
    4. fear of letting providers of care down.

15. List the clinical assessments that would indicate respiratory distress during the weaning process.
    a.

    b.

    c.

    d.

    e.

16. Following laryngectomy, clients are at risk for aspiration. Which of the following assessment findings indicate that interventions to prevent aspiration have been effective? (Select all that apply.)
    1. Adventitious breath sounds in both lung bases
    2. Normal respiratory rate and rhythm
    3. Clear secretions
    4. Ability to cough effectively

17. _____ from the oral cavity, neck, or trachea might alert the nurse to impending carotid rupture following laryngectomy.

18. List the nursing assessments that indicate a return of gastric functioning in the postoperative client.
    a.

    b.

    c.

19. List the critical nursing observations of manifestations of aspiration in a client with vocal cord paralysis.
    a.

    b.

    c.

    d.

20. True or False
    _____ Tracheostomy tubes are universally the same for each client.
    _____ A tracheostomy cuff holds the tube in place.

BEST PRACTICES

21. Place the following steps the nurse follows in order of their occurrence in the event that accidental decannulation occurs in the client with a tracheostomy.
    _____ Auscultate for breath sounds
    _____ Call a respiratory arrest
    _____ Maintain ventilation and oxygenation by bag and mask
    _____ Call for help
    _____ Reinsert the tube, if possible

22. For the client scheduled for an elective tracheostomy, two essential areas for the nurse to discuss with the client preoperatively are the _____ and the _____ _____.

23. A nursing intervention used to minimize postoperative edema in the client who had sinus surgery is to place the client with the HOB _____ _____ _____.

24. Immediately after a nasal fracture occurs, _____ should be applied.

25. True or False
    _____ A tracheostomy provides the best route for long-term airway maintenance.
    _____ A cuffed tracheostomy tube should always be deflated before the client uses the talking tracheostomy adapter.
    _____ Ideally, the tracheostomy tube should be changed at least every 4–6 weeks.
    _____ When a client with a tracheostomy is on a ventilator, the ventilator tubing should be coiled neatly on the bed next to the client.
    _____ If the tumor is limited to the true vocal cord, without causing limitation of the cords, radiation therapy is the best treatment.
    _____ Supraglottic tumors may be treated with radiation therapy or partial laryngectomy, with or without lymph node dissection.

26. Clients with tracheostomy have impaired verbal communication. Interventions to help the client feel safe and able to reach someone for help include: (Select all that apply.)
    1. written list of common needs.
    2. prompt answering of call system.
    3. call button within reach.
    4. paper, pencil, communication board.

KEEPING DRUG SKILLS SHARP

27. If acute laryngeal edema is precipitated by anaphylaxis, _____ is given subcutaneously.

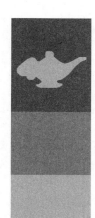

C H A P T E R **61**

Management of Clients with Lower Airway and Pulmonary Vessel Disorders

CHAPTER OBJECTIVES

61.1   Differentiate lower airway disorders and pulmonary vessel disorders from upper airway disorders.
61.2   Describe asthma and its impact on clients in the health care system.
61.3   Identify the causes and risk factors for asthma, chronic obstructive pulmonary disease (COPD), and disorders of the pulmonary vasculature.
61.4   Identify COPD as a complex of diseases.
61.5   Relate the pathophysiology and clinical manifestations of asthma, COPD, and disorders of the pulmonary vasculature.
61.6   Describe the desired outcomes of medical, surgical, and nursing management of asthma, COPD, and disorders of the pulmonary vasculature.
61.7   Describe the immediate nursing assessment for the client with acute respiratory distress.
61.8   Identify self-care strategies for the client with asthma and COPD.
61.9   Identify modifications important in the care of older adults with COPD.
61.10   Identify preventive measures for pulmonary embolism (PE) and venous air embolism.
61.11   Describe diagnostic findings for PE.
61.12   Discuss the importance of anticoagulation therapy for PE.
61.13   Discuss pharmacologic management of the client with pulmonary hypertension.

UNDERSTANDING PATHOPHYSIOLOGY

1.   A late manifestation of hypoxia is:
　　1.   wheezing with exhalation.
　　2.   nasal flaring.
　　3.   use of intercostal muscles.
　　4.   cyanosis.

2.   Characteristics of chronic bronchitis include: (Select all that apply.)
　　1.   decreased ciliary function.
　　2.   destruction of bronchioles.
　　3.   increased number of goblet cells.
　　4.   isolated blebs in the lung periphery.
　　5.   increase in size of submucosal glands in the bronchi.
　　6.   polycythemia.

3.   Which type of emphysema increases the client's risk for spontaneous pneumothorax?
　　1.   Centrolobular
　　2.   Panlobular
　　3.   Paraseptal (panacinar)

4.   The types of emphysema most often associated with a history of smoking include: (Select all that apply.)
　　1.   centrolobular.
　　2.   panlobular.
　　3.   paraseptal (panacinar).

5.   Bronchiectasis is characterized by:
　　1.   inflammation of the trachea and bronchial tree.
　　2.   abnormal dilation of the bronchi.
　　3.   decreased perfusion of the bronchial tree.
　　4.   increased pulmonary vascular resistance.

6. Which of the following clients is at greatest risk for pulmonary embolus?
   1. Client having laparoscopic cholecystectomy
   2. Client having placement of gastric feeding tube
   3. Client having lung biopsy
   4. Client having total abdominal hysterectomy

7. The resulting hypoxemia that occurs following pulmonary embolus (PE) is due to _____ _____.

8. Common clinical manifestations of PE include: (Select all that apply.)
   1. bradycardia.
   2. dyspnea.
   3. anxiety.
   4. chest pain.
   5. tachycardia.
   6. wheezing.

9. *Pulmonary hypertension* is defined as an elevated pulmonary artery pressure above _____ _____ at rest.

10. The underlying pathophysiology which contributes to pulmonary hypertension is _____ _____ _____.

11. Factors which compromise the treatment of older clients with emphysema include: (Select all that apply.)
    1. comorbid conditions.
    2. decreased exercise tolerance.
    3. decreased nutritional status.
    4. smoking history.
    5. drug-drug interactions.

12. True or False
    _____ All pulmonary emboli originate from deep vein thrombus.

APPLYING SKILLS

13. The nurse is assessing a client with emphysema. Which assessment finding would indicate increasing hypoxia?
    1. Decreased breath sounds
    2. Bradycardia
    3. Eupnea
    4. Restlessness

14. The diagnostic measure that is replacing the V/Q lung scan to diagnose pulmonary embolus is _____.

15. Supplemental oxygen would be indicated for the client with asthma when the PaO_2 falls below:
    1. 90 mm Hg.
    2. 80 mm Hg.
    3. 70 mm Hg.
    4. 60 mm Hg.

16. What is an indication to the nurse that a client with asthma is approaching acute respiratory failure? Explain the rationale behind this indicator.

17. An indication that a client with asthma may need supplemental oxygen would be:
    1. PaO_2 of 63 mm Hg.
    2. O_2 saturation of 92%.
    3. respiratory rate of 24.
    4. PaO_2 of 56 mm Hg.

18. The client with a PE is receiving anticoagulant therapy. Which assessment finding would alert the nurse to signs of excess therapy? (Select all that apply.)
    1. Dark yellow urine
    2. Abdominal pain
    3. Dark, tarry stool
    4. Ecchymosis at the injection site

19. A nurse is reviewing the ABGs of a client with primary emphysema for 15 years. The nurse would expect the analysis to reveal that the client has:
    1. uncompensated respiratory acidosis.
    2. compensated respiratory acidosis.
    3. uncompensated respiratory alkalosis.
    4. compensated respiratory alkalosis.

20. The home care nurse is caring for a client with emphysema. Which of the following findings would indicate that treatment goals are being met?
    1. Increase in severity of clinical manifestations
    2. Increase in ability to manage and remove secretions
    3. Increase in complications
    4. Increase in ventilatory problems

21. Anticoagulant therapy is monitored through the International Normalized Ratio (INR). The nurse caring for the client receiving anticoagulant therapy achieves therapeutic levels when the INR is:
    1. 1.
    2. 2.
    3. 2.5–3.
    4. 4.

22. Clients with PE are at risk for developing right-sided heart failure. Assessment findings that would alert the nurse to developing complications include: (Select all that apply.)
    1. increasing dyspnea.
    2. heart murmur.
    3. crackles.
    4. apprehension.
    5. clear breath sounds.
    6. hemoptysis.

BEST PRACTICES

23. The nurse is providing teaching for a client with asthma. The client asks, "What if I have an attack and I don't have my medications with me? What do I do?" The nurse should teach the client to perform _____ in this situation.

24. State the rationale for the following activities with the client who has asthma.

Activity	Rationale
a. Assess severity of dyspnea	
b. Return demonstration of spirometry	
c. Return demonstration of metered dose inhaler (MDI)	
d. Assess medication allergies	
e. Assess medication history	
f. History of triggers	
g. Ability to manage disease	
h. Assess family support	
i. Environmental assessment	

25. The nurse is teaching the client with emphysema about measures to improve his or her general health. The most effective measure would be for the client to:
    1. avoid high altitudes.
    2. move to a warm, dry climate.
    3. stop smoking.
    4. use supplemental oxygen.

26. List multiple measures that can be used to prevent pulmonary embolus.
    a.

    b.

    c.

    d.

27. Explain why the client with a PE who manifests with lower extremity edema should not have the lower extremities elevated.

28. The client with emphysema should be instructed to eat a:
    1. High-carbohydrate, low-fat diet
    2. Low-carbohydrate, moderate-fat diet
    3. High-carbohydrate, high-protein diet
    4. High-protein, low-fat diet

KEEPING DRUG SKILLS SHARP

29. Match the following drugs with their use for quick relief or long-term control of symptoms in asthma and then their mode of action. Answers may be used more than once.

Drug	Use	Action
a. Albuterol nebulizer (Proventil)	_____	_____
b. Cromolyn inhaler (Intal, Nasalcrom)	_____	_____
c. Ipratropium inhaler (Atrovent)	_____	_____
d. Beclomethasone inhaler (Vanceril)	_____	_____
e. Montelukast (Singulair)	_____	_____
f. IV aminophylline	_____	_____
g. Oral prednisone	_____	_____

Uses
1. Long-term control
2. Quick relief

Actions
i. Beta agonist
ii. Anticholinergics
iii. Mast cell stabilizer
iv. Leukotriene inhibitor
v. Steroid, anti-inflammatory
vi. Methylxanthine bronchodilator

30. A nurse administers albuterol through the use of a nebulizer to decrease asthma symptoms. An expected outcome of this intervention would be:
    1. O$_2$ saturation of 92%.
    2. increased anxiety.
    3. a self-report of dyspnea of 8 on a 1–10 scale.
    4. continuous, nonproductive cough.

31. The first line drug of choice for the treatment of pulmonary hypertension is:
    1. calcium channel antagonists.
    2. diuretics.
    3. ACE inhibitors.
    4. peripheral vasodilators.

CONCEPT MAP EXERCISE

The following questions are based on the Concept Map *Understanding Asthma and Its Treatment* in the textbook.

32. Which of the following types of medications are given to the client with asthma to decrease IgE stimulation? (Select all that apply.)
    1. Mast cell stabilizers
    2. Leukotriene modifiers
    3. Anticholinergics
    4. Steroids

33. Clinical manifestations of bronchospasm include: (Select all that apply.)
    1. wheezing.
    2. nonproductive cough.
    3. chest tightness.
    4. shortness of breath.
    5. peak flow variability.

34. Increased mucus secretion is a direct pathophysiologic response to:
    1. IgE stimulation.
    2. mast cell degradation.
    3. airway hyperresponsiveness.
    4. bronchospasm.

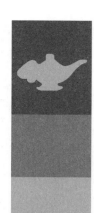

CHAPTER **62**

Management of Clients with Parenchymal and Pleural Disorders

CHAPTER OBJECTIVES

62.1   Examine causes and risk factors for disorders of lung parenchyma and pleura.
62.2   Relate the pathophysiology of lung disorders to clinical manifestations.
62.3   Describe the desired outcomes of medical, surgical, and nursing management of clients with lung disorders.
62.4   Explain nursing interventions for major nursing diagnoses for pneumonia.
62.5   Explain the magnitude of tuberculosis (TB) as a public health concern.
62.6   Describe the screening tests for TB.
62.7   Identify the drug treatment regimen for TB.
62.8   Identify protective equipment for health care workers to use when caring for TB clients.
62.9   Describe the diagnostic studies for clients with lung disorders.
62.10   Describe the nursing management of the client with closed-chest drainage.
62.11   Describe the management of end-stage lung disease including lung transplant.

UNDERSTANDING PATHOPHYSIOLOGY

1. List the common clinical manifestations associated with influenza.
    a.

    b.

    c.

    e.

    f.

    g.

    h.

    i.

    j.

2. List 11 major risk factors for pneumonia:
    a.

    b.

    c.

    d.

    k.

3. Which of the following clinical manifestations of pneumonia may not be present in older adults? (Select all that apply.)
    1. Fever
    2. Dyspnea
    3. Headache
    4. Altered mental status

4. Match each type of pneumonia with the appropriate description.

Type of Pneumonia

_____ a. Segmental

_____ b. Necrotizing

_____ c. Bronchopneumonia

_____ d. Lobar

_____ e. Alveolar

_____ f. Bilateral

_____ g. Interstitial

Description

1. Death of a portion of lung tissue surrounded by viable tissue
2. Accumulation of fluid in lung's distal air spaces
3. Involves inflammatory responses within lung tissue surrounding air spaces and vascular structures
4. Lobes of both lungs
5. Involves terminal bronchioles and alveoli
6. One or more segments of the lung
7. Lobes in both lungs

5. _____ develops when the alveoli become airless from absorption of their air without replacement of the air with breathing and is usually diagnosed by _____ _____.

6. Tubercles heal over a period of months by forming scars and calcified lesions known as _____ _____.

7. List the nine factors that contribute to TB becoming an active disease.
   a.

   b.

   c.

   d.

   e.

   f.

   g.

   h.

   i.

8. True or False

   _____ Fungal respiratory infections produce granulomatous conditions similar to TB.

   _____ Coccidioidomycosis is found mostly in Midwest river valleys.

   _____ A red rash occurs with histoplasmosis.

   _____ Clients with coccidioidomycosis become very ill.

   _____ Infected clients can have histoplasmosis for 1–2 months.

9. List four major types of lung cancer:
   a.

   b.

   c.

   d.

10. The most important risk factor for lung cancer is _____.

11. True/False

   _____ SARS typically begins with a dry cough and other lower respiratory symptoms.

   _____ SARS always becomes a serious illness.

   _____ The SARS virus is transmitted through close person-to-person contact.

12. Match the following types of lung cancer resection with the correct description.

Type of Resection		**Description**
_____	a. Wedge	1. Removal of entire lobe
_____	b. Segmental	2. Removal of entire lung
_____	c. Lobectomy	3. Removal of small localized area
_____	d. Pneumonectomy	4. Removal of one or more segments

13. Lung abscesses usually occur _____ to a bronchial obstruction and produce _____ amounts of sputum.

14. The term _____ in interstitial lung disease (ILD) indicates that the interstitium of the alveolar walls has become thick and non-functional.

15. True/False

    _____ Crackles associated with ILD sound like Velcro being pulled apart.

    _____ The ventilation-perfusion mismatch in ILD causes hypoxemia and CO_2 retention.

16. If there is a high WBC count and the pleural fluid is purulent, the effusion is called an _____ and may require _____ _____.

17. Differentiating transudates and exudates aids in a specific _____ in pleural effusion.

18. True or False

    _____ TB infection is acquired by inhalation of a particle small enough to reach the alveolus.

    _____ A primary TB infection is said to be when the client is exposed for the first time.

    _____ Most clients know when exposure to TB occurred.

    _____ Nontuberculous mycobacteria (NTM) is most prevalent in the northeastern United States.

    _____ Person-to-person transmission of fungal lung infections is virtually unknown.

    _____ Lung cancer is the leading cause of cancer deaths in the United States.

    _____ Lung diseases are among the most common occupational health problems.

_____ Obesity may lead to restrictive lung disorders.

_____ Cystic fibrosis is the most common inherited genetic disease in Caucasians.

_____ The cause of sarcoidosis is unknown.

_____ Clinical manifestations of ILD are insidious and nonspecific.

_____ Clinical manifestations of a subdiaphragmatic abscess include pleuritic pain or pain referred to the shoulder on the same side as the abscess.

_____ A classic manifestation of bilateral paralysis of the diaphragm is decreased dyspnea when the client is lying flat on the back.

APPLYING SKILLS

19. When auscultating the chest of a client with pneumonia, bronchial breath sounds occur over _____.

20. List the respiratory assessments the nurse performs on a client with pneumonia.
    a.

    b.

    c.

21. _____, rather than erythema, indicates a positive TB test.

22. Definitive diagnosis of TB is accomplished with _____ and _____ _____.

23. List the clinical assessments that would alert the nurse to possible hemorrhaging in a client with closed chest drainage.

    a.

    b.

24. Differentiate between intermittent and continuous bubbling in the water-seal compartment.

25. What does rapid bubbling in the water-seal compartment indicate?

26. True or False

    _____ Tidaling may indicate a kink in a drainage tube or lung reexpansion.

    _____ Tidaling is the rise and fall of fluid in the water seal chamber with inspiration and expiration respectively.

    _____ Tidaling may not occur in chest drainage systems that do not use suction.

BEST PRACTICES

27. When caring for an unconscious client with pneumonia, the nurse places the client in a

    _____

    position.

28. Interventions for ineffective breathing patterns in clients with pneumonia include: (Select all that apply.)

    1. elevate HOB.
    2. teach splinting the chest wall during coughing.
    3. administer cough suppressants liberally.
    4. monitor O_2 and other blood gas levels.

29. Decreasing metabolic demands for the client with pneumonia is essential due to decreased O_2–CO_2 exchange. Outcomes of interventions for this problem will include_____ _____ and _____ _____.

30. Explain the rationale for instructing a client with a closed chest drainage to cough and deep breathe.

31. List the three primary nursing goals for providing care for a client with restrictive lung disease.

    a.

    b.

    c.

32. List the interventions that help clear tracheobronchial secretions in a client with cystic fibrosis.

    a.

    b.

    c.

    d.

    e.

33. True or False

    _____ Persons with NTM are isolated to control infection.

    _____ Survival rates are best for non-small cell lung cancer (NSCLC) if treated in the early stages.

    _____ QuantiFERON TB Gold test indicates active TB.

    _____ The lower the height of the water column in the suction chamber, the more suction.

_____ Closed chest drainage systems must always be placed lower than the client's chest.

_____ In most situations, clamping of chest tubes is contraindicated.

_____ Chest tube drainage is usually bloody for the first 2 hours postsurgery and then becomes less bloody.

KEEPING DRUG SKILLS SHARP

34. Vaccination prevents "flu" in high-risk clients if received _____ the start of the winter flu season.

35. When a TB program of treatment fails, how many medications are added?

36. The intravenous antibiotic typically used to treat pulmonary fungal infections is _____ _____.

37. _____ are medications used to control inflammation in clients with ILD.

38. The most important antirejection drug following lung transplant is _____.

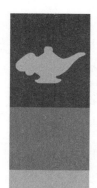

CHAPTER **63**

Management of Clients with Acute Pulmonary Disorders

CHAPTER OBJECTIVES

63.1   Define *acute respiratory failure*.

63.2   Differentiate hypoxemic and ventilatory respiratory failure.

63.3   Identify causes and risk factors of hypoxemic and ventilatory respiratory failure, adult respiratory distress syndrome (ARDS), chest and pulmonary injuries, and other chest trauma.

63.4   Relate the pathophysiology and clinical manifestations of hypoxemic and ventilatory respiratory failure, ARDS, chest and pulmonary injuries, and other chest trauma.

63.5   Describe the desired outcomes of medical and nursing management of hypoxemic and ventilatory respiratory failure, ARDS, chest and pulmonary injuries, and other chest trauma.

63.6   Identify mechanical ventilation as a treatment for acute ventilatory respiratory failure and ARDS.

63.7   Discuss aspects of endotracheal intubation.

63.8   Describe continuous mechanical ventilation and nursing management of the client on mechanical ventilation including the weaning process.

63.9   Identify physiologic changes with and complications of positive pressure ventilation.

UNDERSTANDING PATHOPHYSIOLOGY

1.   The most important function of the respiratory system is to provide the body tissues with _____ and to remove _____.

2.   Compare and contrast hypoxemic versus ventilatory failure.

Hypoxemic	Ventilatory

3. True or False

_____ Failure of alveolar ventilation leads to a ventilation-perfusion mismatch resulting in hypercapnia.

_____ Hallmark manifestations of hypercapnia are headache and dyspnea.

_____ Ventilator-associated pneumonia is a common problem in clients with ARDS.

4. A noncardiogenic cause of pulmonary edema is:
   1. mitral valve stenosis.
   2. shock.
   3. pneumonia.
   4. hypertension.

5. The hallmark of ventilatory failure is an elevated level of _____.

6. The phenomenon of systolic blood pressure falling more than 10 mm Hg during inspiration is called _____.

7. The most common physiologic change that occurs when a client is placed on mechanical ventilation is _____.

8. Which of the following may contribute directly to intensive care unit psychosis?
   1. Respiratory acidosis
   2. Respiratory alkalosis
   3. Elevated vasopressin levels
   4. Cerebral edema

9. Clinical manifestations of oxygen toxicity include: (Select all that apply.)
   1. insomnia.
   2. weakness.
   3. nausea and vomiting.
   4. tachypnea.
   5. increased energy.
   6. hiccoughs.

10. Factors that contribute to the development of ARDS include: (Select all that apply.)
    1. ischemia during shock.
    2. oxygen toxicity.
    3. inhalation of noxious fumes.
    4. inflammation from pneumonia.
    5. positive pressure ventilation.

11. Complete the following critical path that depicts the hallmark of ARDS. (↑ = increases, → = leads to, ↓ = decreases)

Massive _____ by the lungs that _____ movement of fluid into the _____ _____ and _____ _____ spaces which _____ _____ pulmonary edema which _____ and impairs _____.

12. Destruction of the _____ cells results in a decrease in _____ _____ production.

13. Deposition of _____ into the lung contributes to pulmonary fibrosis in Phase 3 ARDS.

14. The two earliest clinical manifestations of ARDS are _____ and _____ _____ 12–24 hours after the initial injury.

15. Major dangers associated with chest injuries are _____ and _____ _____.

16. List the five potential causes of ventilation-perfusion imbalance in clients with chest trauma.
    a.

    b.

    c.

    d.

    e.

17. Clinical manifestations of rib fracture include: (Select all that apply.)
    1. generalized pain and tenderness.
    2. deep respirations.
    3. client's tendency to hold the chest protectively.
    4. clicking sensation during inspiration.

18. Pneumothorax is the presence of _____ _____ in the _____ _____ space that prohibits complete lung expansion.

19. The two classifications of pneumothorax are
_____ and _____
_____.

20. A risk factor for spontaneous pneumothorax is:
    1. thoracentesis.
    2. fall.
    3. motor vehicle accident.
    4. tuberculosis.

21. A clinical manifestation of moderate pneumothorax is:
    1. bradypnea.
    2. dyspnea.
    3. dull pain on the affected side.
    4. symmetrical chest expansion.

22. A clinical manifestation of severe pneumothorax is:
    1. distended neck veins.
    2. increased tactile fremitus.
    3. trachea in midline.
    4. dullness to percussion.

23. A clinical manifestation of a tension pneumothorax is:
    1. mild dyspnea.
    2. bradycardia.
    3. progressive cyanosis.
    4. bradypnea.

24. A risk factor that increases the potential of near drowning is:
    1. alcohol ingestion.
    2. hyperglycemia.
    3. hypoventilation.
    4. eating immediately before swimming.

25. True or False

    _____ Increased volume of fluid in the pulmonary arteries from obstruction of forward flow is the most common cause of pulmonary edema.

    _____ Subcutaneous emphysema is a risk of positive end-expiratory pressure (PEEP).

    _____ Positive pressure ventilation during the inspiratory phase can lead to a decreased blood flow to the splanchnic area and ischemia of the gastric mucosa.

    _____ Clinical manifestations of respiratory muscle fatigue include a respiratory rate of more than 20 breaths per minute.

    _____ An additional benefit of the prone position is better draining of bronchial secretions.

    _____ The most probable cause of shock in the chest-injured client is hypovolemia.

    _____ A flail chest consists of fractures of two or more ribs on the same side and possibly the sternum.

APPLYING SKILLS

26. Which of the following two assessments verify correct endotracheal (ET) tube placement? (Select all that apply.)
    1. Feeling air through the ET tube during exhalation
    2. Client is unable to talk
    3. Auscultation of breath sounds bilaterally
    4. Chest x-ray

27. The amount of air required to seal an ET tube cuff is reflected by the cuff pressure, which is usually maintained at less than _____ mm Hg.

28. All of the following meet diagnostic criteria for ARDS *except*:
    1. delayed onset.
    2. bilateral infiltrates.
    3. ratio of PaO_2 and FiO_2 ≤ 200 mm Hg.
    4. pulmonary artery wedge pressure (PAWP) ≤ 18 mg Hg.

29. List the priority assessments of any client with chest trauma.
    a.

    b.

    c.

30. In the client with flail chest, breath sounds are either _____ or _____
_____ on the affected side.

BEST PRACTICES

31. An intervention aimed at reducing preload is:
    1. oxygen therapy with continuous airway pressure.
    2. diuretic therapy.
    3. antihypertensive drugs.
    4. intra-aortic balloon pump.

32. Which of the following is an expected outcome for intervention for a client with a nursing diagnosis of Impaired gas exchange related to capillary membrane obstruction from fluid?
    1. Capillary refill ≥ 3 seconds
    2. Decreased peripheral edema
    3. O_2 saturation > 90 %
    4. Weight loss

33. State the rationale for keeping the client's legs in a dependent position when he or she has pulmonary edema.

34. Match each type of ventilator with the appropriate description.

	Type of Ventilator		**Description**
_____	a. Pressure-cycled	1.	Terminates when a preset inspiratory time has elapsed
_____	b. Volume-cycled	2.	Triggered to stop when a preset flow rate has been achieved
_____	c. Time-cycled	3.	Delivers a preset tidal volume of inspired gas
_____	d. Flow-cycled	4.	Delivers a volume of gas to the airway using positive pressure during inspiration

35. Match each type of inhalation with the appropriate description.

	Type of Inhalation		**Description**
_____	a. Volume-triggered	1.	Used to manage clients who cannot breathe on their own
_____	b. Flow-triggered	2.	Triggered by the initial negative pressure that begins inspiration
_____	c. Negative pressure	3.	Occurs when the client can initiate a breath
_____	d. Time-triggered	4.	Occurs when the ventilator completes the breath to maximize inhaled gas

36. Differentiate between continuous positive airway pressure (CPAP) and PEEP.

37. Explain high pressure and low pressure alarms on the ventilator.

38. Explain the rationale for placing clients with ARDS in the prone position.

39. Essential nursing activities to keep the family of an ARDS client adequately informed include _____ and _____.

40. The treatment of choice for the client with flail chest is intubation with mechanical ventilation. Indicate below if the therapeutic effect of ventilation is increased or decreased for each of the following parameters.
    a. Hypoxia:

    b. Hypercapnia:

    c. Paradoxical motion:

    d. Pain:

41. True or False

    _____ In the client with acute ventilatory failure, mechanical ventilation is an early intervention.

    _____ One criteria for a weaning trial is PEEP less than 5–8 cm H_2O.

    _____ Mechanical ventilation, ET intubation, and PEEP are usually required to maintain adequate blood oxygen levels.

    _____ Strapping the ribs is the treatment of choice for rib fracture.

KEEPING DRUG SKILLS SHARP

42. Which of the following medications is a beta$_2$ agonist given to reverse bronchospasm?
    1. Ipratropium
    2. Theophylline
    3. Corticosteroid
    4. Albuterol

43. The most common neuromuscular blocking agents given to clients on ventilation are _____ and _____.

44. The actions of nitric oxide include: (Select all that apply.)
    1. selective vasodilation in the pulmonary vascular system.
    2. bronchoconstriction.
    3. reduced pressure in the pulmonary arteries.
    4. increased systemic blood pressure.

45. A desired therapeutic effect of dobutamine in the ARDS client is:
    1. improved cardiac output.
    2. decrease in cardiac output.
    3. decrease in systemic blood pressure.
    4. decrease in preload.

46. Narcotics administered to the client with chest injury to control pain are most effective if administered via:
    1. PO.
    2. IM.
    3. patch.
    4. IV.

47. True or False

    _____ Surfactant therapy has been successful in clients with ARDS.

    _____ Clinical trials have demonstrated the effectiveness of steroid administration in ARDS.

CONCEPT MAP EXERCISES

The following questions are based on the concept map *Understanding ARDS and Its Treatment* in the textbook.

48. Which of the following directly decreases lung compliance?
    1. Ventilation-perfusion mismatch
    2. Decreased surfactant production
    3. Release of vasoactive substances
    4. Atelectasis

49. Hemoptysis is a result of:
    1. ventilation-perfusion mismatch.
    2. increased permeability of alveolar membrane.
    3. damage to alveolar epithelium.
    4. protein movement into the alveoli.

50. Which position improves ventilation and perfusion in the client with ARDS?
    1. Dorsal recumbent
    2. Semi-Fowler's
    3. Sims' lateral
    4. Prone

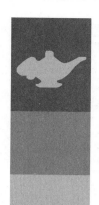

CHAPTER 64

Assessment of the Eyes and Ears

CHAPTER OBJECTIVES

64.1 Clarify misconceptions about the eyes and vision.
64.2 Identify the important aspects of an ophthalmic and otologic health history.
64.3 Relate the client's chief complaint to biographic and demographic health history and current health issues.
64.4 Describe typical clinical manifestations of eye and ear disorders.
64.5 Examine possible systemic manifestations that also involve the ear.
64.6 Identify important assessment questions about manifestations to ask during the review of systems.
64.7 Relate past medical and surgical history and allergies to current clinical manifestations.
64.8 Examine the impact of medication use on clinical manifestations.
64.9 Describe dietary habits that support the health of the eye and the ear.
64.10 Describe social and family history—such as work environment, activities, family eye disorders, loud noise exposure, and swimming—that impact eye and ear health.
64.11 Identify the important aspects of a physical examination of the external and internal eye, external ear and ear canal.
64.12 Examine auditory and vestibular acuity.
64.13 Relate diagnostic testing to clinical manifestations of the eye and ear.

UNDERSTANDING PATHOPHYSIOLOGY

1. A complete ophthalmic history includes: (Select all that apply.)
   1. demographic data.
   2. chief complaint.
   3. clinical manifestations.
   4. mother's breast cancer.
   5. father's heart disease.
   6. alcohol consumption.
   7. appendectomy at age 16.
   8. food consumption.

2. True or False
   _____ The incidence of glaucoma increases with age.
   _____ Color vision problems are more common in women.

_____ The sclera of the eye is normally light yellow in color in Caucasians and white in individuals with darker skin.
_____ The eyeball should be soft on palpation.

3. The four most common preventable causes of permanent vision loss are:
   1. nystagmus.
   2. amblyopia.
   3. diplopia.
   4. glaucoma.
   5. diabetic retinopathy.
   6. "floaters."
   7. age-related maculopathy.
   8. strabismus.

4. True or False
   _____ Reading in the dark is harmful to the eyes.

_____ Cataracts must "ripen" before they can be removed.

_____ Emotional stress does not increase intraocular pressure.

_____ Children will outgrow crossed eyes.

_____ Cataracts are not removed by laser technique.

5. Clinical manifestations of eye disorders are categorized in which three areas?

a.

b.

c.

6. List possible causes of common hearing complaints.

Complaint	Possible Cause
Hearing loss	
Pain	
Ear drainage	
Tinnitus	

7. True or False

_____ Eye pain is often a complaint of pulling or pressure rather than a specific type of pain.

_____ Red eye is the most common abnormal appearance of the eye.

_____ Interference in the vitreous space can cause vision abnormalities.

8. _____ is sensitivity to light.

9. Signs of corneal irritation include: (Select all that apply.)
   1. dryness.
   2. excessive tearing.
   3. burning.
   4. grittiness.
   5. sensation of a foreign body in the eye.
   6. itching.

10. The pain sensation from glaucoma or infection or muscle spasm is described as a _____ _____.

APPLYING SKILLS

11. A thorough ophthalmic assessment is different from the assessment of other body systems because many ophthalmic disorders are _____ _____.

12. State the clinical significance of each disorder when taking a client's ophthalmic history.
Hypertension:

Headaches:

13. During an examination of the eyelids, the nurse notes that the upper lids rest at the top of the iris and the lower lids rest at the bottom, so that the sclerae are not visible. This finding is considered _____.

14. To test the functioning of the trigeminal cranial nerve, the nurse would perform the _____ _____ test.

15. Upon examination of the cornea of an older client, the nurse notes *arcus senilis*. This finding is considered _____.

16. When examining the iris of the eye at an oblique angle, it should _____ and have_____.

17. The pupil should be _____ and _____, have _____, and be _____in size.

18. The MRI is used to image _____, _____, and _____ _____.

19. _____ is used to assess intraocular pressure and screen for glaucoma.

20. Normal range for intraocular pressure is between _____ and _____ mm Hg.

21. List the three areas of assessment during physical examination of the ear.
    a.

    b.

    c.

22. Tophi, deposits of uric acid that form hard nodules in the helix of the ear, are characteristic of:
    1. Meniere's disease.
    2. gout.
    3. glaucoma.
    4. Sjögren's syndrome.

23. Identify the purpose of each of the following tests.

Test	Purpose
Weber test	
Rinne test	
Romberg test	

BEST PRACTICES

24. State the procedure that must be performed prior to application of the tonometer.

25. The nurse should inform a client who believes that vitamins will prevent macular degeneration that _____ _____ _____ _____.

26. Platform posturography is used to _____, _____, and _____ of balance disorders.

27. A client reports clear drainage from his ear. Identify the clinical significance of the drainage and state the appropriate nursing action.

KEEPING DRUG SKILLS SHARP

28. Medications that are ototoxic and can cause hearing loss in nontherapeutic levels include: (Select all that apply.)
    1. aminoglycosides.
    2. antiprotozoal agents.
    3. aspirin.
    4. chemotherapeutic agents.
    5. salicylates.

29. Identify the possible drug interactions that can occur from the use of over-the-counter eye medications.

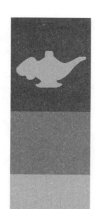

CHAPTER **65**

Management of Clients with Visual Disorders

CHAPTER OBJECTIVES

65.1   Describe the magnitude of the role of vision in our lives.
65.2   Identify the nursing diagnoses related to the loss of vision.
65.3   Identify the causes and risk factors for glaucoma, cataracts, retinal disorders, diabetic retinopathy, macular degeneration, corneal disorders, ocular melanoma, dry eye disorders, refractive disorders, and systemic eye manifestation disorders.
65.4   Relate the pathophysiology and clinical manifestations of visual disorders.
65.5   Identify diagnostic testing for the visual disorders.
65.6   Describe the desired outcomes of medical, surgical, and nursing management of visual disorders.
65.7   Identify treatment modifications for the older client.
65.8   Identify education needs for self-care for the client with visual disorders.

UNDERSTANDING PATHOPHYSIOLOGY

1.   Manifestations that characterize glaucoma include all of the following *except*:
    1.   halos around lights.
    2.   blurred vision.
    3.   visual field loss.
    4.   dry eyes.

2.   Compare and contrast between the various types of glaucoma.

Type	Cause	Manifestations
Primary open angle		
Angle-closure		
Normal tension		
Secondary		

3. List health conditions that may be associated with the development of glaucoma.

   a.

   b.

   c.

   d.

4. Risk factors for the development of cataracts include: (Select all that apply.)
   1. diabetes.
   2. Down syndrome.
   3. living at low altitudes.
   4. retinal detachment.
   5. blunt trauma.
   6. lacerations.
   7. radiation.
   8. chronic use of corticosteroids.
   9. working in dim lighting.
   10. glass-blower or welder without eye protection.

5. True or False

   _____ The leading cause of blindness worldwide is trauma to the eye.

6. Age-related macular degeneration affects _____ vision.

7. Compare and contrast between "dry" and "wet" macular degeneration.

Type	Etiology	Manifestations
Dry		
Wet		

8. List manifestations of dry eye syndrome.

   a.

   b.

   c.

9. Compare and contrast the following common refractive disorders.

Type	Etiology	Manifestations
Myopia		
Hyperopia		
Astigmatism		

APPLYING SKILLS

10. The range for normal intraocular pressure is between _____ and _____ mm Hg.

11. Intraocular pressure is highest upon _____ _____ during a diurnal cycle.

12. True or False

_____ Clients with cataracts will experience blurred vision, photophobia, and glare.

_____ Cataracts cause a dull, aching pain, especially at night.

_____ Secondary glaucoma can be a result of edema or eye injury.

_____ Wound leaks may be a complication of cataract surgery.

_____ Visual acuity following cataract surgery will be greatly improved.

13. A client reports a shadow or "curtain falling across the field of vision." This is a classic manifestation of _____ _____.

14. Identify the common ocular manifestations for each of the following systemic disorders:
    a. Graves' disease:

    b. Rheumatoid arthritis/connective tissue disorder:

    c. Systemic lupus erythematosus (SLE):

    d. Myasthenia gravis:

    e. Multiple sclerosis:

    f. Hypertension:

    g. AIDS:

    h. Lyme disease:

BEST PRACTICES

15. Nursing interventions to assist the client in coping with vision loss due to glaucoma include: (Select all that apply.)
    1. recognizing that the client is experiencing grief over the loss and will be anxious during examinations fearing discovery of more problems.
    2. counseling the client to prepare to accept further vision loss even with treatment.
    3. assisting the client in identifying effective coping skills used in the past.
    4. maintaining professional relationship with the client, using therapeutic communication to express empathy.
    5. allowing the client to verbalize feelings regarding visual problems/loss.

16. It imperative for the nurse to intervene to calm an anxious client with glaucoma, because increased anxiety may raise _____ _____, which may increase intraocular pressure even though the two pressures are independent of each other.

17. Nursing interventions for the client with glaucoma should include all of the following *except*:
    1. determine the client's level of understanding.
    2. use diagrams or pictures to help illustrate important points.
    3. written information should be in colored ink so the client may read it more easily.
    4. validate the client's ability to administer eye drops through a return demonstration.

18. State the rationale for the nurse instructing a client to promptly report any nausea or vomiting after cataract removal.

19. List two nursing actions following retinal detachment surgery.
    a.

    b.

20. Nursing interventions following retinal detachment surgery include: (Select all that apply.)
    1. evaluating the home environment for needed support.
    2. instruct client to clean the eye with warm compresses.
    3. instruct client to wear an eye shield or glasses during the day.
    4. instruct client that there are no restrictions on lifting.
    5. instruct the client that he or she can travel by air.

21. True or False
    _____ LASIK is the surgical procedure for nearsightedness or astigmatism that peels back a layer of the cornea and then puts it back in place.
    _____ A scleral buckle is used to hold the new intraocular lens (IOL) in place until healed.
    _____ An IOL does not provide the same visual acuity as the natural lens of the eye.
    _____ Return of vision with corneal transplant surgery will take 6–12 months.
    _____ A laser beam can burn the edges of a retinal tear to halt its progression.
    _____ Scleral buckling uses silicone bands to hold a retinal tear in place.

KEEPING DRUG SKILLS SHARP

22. _____ help to reduce IOP for the client with glaucoma by acting to constrict the pupil, which opens the canal of Schlemm and aids in drainage of aqueous humor.

23. _____ are prescribed for clients with narrow-angle glaucoma because they reduce the production of aqueous humor and thereby reduce IOP.

24. True or False
    _____ Use of beta-blockers and steroids will help to correct cataracts.
    _____ Mydriacyl is used preoperatively to dilate the eyes for removal of a cataract.
    _____ To facilitate the removal of a cataract, the physician may order Cyclogyl, a paralyzing agent for the ciliary muscles.

25. Research has shown that all of the following supplements may help to delay macular degeneration *except*:
    1. high-dose vitamin C.
    2. high-dose vitamin E.
    3. beta carotene.
    4. iron.
    5. zinc.

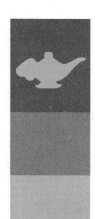

CHAPTER **66**

Management of Clients with Hearing and Balance Disorders

CHAPTER OBJECTIVES

66.1 Explain the magnitude of hearing impairment in clients in the U.S.

66.2 Identify the causes and risk factors of hearing impairment, otalgia, and balance disorders.

66.3 Describe the types of hearing loss.

66.4 Identify diagnostic measures to discover hearing, otalgia, or balance disorders.

66.5 Relate the pathophysiology and clinical manifestations of hearing impairment, otalgia, and balance disorders.

66.6 Describe the desired outcomes of medical, surgical, and nursing management of clients with hearing impairment, otalgia, and balance disorders.

UNDERSTANDING PATHOPHYSIOLOGY

1. _____
   is the nation's primary disability, affecting 1 in 15 Americans.

2. Compare and contrast the main types of hearing loss.

Type	Cause	Results
Conductive		
Sensorineural		
Mixed hearing loss		

3. The most common cause of obstruction of the ear is _____ _____ _____.

4. _____ is a common disorder of the middle ear.

5. Manifestations that occur with rupture of the tympanic membrane include: (Select all that apply.)
   1. brief, intense pain.
   2. reduction of pressure or pain.
   3. temporary hearing loss.
   4. vertigo.

6. _____ is a type of sensorineural hearing loss that affects older people.

7. Causative factors for sudden hearing loss include all of the following *except*:
   1. excess cerumen.
   2. rapid infectious processes (meningitis).
   3. ototoxic agents.
   4. trauma.
   5. metabolic disturbances.
   6. immunologic disorders.

8. Common manifestations of hearing loss in a client include: (Select all that apply.)
   1. failure to respond to oral communication.
   2. inappropriate response to oral communication.
   3. soft speech.
   4. constant need for clarification of conversation.
   5. listening to radio or television at increasing volume.

9. Sources of infection that can result in otalgia include: (Select all that apply.)
   1. insertion of unclean articles into ear.
   2. insertion of anything sharp into ear canal.
   3. instilling contaminated solutions into ear.
   4. swimming in polluted water.
   5. recent upper respiratory infection.
   6. allergies.

10. True or False
    _____ Bullous myringitis is an inflammatory disease that forms blisters on the tympanic membrane.

    _____ Serous otitis media is associated with damage to the pinna.

    _____ Drainage from mastoiditis travels through the middle ear and out the tympanic membrane.

    _____ Cholesteatoma, a type of conductive hearing loss, results from large deposits of cholesterol in the middle ear.

    _____ Perichondral hematomas can develop into "cauliflower ear."

    _____ Pain from disorders of the tympanic membrane is more painful than disorders of the middle ear.

11. Compare and contrast common types of peripheral vestibular disorders.

Disorder	Cause	Manifestations
Benign paroxysmal positional vertigo		
Labyrinthitis		
Meniere's disease		

12. List the four components necessary to maintain balance.

    a.

    b.

    c.

    d.

APPLYING SKILLS

13. A nurse is assessing a client with hearing loss using the Rinne and Weber tests. State the findings the nurse could expect for each test if there is hearing loss.

    a.   Rinne test:

    b.   Weber test:

14. Identify the method of assessment the nurse uses to determine if pain reported by a client is from external otitis or from otitis media.

15. A client experiencing a middle ear infection may report all of the following sensations *except*:

    1. bubbling.
    2. popping.
    3. crackling.
    4. sense of fullness.
    5. pain.
    6. total hearing loss.

16. The nurse should be aware that a _____ _____ may appear to be vertigo, because the temporary loss of blood flow to the brain can cause manifestations similar to balance disorders.

BEST PRACTICES

17. The major nursing responsibility for a client with tinnitus includes: (Select all that apply.)

    1. perform a thorough history.
    2. assess onset.
    3. assess level of intensity.
    4. assess frequency and constancy.

18. Identify an outcome and interventions for the nursing diagnosis Impaired verbal communication related to effects of hearing loss.
    Outcome:

    Interventions:

19. A client may have trouble coping with the loss of hearing. Appropriate nursing interventions to assist the client include all of the following *except*:

    1. teaching the client to inform others of hearing impairment.
    2. instructing the client to request that others communicate by using techniques that improve comprehension.
    3. instructing the client to limit social contact with others outside of family.
    4. teaching the client to avoid noisy areas that impair hearing.

20. Appropriate postoperative instructions for a client who has undergone a stapedectomy include which of the following? (Select all that apply.)

    1. Lie on nonoperative ear with HOB elevated
    2. Surgical packing in ear should not be disturbed
    3. Exercise regularly
    4. Blow nose gently, one nostril at a time
    5. Sneeze with mouth closed
    6. No airplane travel for 1 month

21. List two nursing actions to be completed prior to instilling antibiotic solution into the ear.

    a.

    b.

22. A critical teaching point the nurse should stress to the client receiving antibiotics for an ear infection is that the client must _____ _____ the prescription after the manifestations have cleared.

23. A 23-year-old college student has been admitted due to a complicated sinus infection that also involves his ears. He calls to the nurse's station complaining of discomfort that will not allow him to rest. In addition to medications ordered for pain, interventions the nurse can implement at the bedside to relieve ear pain include: (Select all that apply.)
    1. application of cool compress to ear.
    2. soft diet.
    3. quiet environment.
    4. positioning client with affected ear down.

KEEPING DRUG SKILLS SHARP

24. Because the cause is usually viral infection of the inner ear, _____ are often administered to clients who experience sudden hearing loss.

25. An ear solution of _____ is often prescribed because it is a drying agent that cleans the ear of debris and infection.

26. Methods used to remove a live insect from the ear canal include: (Select all that apply.)
    1. mineral oil.
    2. mineral water.
    3. lidocaine.
    4. ether-soaked cotton ball.

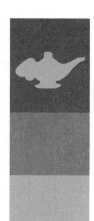

CHAPTER 67

Assessment of the Neurologic System

CHAPTER OBJECTIVES

67.1   Identify the complexity of a neurologic assessment.
67.2   Discuss the components of a neurologic history.
67.3   Identify the clinical manifestations often associated with neurologic functioning.
67.4   List the specific questions to ask the client to elicit information about the clinical manifestations.
67.5   Discuss appropriate questions for the client in the review of systems.
67.6   Identify client neurologic risks based on medical and surgical history.
67.7   Discuss allergies, medications, and dietary habits that might influence neurologic functioning.
67.8   Discuss the interaction of herbal medications taken for neurologic problems with prescription drugs.
67.9   Relate the need for B vitamins to peripheral nerve functioning.
67.10 Identify social and family health history factors that would contribute to a risk for neurologic disorders.
67.11 Perform a physical assessment of all aspects of the neurologic system.
67.12 Describe diagnostic testing including the appropriate use for each test to detect abnormalities of the neurologic system.

UNDERSTANDING PATHOPHYSIOLOGY

1. Pain is a common complaint of the client with a neurologic problem. The client should be asked: (Select all that apply.).
    1. are headaches present?
    2. does the pain radiate?
    3. are you dizzy?
    4. are there any relieving factors?
    5. have you been injured?
    6. have you had panic attacks?

2. Impaired consciousness may be a manifestation of neurologic disease. The client is unable to answer questions. The best source of information to assess onset and duration of this problem would be _____.

3. The absence of superficial reflexes on one side of the body may be due to the effects of _____ _____.

4. Childhood diseases that can cause a neurologic sequelae include all of the following *except*:
    1. rubella.
    2. rubeola.
    3. cytomegalovirus infection.
    4. herpes simplex.
    5. chicken pox.
    6. influenza.
    7. meningitis.

APPLYING SKILLS

5. Identify the clinical significance for each of the areas of the neurologic history.

Area	Clinical Significance
Growth and development	
Family health history	
Psychosocial history	

6. _____ is the most sensitive indicator of changes in the neurologic status of a client.

7. An 82-year-old nursing home resident has been admitted to the hospital due to changes in her level of consciousness. As part of her neurologic examination, the nurse will assess her orientation to: (Select all that apply.)
    1. time.
    2. place.
    3. person.
    4. event/situation.

8. A nurse assess intellectual performance of a client by asking him or her to count by _____ or _____.

9. List the four assessment techniques to examine the head, neck, and spine of a client with a possible neurologic problem.
    a.

    b.

    c.

    d.

10. _____ are dark circles around the eyes caused by periorbital ecchymosis from an anterior basal skull fracture.

11. A 32-year-old computer programmer has come to the clinic with complaints of fatigue, fever, and malaise. When assessing the neurologic system the nurse will ask him to flex his neck, with the chin touching the chest. This technique is used to check for _____ _____, a manifestation of meningitis.

12. Compare and contrast each of the cranial nerves. Identify the function and testing method for each during physical examination of the client.

Cranial Nerve	Function	Testing Method	Indication of Dysfunction
I			
II			
III, IV, VI			
V			
VII			
VIII			
IX, X			
XI			
XII			

13. A 52-year-old school teacher has come to the clinic with complaints of dizziness. Identify the technique the nurse will use to assess proprioception as part of the physical examination.

14. Compare and contrast testing of the following types of discrimination.

Type	Method of Testing
Stereognosis	
Graphesthesia	
Extinction phenomenon	
Two-point simulation	

15. A positive _____ reflex in an adult client indicates significant neurologic problems with transmission of impulses through the spinal cord to higher neuro areas.

16. True or False

_____ Patellar reflex is tested by tapping the inside aspect of the arm.

_____ The "snout reflex" is normal in infants but abnormal in adults.

_____ A positive result for testing for the "sucking reflex" is abnormal in adults.

_____ To check for the "chewing reflex," the client is offered a small piece of soft food and observed.

_____ Placing an object in the palm of the hand and curling fingers around it is a positive result of the grasp reflex.

17. Doppler ultrasonography can be used to measure

_____.

18. EEG is a measurement of the electrical activity of the cerebral cortex and a defining criteria for

_____.

BEST PRACTICES

19. Clinical manifestations of possible neurologic disorders are assessed when the nurse takes the health history. List each manifestation and the focus of the assessment.

20. True or False

_____ Skull x-ray studies reveal fractures, erosion, or calcification.

_____ CT scanning is very useful in acute trauma situations because of the ability to identify injuries quickly.

_____ MRI evaluates similar disorders to the CT and has few, if any, advantages over the CT.

_____ Neuropsychological tests help a neurologic assessment by gauging intelligence, emotions, language, and personal adjustment.

_____ Positron emission tomography can visualize physiologic function of specific body tissues.

_____ The primary assessment during a lumbar puncture is cerebrospinal fluid and pressure.

KEEPING DRUG SKILLS SHARP

21. State the rationale for documenting the use of over-the-counter medications and herbal remedies when assessing a client with neurologic problems.

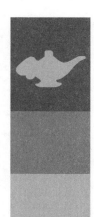

CHAPTER **68**

Management of Comatose or Confused Clients

CHAPTER OBJECTIVES

68.1 Define *consciousness, coma,* and *confusion.*
68.2 Define types of confusion.
68.3 Identify the causes and risk factors for disorders of consciousness and confusional states.
68.4 Relate the pathophysiology and clinical manifestations for disorders of consciousness and confusional states.
68.5 Define *level of consciousness.*
68.6 Identify diagnostic testing appropriate for disorders of consciousness and confusional states.
68.7 Describe the desired outcomes of the medical and nursing management for disorders of consciousness and confusional states.

UNDERSTANDING PATHOPHYSIOLOGY

1. _____ place pressure on brain stem or structures within the posterior cranial fossa.

2. _____ impair wakefulness by reducing supply of oxygen and glucose, allowing waste products to accumulate in the brain.

3. True or False

    _____ Most metabolic comas originate in systems outside the brain.

4. Asterixis is a manifestation of a _____ _____ coma.

5. When muscle groups are not used during periods of immobility, _____ develop.

6. List the three memory impairments that occur with dementia.
    a.

    b.

    c.

7. For each clinical manifestation of confusion, provide an example of a client behavior.

Manifestation	Example of Client Behavior
Disorder of attention	
Fluctuations in cognition	
Loss of memory for recent events	
Perceptual errors	
Hallucinations	
Illusions	
Delusions	

8. State the rationale for using the term "patient" when referring to a client who is comatose.

APPLYING SKILLS

9. A patient is in a comatose state, receiving enteral feedings. The nurse notes small, frequent liquid stools, which may indicate _____ _____.

10. Conditions a patient must exhibit to be considered "in a coma" include: (Select all that apply.)
   1. no response to verbal stimuli.
   2. varying responses to painful stimuli.
   3. no voluntary movements.
   4. altered respiratory patterns.
   5. altered pupillary responses to light.
   6. repeated blinking.

11. The presence of the _____ _____ reflex in the comatose patient indicates that brain stem functioning is preserved.

12. Initial assessment of a comatose patient includes: (Select all that apply.)
   1. level of consciousness.
   2. presence/absence of neurologic manifestations.
   3. pupil size and reactivity to light.
   4. deep tendon reflexes.
   5. response to noxious stimuli.
   6. evidence of trauma.
   7. lab values if metabolic coma is suspected.
   8. history from significant other.

13. Absence of pupillary, corneal, or oculovestibular responses in the comatose patient is highly predictive of _____.

14. The _____ Scale is the most common neurologic assessment tool used in clinical practice.

15. Characteristics of confusion include all of the following *except*:
   1. alterations in thought.
   2. attention deficit.
   3. loss of long-term memory.
   4. irritability alternating with drowsiness.

BEST PRACTICES

16. State the appropriate action for prevention the complication of corneal abrasions in the comatose patient.

17. True or False

_____ Comatose patients may have sips of water and ice chips in high Fowler's position.

_____ After suctioning the trachea, the nurse may use the same suction catheter for oral or pharyngeal suctioning but not vice versa.

_____ If the patient has facial paralysis, position him or her with the affected side up.

_____ Dried mucus may form, break off, and be aspirated in the comatose patient.

_____ Suctioning of a comatose patient is limited to no more than 30 seconds of suctioning time to prevent hypoxia.

18. The nurse should place the recovering comatose patient in the _____ position to test the gag reflex.

19. State the appropriate nursing action for switching a patient from tube feedings to oral feedings.

20. After checking the residual volume of a tube feeding on a comatose patient, the nurse notes 75 ml residual volume. State the action the nurse should take after making this observation.

21. An 82-year-old client has been admitted to the hospital for treatment. After assisting the client to her room, the nurse notices her wandering around the hallways. The client is assisted back to her room. Nursing interventions to assist this confused client would include: (Select all that apply.)
    1. reorient client as often as necessary.
    2. placing clocks and calendars in the hospital room.
    3. using familiar objects from home.
    4. reducing unfamiliar noises.
    5. using bright lighting.
    6. allowing restful sleep at night without unnecessary interruptions.
    7. administering sedatives.

22. Compare and contrast management and delegation of tasks for providing an enteral feeding to a comatose patient.

Task	Responsibility	Can RN Delegate?
Verification of physician order		
Verification of placement of feeding tube		
Reconstitution of feeding		
Preparation of feeding		
Priming the feeding pump		
Irrigation of feeding tube		
Tube site care		
Monitoring fluid/nutritional balance		

23. Family processes are very disrupted during an illness that produces a coma in a patient. It is important for the family to see _____, _____ nursing care to assist families to _____ with the illness of a family member. Not only is it important to _____ the family, but also to _____ with the patient.

24. Seizures from an overdose of cocaine are treated with _____.

25. Identify the nursing action that should be performed prior to administering a diuretic to a comatose patient.

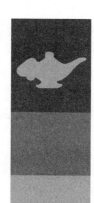

CHAPTER 69

Management of Clients with Cerebral Disorders

CHAPTER OBJECTIVES

69.1   Identify specific cerebral disorders.
69.2   Differentiate seizures and epilepsy.
69.3   Identify the causes and risk factors for cerebral disorders.
69.4   Relate the pathophysiology and clinical manifestations of cerebral disorders.
69.5   Identify specific types of seizures, brain tumors, and headaches and related manifestations.
69.6   Identify diagnostic testing for specific cerebral disorders.
69.7   Describe the desired outcomes for the medical, surgical, and nursing management for specific cerebral disorders.
69.8   Identify important modifications in health care for the older client.
69.9   Describe emergency care for the client with status epilepticus.
69.10   Discuss specific nursing activities for the client with craniotomy.
69.11   Differentiate nursing activities for the client with pituitary surgery versus craniotomy for other benign or malignant tumors.
69.12   Identify the grading scales for the client with subarachnoid hemorrhage.

UNDERSTANDING PATHOPHYSIOLOGY

1. A _____ is a sudden, abnormal electrical discharge from the brain.

2. _____ is a chronic disorder of recurrent seizures.

3. Identify the mechanism for development of severe hypoxia and lactic acidosis in brain tissue during seizures.

4.   For each area of the brain, identify the clinical manifestations of seizure activity originating in that area.

Area of Brain	Manifestations
Motor cortex	
Parietal region	
Occipital region	
Posterior temporal area	
Anterior temporal lobe	

5.   Tonic-clonic seizures, formerly known as "grand mal" seizures, follow a pattern of manifestations. Place the manifestations in the correct order according to this pattern.

    _____   Tonic phase

    _____   Postictal phase

    _____   Aura

    _____   Sudden loss of consciousness

    _____   Clonic phase

6.   True or False

    _____   Most primary brain tumors do not metastasize out of the brain to other areas.

    _____   Brain tumors are space-occupying lesions and the compression of tissue causes a decrease in intracranial pressure.

    _____   Astrocytomas are the most common type of glial cell tumor.

    _____   Oligodendrogliomas are slow-growing and calcify, making them recognizable on x-ray studies.

    _____   A meningioma is a rapidly growing malignant tumor of the spinal cord.

    _____   Acoustic neuromas affect the sense of balance and can cause dizziness, tinnitus, and unilateral hearing loss.

7. For each area of the brain, identify the clinical manifestations that would develop due to a brain tumor in that area.

Area of Brain	Manifestations
Frontal lobe	
Temporal lobe	
Parietal lobe	
Occipital lobe	
Cerebellar	
Brain stem	
Pituitary/hypothalamus	
Ventricle	

8. Conditions that can accelerate development of an intracranial aneurysm include all of the following *except*:
   1. hypotension.
   2. atherosclerosis.
   3. aging.
   4. alcohol abuse

9. Compare and contrast the common types of headaches.

Type	Etiology	Manifestation
Tension		
Cluster		
Migraine		

APPLYING SKILLS

10. A major diagnostic tool for assessment of clients with suspected epilepsy is _____.

11. A client has been admitted to the hospital with a possible seizure disorder. While he is undergoing diagnostic testing, the nursing staff is instructed to closely observe any clinical manifestations during the seizure. State the rationale for observing a client during a seizure.

12. Explain how the nurse can differentiate between actual seizures and "pseudoseizures" which occur in clients with psychiatric disorders.

13. The nurse is observing a client during a seizure. To distinguish the potential type of seizure, she notes specific manifestations that could be absence, myoclonic, clonic, or tonic in nature. List characteristics of each that the nurse would observe.

14. The clinical manifestation of sudden, severe headache accompanied by vomiting may indicate that a client is experiencing an _____.

15. The hallmark of a ruptured aneurysm is the presence of _____ in the CSF.

16. A 22-year-old college student is rushed to the emergency room with suspected meningitis. While completing a full physical exam and neurologic assessment, the clinician should be alert to the classic manifestations listed below. Describe what the client would present with clinically if she had developed meningitis.
    a. Nuchal rigidity:

    b. Brudzinski's sign:

    c. Kernig's sign:

BEST PRACTICES

17. List four nursing management goals for clients with seizures:
    a.

    b.

    c.

    d.

18. During an actual seizure, the priorities of care include: (Select all that apply.)
    1. maintaining an airway.
    2. protecting the client from injury.
    3. observing the seizure.
    4. restraining the client.
    5. administering anticonvulsant medications.

19. When managing the airway of a client during a generalized seizure, what is one activity that the nurse should *not* use to manage the airway?

20. Seizure precautions include: (Select all that apply.)
    1. no oral temperatures.
    2. padded bedrails.
    3. oxygen equipment at bedside.
    4. no nasal suction.
    5. fall risk precautions

21. Identify the nursing responsibilities for the preoperative neurosurgery client.

22. A client who is postoperative from removal of a pituitary tumor has a "moustache" dressing in place. The nurse notes clear fluid on the pad. State the action the nurse should perform after making this observation.

23. For a client with a seizure disorder, prior to discharge, the nurse should emphasize which of the following client teachings? (Select all that apply.)
    1. How anticonvulsants prevent seizures
    2. Limiting physical activity
    3. The importance of taking medications regularly
    4. Care during a seizure
    5. Wearing a life jacket when in or near water
    6. No driving for at least 6 months
    7. Cooking only with others present

24. Assessing the client with a subarachnoid hemorrhage, the nurse is observing for rebleeding. Doing so, she notes serial trends in the data. The most sensitive indicator of neurologic change is _____. Secondly, the nurse needs to keep the _____ _____ low to reduce the rebleeding risk.

KEEPING DRUG SKILLS SHARP

25. Explain what modifications should be made for the older adult taking anticonvulsant medications.

26. Anticonvulsant medications should be resumed _____ after surgery to obtain therapeutic levels of the medication.

27. State the rationale for contraindicating alcohol consumption for clients taking anticonvulsant medications.

28. The medication _____ is given to terminate status epilepticus and prevent exhaustion.

29. The medication _____ is administered to treat the decreased secretion of ADH after pituitary surgery.

30. Identify the technique used to facilitate delivery of chemotherapy through the blood-brain barrier.

31. _____ are administered to reduce cerebral edema in the treatment of brain abscesses.

32. _____ is the most frequently used chemotherapy agent for brain tumors.

33. Drug absorption is impaired during a migraine due to reduced _____.

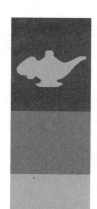

CHAPTER **70**

Management of Clients with Stroke

CHAPTER OBJECTIVES

70.1   Identify the major causes of strokes.
70.2   Differentiate ischemic and hemorrhagic strokes.
70.3   Relate the term *brain attack* to stroke.
70.4   Identify causes and risk factors for strokes and transient ischemic attacks (TIAs).
70.5   Explain the process of thrombosis, embolism, and hemorrhage.
70.6   Relate the pathophysiology and clinical manifestations of stroke and TIAs.
70.7   Describe deficits following stroke.
70.8   Identify specific diagnostic findings for stroke.
70.9   Describe the desired outcomes of medical, surgical, nursing, and interdisciplinary rehabilitation management of stroke and TIAs.
70.10   Identify specific complications of stroke, along with assessment and treatment.
70.11   Identify the major nursing diagnoses in the self-care of the stroke client.
70.12   Describe public education necessary for stroke prevention.

UNDERSTANDING PATHOPHYSIOLOGY

1. Identify the causes for the two major types of strokes.
   a. Ischemic:

   b. Hemorrhagic:

2. The _____ type of stroke has a higher incidence.

3. The degree of damage to brain tissue from stroke is determined by the length of time the area was deprived of _____.

4. Identify the mechanism that leads to the development of a thrombus in a blood vessel, which can cause a stroke.

5. Clients with _____ are at greatest risk for development of a thrombotic stroke.

6. Intracerebral hemorrhage results from effects of _____ on blood vessels, causing them to rupture.

7. List the modifiable risk factors for stroke:
   a.

   b.

   c.

   d.

   e.

8. The brain requires a mean arterial pressure of _____ mm Hg to maintain adequate blood flow.

9.   The most common site of ischemic stroke is the
     _____.

10. Explain why *right*-sided hemiplegia affects
     speech.

11. Differentiate between dysarthria and aphasia.

12. Differentiate between a stroke and a TIA and ex-
     plain how they are related.

13. Identify the characteristics of each type of aphasia due to stroke.

Type	Characteristics
Wernicke's	
Broca's	
Global	

APPLYING SKILLS

14. Compare and contrast the early warning manifestations of the major types of strokes.

Type of Stroke	Warning Manifestations
Ischemic	
Thrombotic	
Embolic	
Hemorrhagic	

15. Manifestations of unilateral neglect after a stroke include: (Select all that apply.)
    1. attention to only one side of the body.
    2. failure to respond to stimuli on one side of the body.
    3. use of only lower extremities.
    4. orienting the head and eyes to one side.

16. List the pertinent information the nurse should include when completing an *initial* assessment of a client who has suffered a stroke:
    a.

    b.

    c.

    d.

    e.

    f.

    g.

    h.

BEST PRACTICES

17. Identify the difficulties of nurse-client communication for each type of aphasia.
    a. Acoustic aphasia:

    b. Visual aphasia:

18. Appropriate nursing actions to communicate with an aphasic client who has suffered a stroke include: (Select all that apply.)
    1. speak slowly and clearly.
    2. do not shout.
    3. do not press for a response.
    4. use a picture board.

19. For a client with dysphagia, the nurse would teach all of the following steps to prevent choking or aspiration *except*:
    1. opening the mouth properly.
    2. leaving lips slightly open after food is placed inside mouth.
    3. keeping the head slightly flexed forward during swallowing.
    4. have clients check for food on the paralyzed side of the mouth after swallowing using the tongue and turning the head to the affected side.

20. Identify the priority action for emergency care of the client with stroke.

21. State the rationale for reducing elevated temperatures in the client who is experiencing a stroke.

22. The nurse is assisting a client with ROM exercises to improve his strength after suffering a stroke. He doesn't understand how having the nurse "do all the work of the muscles really helps." List the benefits of *passive* ROM:
    a.

    b.

    c.

23. Identify an appropriate nursing action to assist a client in the prevention of hip contractures after a stroke.

24. Further evaluation of a TIA includes which of the following? (Select all that apply.)
    1. Auscultation for carotid bruit
    2. CT to rule out stroke
    3. Cerebral angiogram
    4. ECG
    5. Doppler studies of the basilar arteries
    6. TTE and TEE

25. The major assessment following a carotid endarterectomy is _____.

KEEPING DRUG SKILLS SHARP

26. State the rationale for performing a non-contrast CT scan of the head prior to beginning thrombolytic therapy.

27. Contraindications for beginning thrombolytic therapy include: (Select all that apply.)
    1. current use of oral anticoagulants.
    2. use of intravenous dextrose solution.
    3. platelet count less than 100,000/mm^3.
    4. blood glucose less than 50 mg/dl or greater than 400 mg/dl.
    5. recent myocardial infarction.
    6. diabetes mellitus.
    7. rapidly improving neurologic signs.

28. A treatment window of _____ hours from onset of stroke manifestations creates the sense of urgency when treating clients with stroke.

29. After a thrombolytic infusion, the nurse should wait _____ hours before beginning administration of anticoagulants and antiplatelet medications.

30. Activated partial thromboplastin time (aPTT) should be at _____ times the control value for anticoagulation to be effective.

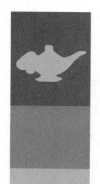

CHAPTER **71**

Management of Clients with Peripheral Nervous System Disorders

CHAPTER OBJECTIVES

71.1 Identify the magnitude of lower back pain as a common health problem.

71.2 Describe the causes and clinical manifestations of lower back pain, cervical disk disorders, postpolio syndrome, spinal cord disorders, UMN/LMN disorders, cranial nerve disorders, peripheral nerve disorders, and nerve trauma disorders.

71.3 Differentiate specific back injuries.

71.4 Relate pathophysiology and clinical manifestations of lower back pain, cervical disk disorders, postpolio syndrome, spinal cord disorders, UMN/LMN disorders, cranial nerve disorders, peripheral nerve disorders, and nerve trauma disorders.

71.5 Identify the diagnostic testing appropriate for initial and follow-up testing of the spine.

71.6 Describe the desired outcomes of medical, surgical, and nursing management for lower back pain disorders, cervical disk disorders, postpolio syndrome, spinal cord disorders, UMN/LMN disorders, cranial nerve disorders, peripheral nerve disorders, and nerve trauma disorders.

71.7 Identify self-care education needs for the client with lower back pain and cervical disk disorders.

UNDERSTANDING PATHOPHYSIOLOGY

1. Provide examples for each of the three groups of problems leading to the development of low back pain.

Cause	Example
Biomechanical and destructive	
Destructive origins	
Degenerative	
Other	

2. Identify the mechanism for increased damage to intervetebral disks due to normal aging.

   c. Spondylosis:

   d. Spinal stenosis:

3. True or False

   _____ Lumbar disks are more likely to rupture than cervical disks.

   _____ Ruptured intervetebral disks may occur at any level of the spine.

   _____ Factors increasing risk of disk injury include extended sitting, aerobic exercise, and high cholesterol.

4. For each spinal disorder, identify the cause and resulting body changes.
   a. Lordosis:

   b. Spondylothesis:

5. Any lesion that destroys the upper motor neuron will result in _____ _____.

6. _____ and _____ are the most common spinal cord tumors. Both are benign and operable.

7. Trigeminal neuralgia, or tic douloureux, is an irritation of the _____ cranial nerve and is characterized by intense pain of sudden onset along the maxilla and mandible.

8. Bell's palsy affects the motor aspects of the _____ cranial nerve and presents as _____ of the facial muscles of expression.

9. Peripheral neuropathy causes different clinical manifestations, depending on the type of nerves affected. For each type of nerve, identify the ways in which the manifestation will present in the client.

Type	Manifestation
Motor nerves	
Sensory nerves	
Autonomic nerves	

10. Repetitive motion of the wrists can result in _____ syndrome, which occurs when the median nerve is compressed.

11. True or False

_____ The peroneal nerve, a branch of the sciatic nerve, is commonly subjected to injury.

_____ Full function of the fingers is possible after surgery for Dupuytren's contracture.

_____ Diabetic neuropathy is a type of peripheral neuropathy caused by disease.

_____ No known cure is available for Bell's palsy.

APPLYING SKILLS

12. State the rationale for evaluating occupation and working equipment of a client with low back pain.

13. The nurse should assess both the surgical site of the spine of a spinal fusion client and the _____ site on a postoperative client.

14. A critical nursing assessment for a client who is postoperative from cervical disk surgery is to check the site for excessive _____ that may compromise breathing.

15. Label the assessment techniques for carpal tunnel syndrome.

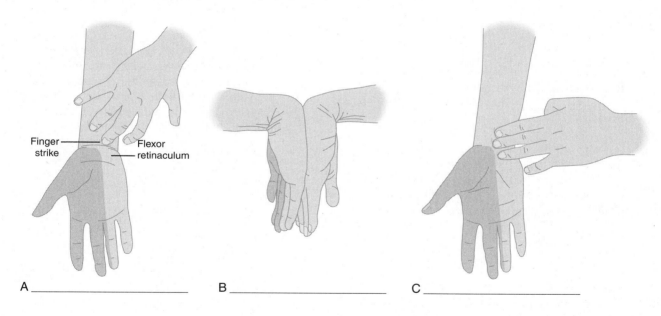

Finger strike — Flexor retinaculum

A _____   B _____   C _____

16. A client returns after surgical correction to relieve pressure from carpal tunnel syndrome. State the rationale for delaying assessment of sensation of the fingers after surgery.

17. After spinal surgery, if the client develops
_____,
_____,
_____, or
_____, the physician should be notified immediately because surgical decompression may be needed.

BEST PRACTICES

18. A client calls for the nurse with complaints of discomfort due to his sciatica. State the appropriate nursing intervention to assist him and reduce the discomfort.

19. Important client teaching points the nurse should discuss to assist in resolving low back pain include: (Select all that apply.)
    1. using good body mechanics.
    2. keeping objects close to the body when lifting.
    3. locking knees when lifting.
    4. avoiding twisting when lifting.

20. Identify an effective intervention for preventing future low back injuries.

21. Clients who have undergone spinal surgery are turned in their beds with the _____ _____ maneuver in the postoperative period.

22. A postoperative spinal fusion client is uncomfortable from prolonged bed rest and asks for assistance from the nurse. Identify the action the nurse should *avoid* to prevent complications from immobility in this client.

23. Normal protocol for postoperative voiding calls for the client being able to void sufficiently within _____ hours after spinal surgery.

24. Many clients who undergo cervical disk surgery complain of discomfort when swallowing or talking. Nursing actions to improve comfort include: (Select all that apply.)
    1. soft diet.
    2. throat lozenges.
    3. viscous lidocaine solution.
    4. cool, dry air.
    5. minimal talking.

KEEPING DRUG SKILLS SHARP

25. To reduce pain and spasms from low back pain, all of the following medications may be prescribed except:
    1. NSAIDs.
    2. beta blockers.
    3. COX-2 inhibitors.
    4. muscle relaxants.

26. A PCA pump filled with _____ is the best way to control postoperative pain for the spinal surgery client.

27. Why is use of Capsaicin topical cream indicated for the postpolio client?

28. A postpolio syndrome client complains of significant discomfort from overuse, pain, and cramps in her muscles. She doesn't understand why she "must suffer" with these pains and wants to take strong medications to "take all the pain away." Her physician has cautioned against this. State the rationale for the physician's advice against pain medication.

29. _____ is prescribed for treatment of trigeminal neuralgia because it dampens the reactivity of the neurons within the trigeminal nerve, reducing pain stimuli.

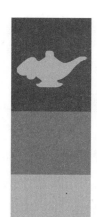

CHAPTER **72**

Management of Clients with Degenerative Neurologic Disorders

CHAPTER OBJECTIVES

72.1   Identify degenerative neurologic disease as a significant health challenge for clients, families, and health care providers.

72.2   Define *dementia*.

72.3   Differentiate types of dementia.

72.4   Describe the causes and risk factors for degenerative neurologic diseases.

72.5   Relate the pathophysiology and clinical manifestations of the degenerative neurologic diseases.

72.6   Describe the stages of Alzheimer's dementia.

72.7   Identify the diagnostic testing for degenerative diseases.

72.8   Describe management of Parkinsonian and myasthenic crises.

72.9   Describe the desired outcomes of medical and nursing management for degenerative neurologic disorders.

72.10   Identify the prognoses for the degenerative diseases.

UNDERSTANDING PATHOPHYSIOLOGY

1.   Compare and contrast the major types of dementia.

Type	Characteristics
Alzheimer's disease	
Multi-infarct disease	
Lewy body dementia	
Pick's disease	

2. Describe the stages of Alzheimer's disease and the manifestations of each stage.

Stage	Manifestations
Preclinical	
Mild Alzheimer's	
Moderate Alzheimer's	
Severe Alzheimer's	

3. A client with Huntington's disease (HD) has a _____ % chance of passing his disease on to future children.

4. Areas of the body most affected by multiple sclerosis include all of the following *except* the:
   1. optic nerves.
   2. cerebellum.
   3. cerebrum.
   4. cervical spinal cord.

5. Although clinical manifestations may vary due to the random distribution of the multiple sclerosis (MS) plaques on nerves, they can include: (Select all that apply.)
   1. bowel and bladder dysfunction.
   2. hair loss.
   3. vision loss from optic neuritis.
   4. weakness.
   5. uncoordination.
   6. constipation.
   7. fatigue.
   8. insomnia.

6. During the recovery phase of Guillain-Barré syndrome (GBS), remyelination occurs in a _____ _____ pattern.

7. The cause of muscle weakness in myasthenia gravis (MG) is loss of _____ at the neurotransmitter junction.

8. Although amyotrophic lateral sclerosis (ALS) involves degeneration of both upper and lower motor neurons, it does not affect _____ _____.

9. Progressive muscle weakness from ALS will eventually lead to _____ _____.

10. Compare and contrast between a myasthenic crisis and a cholinergic crisis in the client with MG.
    Myasthenic crisis:

    Cholinergic crisis:

APPLYING SKILLS

11. Assessing pain or discomfort in the client with advanced Alzheimer's disease (AD) is difficult due to communication problems. Behaviors that would indicate discomfort include: (Select all that apply.)
    1. noisy breathing.
    2. negative vocalizations (mutterings).
    3. sad or frightened facial expression.
    4. frowning.
    5. tense body language.
    6. motionlessness.

12. List the six cardinal features of Parkinson's disease:
    a.

    b.

    c.

    d.

    e.

    f.

13. Identify a classic feature of MG.

14. A common test for MG is to ask the client to hold an upward gaze for 3 minutes. If the test is positive, a manifestation of _____ of the upper eyelid will be observed.

15. A client suspected of having MG is to undergo a Tensilon test. After injecting Tensilon IV into the client, a positive result would be _____ _____ in muscle strength.

BEST PRACTICES

16. A nursing diagnosis of Risk for injury related to impaired judgment has been developed for a client with AD. List the appropriate interventions to prevent injury to the client:
    a.

    b.

    c.

    d.

    e.

17. A nurse caring for a client with MS develops the nursing diagnosis of Impaired physical mobility related to weakness, contractures, and spasticity. List the appropriate interventions for this client:
    a.

    b.

    c.

    d.

    e.

18. Upon entering the room of a client who has been diagnosed with AD, the nurse notes manifestations of increased frustration. The client is pacing the room and shaking his fist at the air. Interventions the nurse can implement to help the client include all of the following *except*:
    1. increase environmental stimuli.
    2. approach the client calmly.
    3. do not place any demands on the client.
    4. gently distract the client.
    5. use multiple sensory methods, but not all at the same time.

19. An 84-year-old female client diagnosed with early stages of AD has begun to show manifestations of skin breakdown in the perineal area due to incontinence. Nursing interventions for incontinence appropriate to her age and physical/mental condition include: (Select all that apply.)
    1. schedule voiding and defecation times.
    2. monitor client for nonverbal clues of needing to void/defecate.
    3. post bright, clear signs indicating where bathroom is located.
    4. use an indwelling catheter to reduce risk of infection.
    5. use disposable undergarments in later stages of AD.

20. A 79-year-old client diagnosed with Parkinson's disease suddenly stops moving in the middle of walking to the bathroom. This phenomenon called "freezing" can be corrected through which nursing actions? (Select all that apply.)
    1. Have the client step over an imaginary line to get moving again.
    2. Assist the client to rock to get momentum.
    3. Toss small scraps of paper in front of the client to encourage walking.
    4. Gently push the client forward.

21. Nursing interventions to assist the client with HD who is experiencing problems eating due to dysphagia include: (Select all that apply.)
    1. diets that include easy-to-swallow foods.
    2. two large meals a day.
    3. have the client sit upright.
    4. have the client keep chin down toward the chest while swallowing.
    5. have the client hold his or her breath before swallowing and cough to clear the throat afterward.

KEEPING DRUG SKILLS SHARP

22. Identify the primary indication for prescribing medications such as tacrine, donepezil, and rivastigmine for clients with AD.

23. Explain how Sinemet (combination of levodopa and carbidopa) works to correct manifestations of Parkinson's disease.

24. The dopamine blocker _____ helps control the abnormal movements that result from HD by altering neurotransmission of signals for movement.

25. The standard therapy to treat an acute exacerbation of MS is administration of _____ _____ to reduce inflammation.

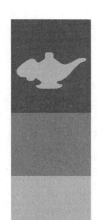

CHAPTER **73**

Management of Clients with Neurologic Trauma

CHAPTER OBJECTIVES

73.1 Define increased *intracranial pressure (IICP)* and its components, *mean arterial pressure (MAP)* and *cerebral perfusion pressure (CPP)*.

73.2 Differentiate cerebral edema and brain swelling.

73.3 Define *traumatic brain injury (TBI)* and *spinal cord injury (SCI)*.

73.4 Identify the causes and risk factors for IICP, TBI, and SCI.

73.5 Relate the pathophysiology and clinical manifestations of IICP, specific types of TBI, and SCI according to level of injury.

73.6 Explain Cushing's triad.

73.7 Identify specific herniation syndromes as a consequence of IICP.

73.8 Describe the desired outcomes of medical, surgical, and nursing management for clients with IICP and herniation, TBI, and SCI.

73.9 Describe specific mechanisms of injury in TBI.

73.10 Describe specific types of brain injuries in TBI.

73.11 Describe specific types of SCI.

73.12 Identify the initial management of the client with head injury and spinal cord injury.

73.13 Describe rehabilitation and self-care for the head-injured client.

73.14 Identify modifications of care for the older head-injured client.

73.15 Describe spinal shock and autonomic dysreflexia.

73.16 Identify clinical syndromes that cause partial paralysis.

73.17 Identify diagnostic tests that confirm spinal cord injuries.

73.18 Identify potential complications of TBI and SCI.

UNDERSTANDING PATHOPHYSIOLOGY

1. To maintain a balance between the brain tissue, blood, and cerebrospinal fluid, intracranial pressure should not exceed _____ mm Hg.

2. List the common causes for IICP:
    a.

    b.

    c.

    d.

    e.

    f.

3. List the three mechanisms that compensate for IICP:
    a.

    b.

    c.

4. List the two initial manifestations of IICP:
   a.

   b.

5. Cushing's triad is a late response to IICP. The manifestations are _____, _____, and _____.

6. The leading cause of traumatic head injuries is _____.

7. Identify the characteristics of each type of common brain injury.

Injury	Characteristics
Concussion	
Open head injury	
Closed head injury	
Contusions	
Subdural hematoma	

8. Herniation into the brain stem is a result of severe IICP. Define each herniation syndrome and list manifestations of each.
   a. Transcalvarial:

   b. Central:

   c. Lateral transtentorial:

   d. Cingulate:

   e. Infratentorial:

9. Spinal cord injuries occur most often in _____ between the ages of _____ and _____.

10. _____ are the most common type of spinal cord injury.

11. Clinical manifestations of spinal cord damage *below* the level of injury include loss of: (Select all that apply.)
    1. voluntary movement.
    2. sensation of pain, temperature, pressure, and proprioception.
    3. bowel and bladder function.
    4. spinal and autonomic reflexes.

12. A spinal cord injury to the cervical area results in _____.

13. Injuries to the thoracic or lumbar spinal segments produce _____.

14. Clinical manifestations of autonomic dysreflexia include: (Select all that apply.)
    1. sudden onset of severe hypertension.
    2. throbbing headache.
    3. profuse diaphoresis.
    4. flushing of the skin above level of the lesion.
    5. blurred vision.
    6. nausea.
    7. bradycardia.

15. When the spinal cord is damaged, the immediate response is "spinal shock" with the loss of all of the following *except*:
    1. skeletal muscle function.
    2. bowel and bladder tone.
    3. vision.
    4. sexual function.
    5. autonomic reflexes.

APPLYING SKILLS

16. A young client is admitted to the emergency department with a head injury. The Glasgow Coma Scale is used for the initial assessment. Client characteristics that might invalidate the GCS score include: (Select all that apply.)
    1. the client is intubated and cannot speak.
    2. the client does not communicate in English.
    3. the client has a hearing loss.
    4. eyes are swollen and closed.
    5. the client is blind or aphasic.
    6. the client is hemiplegic.

17. A client arrives via ambulance in the emergency department from an accident. Upon assessment, the nurse notes ecchymosis around the eyes and drainage of clear fluid from the ear. These manifestations are consistent with the injury _____

_____.

18. Explain why the description of the accident causing a head injury is critical to care.

19. A client has been diagnosed with Brown-Séquard syndrome. Upon assessment, the nurse would expect to find all of the following clinical manifestations *except*:
    1. ipsilateral motor paralysis (same side as lesion).
    2. ipsilateral motor paralysis (opposite side of lesion).
    3. loss of vibratory and position sense.
    4. contralateral loss of pain and temperature sensation (opposite side).

20. When completing an assessment of a client with an SCI, levels of sensation are documented according to _____

_____.

BEST PRACTICES

21. List the immediate interventions that should be implemented to decrease ICP and state the rationale for each:
    a.

    b.

    c.

22. A client with traumatic brain injury is at risk for ineffective airway and aspiration. Nursing actions to protect the airway include: (Select all that apply.)
    1. clearing mouth and oropharynx of foreign bodies.
    2. suctioning oropharynx and trachea to remove secretions.
    3. placing the client in supine position to facilitate drainage of secretions.
    4. using humidified oxygen or intubation as needed to maintain PaO$_2$ within parameters.

23. List the emergency interventions that should be implemented to correct autonomic dysreflexia:
    a.

    b.

    c.

    d.

    e.

24. When turning a client with a suspected spinal injury, the nurse should use the _____ _____ maneuver to maintain straight body alignment.

25. Clients with SCI have altered thermoregulation due to loss of hypothalamic control of the sympathetic nervous system. Nursing actions to maintain normothermic status include: (Select all that apply.)
    1. rectal or core temperature monitoring every 24 hours.
    2. palpation of skin surfaces for areas of warmth or coolness.
    3. control of environmental temperature.
    4. use of bed linens and eliminating drafts in room.

26. For each rehabilitation goal for the client with SCI, identify appropriate nursing interventions.
    a. Promote mobility:

    b. Reduce spasticity:

    c. Improve bladder control:

    d. Improve bowel control:

    e. Prevent pressure ulcers:

    f. Reduce respiratory dysfunction:

    g. Control pain:

    h. Promote psychological adjustment:

27. True or False
    _____ PERRLA includes an assessment of the shape of the pupil.
    _____ Glasgow Coma Scale score of 9 or lower indicates a nonserious injury.
    _____ The IICP client should be positioned in a supine position with the HOB at 30 degrees unless contraindicated.
    _____ Plateau waves on the ICP monitor require intervention.
    _____ An acute subdural hematoma produces symptoms gradually.
    _____ Diffuse axonal head injury is the most serious type of head injury.
    _____ Initial care of the SCI client includes neck stabilization without flexion.
    _____ An alternating pressure mattress eliminates the need to turn the SCI client.

28. In the emergency department, a cervical spine–injured client is immediately placed in _____ _____.

29. A collaborative problem in the care of the SCI client is Risk for thrombophlebitis. List the outcome for this problem along with two interventions.

   Outcome:

   Intervention #1:

   Intervention #2:

30. The nursing diagnosis of Constipation related to paralysis is common with SCI clients. List the outcome for the diagnosis and two interventions.

   Outcome:

   Intervention #1:

   Intervention #2:

KEEPING DRUG SKILLS SHARP

31. State the rationale for controlling seizure activity prophylactically with phenytoin or carbamazepine in the client with IICP.

32. If a client with IICP begins shivering from a fever, _____ would be administered to prevent shivering, which would increase metabolism.

33. True or False

   _____ Clients with severe traumatic brain injury are not candidates for barbiturate therapy (undergo a prophylactic barbiturate coma).

   _____ A client undergoing barbiturate therapy should have respirations monitored with pulse oximetry and incentive spirometer every 4 hours.

   _____ Barbiturate therapy can cause hypothermia.

   _____ Even when a client is in a coma, the pupils dilate if the brain stem is compressed.

34. State the indication for each type of medication used to treat acute SCI.

Medication	Indication for Use
Vasoactive agents	
Steroids	
Thyrotropin-releasing hormone	
H_2 receptor blocking agents	

35. _____ is used for neurogenic bladder control to stimulate contractions and _____ to reduce the contractions.

36. Pain control for the client with SCI includes analgesics, which may need to be supplemented with other medications such as _____ _____ to control neuropathic pain.

37. Heterotopic ossification is the formation of bone in abnormal locations. Clients with SCI who develop this complication are treated with _____ _____.

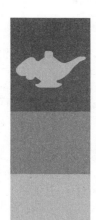

CHAPTER 74

Assessment of the Hematopoietic System

CHAPTER OBJECTIVES

74.1 Distinguish biographic and demographic data significant to the hematopoietic and immune system.
74.2 Relate the chief complaint and clinical manifestations to the client's current health status.
74.3 Describe the common clinical manifestations of hematopoietic system disorders.
74.4 Identify specific questions to elicit client information about the clinical manifestations.
74.5 Relate past medical and surgical history to the development of hematopoietic conditions.
74.6 Describe the food and drug allergy relationship to hematopoietic disorders.
74.7 Identify medication intake that has an impact on the hematopoietic system.
74.8 Identify interactions of herbal medicines with prescription medications.
74.9 Describe an adequate dietary intake to support the hematopoietic and immune systems.
74.10 Relate social history factors such as stress levels, occupational exposures, and lifestyle choices to predisposition to hematopoietic disorders.
74.11 Explore the possibility of familial tendencies to hematopoietic disorders.
74.12 Describe important aspects of the physical examination of the hematopoietic system including a lymph node assessment.
74.13 Discuss basic hematologic laboratory tests.
74.14 Relate diagnostic testing to specific hematologic disorders.

UNDERSTANDING PATHOPHYSIOLOGY

1. The focus of the health history for a client with hematopoietic and immune system problems depends on _____ _____.

2. List the two groups of individuals that have a diminished immune response:
   a.

   b.

3. Which of the following clinical manifestations may be found in a client that presents with anemia? (Select all that apply.)
   1. Epistaxis
   2. Recurrent infections
   3. Fatigue
   4. Chronic diarrhea

4. List the major allergic triggers:
   a.

   b.

   c.

   d.

5. Explain why clients who have had a partial or total gastrectomy may develop anemia.

333

6. What physiologic response occurs when clients live at altitudes above 10,000 feet?

7. Which of the following clinical manifestations is/are most likely to occur with severe anemia? (Select all that apply.)
   1. Weakness
   2. Fatigue
   3. Exertional dyspnea
   4. Ringing in the ears

8. Clients with immunodeficiencies are most likely to present with a history of:
   1. recurrent infections.
   2. pruritus and ruddy skin.
   3. petechiae and purpura.
   4. scleral jaundice.

9. Fever is a manifestation of many illnesses and may not occur due to immunosuppression. Immunodeficiencies may result from:
   a.

   b.

   c.

   d.

10. Abnormal assessment findings of the eyes, ears, nose, and mouth related to blood disorders are:

11. True or False
    _____ The type of allergen and individual sensitivity pattern may cause varied clinical manifestations.

    _____ Strict vegetarians are not at greater risk for iron deficiency anemia than people who eat nonvegetarian diets.

    _____ Clients who abuse alcohol may be at risk for bleeding disorders.

    _____ The RBC count varies with age and gender.

    _____ Bleeding disorders manifest with petechiae, purpura, and ecchymoses.

    _____ During the assessment of client medications, it is important to ask about corticosteroid use or previous use of cytotoxic agents because they can mask infection.

APPLYING SKILLS

12. Which of the following responses from a client may alert the nurse to a possible immunodeficiency?
    1. "It takes a long time for me to heal even the smallest wound."
    2. "I have occasional diarrhea."
    3. "I rarely get a cold."
    4. "I haven't had an infection that required an antibiotic for over a year."

13. List the nine areas to assess with regard to family health history when conducting the hematopoietic assessment:
    a.

    b.

    c.

    d.

    e.

    f.

    g.

    h.

    i.

14. List the portions of the lymphatic system that are accessible for a physical examination:
    a.

    b.

    c.

15. List the four specific blood tests that are generally needed to diagnose hematopoietic disorders:

    a.

    b.

    c.

    d.

17. List the four laboratory studies used to pinpoint bleeding disorders:

    a.

    b.

    c.

    d.

16. Anemia and sickle cell crisis can produce respiratory manifestations such as _____ and _____.

18. Identify the following laboratory tests as low, normal, or high (See Table 74-5).

Laboratory Test	Low, Normal, High
a. RBC woman 3.7	
b. RBC man 4.9	
c. Hemoglobin woman 12.6	
d. Hemoglobin man 12.6	
e. Hematocrit woman 50%	
f. Hematocrit man 40%	
g. WBC 12,000	
h. Neutrophils 60%	
i. Eosinophils 6%	
j. Basophils 0.5%	
k. Lymphocytes 50%	
l. Monocytes 6%	
m. Platelets 200,000	

19. True or False

    _____ Some hematologic tests are age-specific and gender-specific.

    _____ When conducting a symptom analysis it is important to ask about onset and timing.

BEST PRACTICES

20. Explain why it is important to ask a client if he or she has donated blood or blood components recently.

21. Relate occupational exposure to possible hematopoietic disorders.

22. An important assessment of the cardiovascular system to anticipate when the client has anemia is _____.

23. A test that is used to detect antigen-antibody reactions between serum antibodies and RBCs and to find hemolytic disease in newborns is the _____.

KEEPING DRUG SKILLS SHARP

24. Certain over-the-counter medications can aggravate _____.

25. Explain why it is important to assess client use of herbal preparations. Give three examples.

26. Some medications such as _____, _____, and _____ _____ have the side effect of myelosuppression.

27. True or False

    _____ Tissue plasminogen activator (t-PA) can cause a decrease in bleeding time.

    _____ Ephedra might reduce the effect of prednisone.

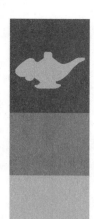

CHAPTER **75**

Management of Clients with Hematologic Disorders

CHAPTER OBJECTIVES

75.1   Recognize anemia as a pathologic process symptomatic of other underlying disorders.

75.2   Relate the condition of anemia to hypoxia.

75.3   Identify major causes and risk factors for development of anemia, white blood cell disorders, platelet disorders, spleen disorders, and clotting disorders.

75.4   Describe the three major classifications of anemia.

75.5   Describe the classifications of white cell disorders.

75.6   Relate the lack of red blood cells to the subsequent clinical manifestations of the various types of anemia.

75.7   Relate laboratory findings to specific types of anemia, white blood cell disorders, platelet disorders, spleen disorders, and clotting disorders.

75.8   Describe the desired outcomes for medical intervention for clients with anemia, white blood cell disorders, platelet disorders, spleen disorders, and clotting disorders.

75.9   Explain blood transfusions as a therapeutic intervention for anemia, including appropriate types, risks, ethical issues, preparation, blood compatibility, appropriate infusion method, monitoring, and the urgent nature of transfusion reaction manifestations and subsequent care.

75.10   Explain the desired outcomes for nursing assessment and interventions for the client with anemia, white blood cell disorders, platelet disorders, spleen disorders, and clotting disorders.

75.11   Modify nursing care according to the age of the client.

UNDERSTANDING PATHOPHYSIOLOGY

1. Which of the following is essential for RBC production?
   1. Manganese
   2. Vitamin A
   3. Vitamin C
   4. Folic acid

2. Which of the following depicts a compensatory mechanism for tissue hypoxia?
   1. A shift in oxygen-hemoglobin dissociation curve to the left
   2. Redistribution of blood from tissues of low O_2 needs to tissues of high O_2 needs
   3. Decreased cardiac output
   4. Decreased rate of RBC production

3. List the four factors that determine the severity of clinical manifestations associated with anemia:
   a. Severity of blood loss
   b. speed of blood loss
   c. chronic anemia - how frequent
   d. other comorbid conditions

4. Transport of oxygen is impaired with anemia for two reasons. List the two reasons and state the outcome of impaired oxygen transport.
   a. ↓ hemoglobin

   b. ↓ RBC's

   c. hypoxia

5. The most common etiologic factor in men for iron-deficiency anemia is __blood loss__ __most often from GI tract.__

6. Thalassemia disrupts the synthesis of __globin__ _____.

7. Megaloblastic anemias result in defective __RBC's__ _____ and are caused by deficiencies of __Vit. B12__ and __folic acid__.

8. A common GI symptom associated with pernicious anemia is:
   1. weight gain.
   2. increased appetite.
   3. abdominal distention.
   4. flatulence.

9. A failure of bone marrow to replace RBCs results in __hemolytic__ anemia.

10. Sickling of RBCs occurs when there is low __oxygenation__.

11. The cause of polycythemia vera (PV) is excessive activation of __pluripotent stem cells__.

12. The most common clinical manifestation of hemochromatosis is __joint pain__.

13. The means used to rid the body of excess iron in hemochromatosis is __phlebotomy__.

14. Agranulocytosis is characterized by a profound decrease in __Neutrophils__.

15. The most common presenting complaint in multiple myeloma is __bone pain__ _____.

16. List the four factors essential for normal clot formation:
    a. intact blood vessels
    b. adequate # of functioning platelets
    c. sufficient amts of 12 clotting factors
    d. well controlled fibrinolytic system

17. The most common thrombocytopenic disorder is __Idiopathic thrombocytopenic purpura__

18. Prothrombin synthesis is dependent on __Vit. K__ to act as a catalyst.

19. List the four primary causative factors of disseminated intravascular coagulation (DIC):
    a. infection
    b.
    c.
    d.

20. List the eight primary manifestations of acute DIC:
    a.
    b.
    c.
    d.
    e.
    f.
    g.
    h.

21. Hemophilia is most often found in _____
_____.

22. True or False

_____ Anemia is a disease with a number of underlying pathologic processes leading to an abnormality in RBC numbers.

_____ Older adults are at increased risk for anemia.

_____ Clients with mild anemia typically present with complaints of exertional dyspnea.

_____ People whose diets lack meat are at greatest risk for iron-deficiency anemia.

_____ Iron-deficiency anemia is the most prevalent hematologic disorder worldwide.

_____ Infants, children, and all adolescents are high risk for iron-deficiency anemia.

_____ A lack of interest in food preparation contributes to a higher prevalence of iron-deficiency anemia in older adults.

_____ Iron is used in the bone marrow to form iron compounds called *heme* that are responsible for synthesis of the molecule responsible for transport of oxygen.

_____ Thalassemia is thought to be a response to endemic malaria.

_____ Due to diminished sensitivity and nerve damage, clients with pernicious anemia are at high risk for injury.

_____ Folic acid deficiency can occur during pregnancy due an increased demand for folate.

_____ Sickle cell anemia is a hereditary hemoglobinopathy.

_____ Sickle cell anemia is the most common anemia worldwide.

_____ The peak incidence of PV is in the group 50 to 70 years of age.

_____ Clinical manifestations of PV are related to hypoxia.

_____ The most common cause of agranulocytosis is drug or chemical toxicity or hypersensitivity.

_____ If left untreated, clients with agranulocytosis develop overwhelming infection and septicemia and die.

_____ Multiple myeloma is a malignancy of the plasma B-cell.

_____ The Epstein-Barr virus (EBV), which causes 85% of infectious mononucleosis, is a herpes virus.

_____ Splenectomy cures secondary hypersplenism.

_____ Hypoprothrombinemia is a congenital or acquired deficiency of the clotting factor VIII.

_____ DIC is a loss of balance between the clotting and lysing systems in the body.

APPLYING SKILLS

23. Which of the following statements by a client with anemia indicate that he or she needs further teaching about iron supplement therapy?
   1. "I should take one 325 mg tablet orally 3–4 times a day."
   2. "When possible, I should take my pills with milk to increase absorption."
   3. "My stools may look black."
   4. "I may experience constipation when taking this drug."

24. A client has a nursing diagnosis of Activity intolerance related to decreased blood supply or low Hgb levels. A nurse would know that the outcome of activity tolerance has been met when the client:
   1. has difficulty sitting up.
   2. participates in ADLs without dyspnea.
   3. walks short distances with a heart rate of 110 bpm.
   4. complains of shortness of breath while bathing.

25. A nurse provides teaching to a client with a nursing diagnosis of Imbalanced nutrition, less than body requirements related to disease, treatment, or lack of knowledge of adequate nutrition. Which statement made by the client indicates that teaching has been effective?
   1. "I should eat a diet high in proteins and fats."
   2. "I should eat three regularly scheduled meals daily."
   3. "I should eat egg whites instead of the yolk."
   4. "Liver is the richest source of iron."

26. Complete the table for the laboratory values for iron deficiency anemia and indicate if the value is increased or decreased.

Laboratory Value	Increased or Decreased
1. Hgb	
2. RBC	
3. MCV	
4. MCH	
5. MCHC	
6. Serum iron	
7. Total iron binding capacity	

27. The nurse is teaching the client with pernicious anemia about adherence to the treatment regimen. Which statement indicates understanding of the teaching?
    1. If I follow the treatment that is prescribed, I will not have as much nerve pain.
    2. I will take vitamin B$_{12}$ for a month and my treatment will be complete.
    3. Symptoms of my disease are not serious and will not get worse than they are right now.
    4. My constipation will disappear if I increase my fiber and water intake.

28. The two primary indications for splenectomy are _____ and _____ _____.

29. True or False

    _____   In folic acid deficiency, the Schilling test is abnormal.

    _____   African-American parents should be encouraged to have themselves and their children tested for the presence of Hb-S.

BEST PRACTICES

30. List the eight interventions that are used to control the causes of anemia:
    a.

    b.

    c.

    d.

    e.

    f.

    g.

    h.

31. When clients with severe chronic anemia have responded poorly to other forms of therapy, _____ is an appropriate intervention.

32. Explain the procedure that is initiated if the nurse suspects a transfusion reaction.

33. The infusion set for blood administration usually contains a _____ mm filter to _____. The tubing should be changed every _____ hours to avoid septicemia.

34. Explain the rationale for encouraging activity, such as walking, for the client with multiple myeloma.

35. A critical nursing intervention for clients with DIC and their families is to provide _____ _____.

36. True or False

_____ Because most of the care for clients with anemia occurs in an outpatient clinic or the client's home, teaching is critical to effective management.

_____ Blood components that contain a significant volume of plasma or other diluents are infused at a slow rate through a large gauge needle.

_____ Blood components not used can be returned to inventory for up to 3 hours out of monitored storage.

_____ An estimated 40% of transfusion reactions are due to labeling errors.

_____ Blood warmers are used to promote comfort for the client and have no therapeutic value.

_____ Autologous blood donations are tolerated well by most clients, including those with heart disease, every 3 days with a Hb of 11 or higher.

_____ Sickle cell crisis is a medical emergency and requires immediate attention.

_____ Teaching clients with sickle cell disease to avoid dehydration is one way to avoid crisis.

_____ The treatment of choice for multiple myeloma is bone marrow suppression using chemotherapy.

KEEPING DRUG SKILLS SHARP

37. A positive response to iron therapy is evidenced by an increase in _____ in _____ days.

38. What multidrug combinations are used to treat neurologic complications of pernicious anemia?

39. The drug of choice for acute pain control in sickle cell crisis is _____.

40. Which of the following drugs is used to treat deep bone pain in clients with sickle cell disease?
    1. Morphine elixir
    2. NSAIDs
    3. Acetaminophen
    4. Tricyclic antidepressants

41. The drug of choice to treat hyperuricemia in clients with PV is _____.

42. True or False

_____ Clients with a history of a transfusion reaction may receive Benadryl prophylactically.

_____ Recommended daily iron intake for women is 10 mg/daily.

_____ Persons with pernicious anemia require vitamin B_{12} supplementation for life.

_____ Folic acid deficiency can occur with long-term use of Dilantin.

_____ Hydroxyureas are the drug of choice in the treatment of all clients with sickle cell disease.

_____ Infectious mononucleosis is aggressively treated with antibiotics and steroids.

_____ Clients with hemophilia should be taught to take aspirin to decrease joint pain.

CONCEPT MAP EXERCISE

The following questions are based on the concept map *Understanding DIC and Its Treatment* in your textbook.

43. Which of the following treatments in DIC is instituted first?
    1. Administration of platelets
    2. Administration of fresh frozen plasma
    3. Administration of heparin
    4. Treatment of the underlying problem

44. The pathophysiologic process that leads to tissue necrosis is:
    1. consumption of clotting factors.
    2. endothelial damage.
    3. occlusion of small blood vessels.
    4. inhibition of platelet function.

45. A factor that directly contributes to the intrinsic pathway of coagulation is:
    1. activation of fibrinolytic system.
    2. consumption of clotting factors.
    3. increased tissue thromboplastin.
    4. endothelial damage.

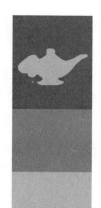

CHAPTER **76**

Management of Clients with Immune Disorders

CHAPTER OBJECTIVES

76.1   Identify hypersensitivity as a manifestation of an immune disorder.
76.2   Identify causative agents and risk factors for hypersensitivity reactions.
76.3   Relate the pathophysiology, including types of reactions and clinical manifestations of hypersensitivity.
76.4   Identify diagnostic tests for allergies.
76.5   Describe the desired outcomes for medical and nursing management of the allergic client.
76.6   Describe specific allergic disorders and treatment.

UNDERSTANDING PATHOPHYSIOLOGY

1. Which of the following statements are true regarding allergy?
   1. Allergy involves immunoglobulin E (IgE) formation.
   2. *Hypersensitivity* and *allergy* are not synonymous.
   3. Allergy represents a decreased response to an allergen.
   4. Over 50% of the population has allergies.

2. Factors that influence manifestations of allergies include: (Select all that apply.)
   1. gender.
   2. exposure to secondhand smoke.
   3. noise pollution.
   4. age.

3. List four routes by which an allergen can enter the body:
   a.

   b.

   c.

   d.

4. Factors that influence the likelihood of developing an allergy include: (Select all that apply.)
   1. exposure later in life rather than earlier.
   2. the type of allergen.
   3. the allergen load.
   4. having January as a birth month.

5. Arrange the following pathophysiologic events in the order in which they occur in an immediate reaction.

   _____ Increased vascular permeability

   _____ IgE production in response to allergen

   _____ Degranulation of mast cells and basophils

   _____ Activation of mast cells and basophils

   _____ Release of histamine, leukotrienes

6. The cells responsible for delaying an inflammatory response after mast cells have been activated are the _____ cells.

7. List the four main types of hypersensitivity reactions:
   a.

   b.

   c.

   d.

8. Which of the following is associated with an anaphylactic hypersensitivity reaction?
   1. Chills and fever
   2. Hypertension
   3. Coughing
   4. Hives

9. Arrange the following pathophysiologic events in the order in which they occur in a cytotoxic reaction.

   _____ Tissue injury

   _____ Antibody binding

   _____ Cell destruction of cell where antigen is bound

   _____ Activation of the complement system

10. Clinical manifestations associated with a blood transfusion reaction include: (Select all that apply.)
    1. hypertension.
    2. glucosuria.
    3. bradycardia.
    4. urticaria.

11. A localized area of tissue necrosis that results from immune complex hypersensitivity is called a _____ reaction.

12. A typical clinical manifestation of contact dermatitis reaction is:
    1. hypotension.
    2. hematuria.
    3. vesicular lesions.
    4. pain.

13. List three factors that are considered in the diagnosis of allergic disease:

    a.

    b.

    c.

14. List the two classifications for adverse food reactions:

    a.

    b.

15. Food intolerances:
    1. occur most often in young- and middle-aged adults.
    2. are less prevalent than food allergies.
    3. result in food-induced anaphylaxis.
    4. are commonly manifested by diarrhea and vomiting.

16. Match each allergen associated with allergic rhinitis with the appropriate time of occurrence.

Allergen	Most Frequent Time of Occurrence
_____ a. Animal dander	1. Spring
_____ b. Ragweed	2. Summer
_____ c. Tree pollen	3. Fall
_____ d. Grasses	4. Winter
	5. Year-round

17. Arrange the following pathophysiologic events in the order in which they occur in allergic rhinitis.

_____ Watery nasal discharge, sneezing, and nasal itching

_____ Mediator release

_____ Allergen exposure

_____ Binding of IgE to receptors on mast cells and basophils

_____ Increased production of IgE

_____ Nasal swelling

18. True or False

_____ It is believed that environmental factors acting either before or after birth contribute to the increasing prevalence of allergic disease.

_____ Due to a direct correlation between higher concentrations of allergens and the intensity of the response, subsequent lower concentrations can induce more severe reactions when reexposure occurs.

_____ Blood transfusions are associated with anaphylactic hypersensitivity reactions.

_____ Serum sickness develops 21 to 28 days after injection with a foreign serum.

_____ A positive skin test reaction indicates antibody response to a previous exposure to an antigen.

_____ The distinguishing factor between food allergies and food intolerances is a specific IgE mediated response.

APPLYING SKILLS

19. The allergy test used for the diagnosis of asthma is:
    1. blood assays for IgE.
    2. skin testing.
    3. radioallergosorbent test (RAST).
    4. pulmonary function tests.

20. Negative results of a skin test may indicate: (Select all that apply.)
    1. the client is immunocompromised.
    2. the client has taken antihistamines within 72 hours.
    3. the antigen was likely introduced subcutaneously.
    4. antibodies did not form to the antigen.

21. A radioallergosorbent test:
    1. is more sensitive than skin testing.
    2. is less time-consuming and costly.
    3. involves blood incubated with a paper disc bound with allergen.
    4. is most widely used due to increased sensitivity and specificity.

BEST PRACTICES

22. List the four nursing interventions to be initiated if the nurse suspects a transfusion reaction:
    a.

    b.

    c.

    d.

23. State the most important nursing intervention to prevent a serum sickness.

24. An indication that a client has understood teaching about skin care measures is that the nurse observes the client:
    1. bathing in hot water.
    2. scratching his or her skin.
    3. applying Alpha Keri after bathing.
    4. bathing with a strong antibacterial soap.

25. List appropriate nursing interventions for itching and discomfort at the injection site for a skin test:
    a.

    b.

26. Explain the rationale for having clients wait 30–40 minutes after receiving immunotherapy injections.

27. The most important component of therapy for the client with allergic rhinitis is _____ _____.

28. The standard of diagnosis for food allergies is the _____ _____.

29. The nurse will know that outcomes are achieved for the diagnosis of Readiness for enhanced self-care if the client: (Select all that apply.)
    1. uses a spacer with an inhaler.
    2. uses proper injection technique.
    3. carries an Epi-Pen.
    4. wears an Medic Alert bracelet.

KEEPING DRUG SKILLS SHARP

30. Which of the following types of medication may be administered to a client with severe serum sickness reaction?
    1. Analgesic
    2. Antihistamine
    3. Steroids
    4. Diuretic

31. Explain why newer over-the-counter antihistamines are safer to use than traditional antihistamines such a diphenhydramine (Benadryl).

32. A beta$_2$ agonist used to control bronchospasm in asthma is:
    1. fluticasone (Flovent).
    2. cromolyn sodium (Intal).
    3. ipratropium (Atrovent).
    4. albuterol (Ventolin).

33. List the three types of medications commonly used to treat atopic dermatitis:
    a.

    b.

    c.

34. The primary drug for the treatment of urticaria is an _____.

35. True or False
    _____ The administration of penicillin can initiate a serum-sickness–like reaction.
    _____ Oral sympathomimetics such as pseudoephedrine should be used with caution in clients with heart disease and hypertension.

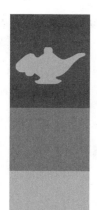

CHAPTER 77

Management of Clients with Rheumatic Disorders

CHAPTER OBJECTIVES

77.1 Explain the rising incidence of rheumatic disorders.

77.2 Relate the concept of autoimmunity to rheumatic disorders.

77.3 Describe the etiology and risk factors for rheumatoid arthritis, connective tissue disorders, and myopathies.

77.4 Relate the pathophysiology and clinical manifestations of rheumatoid arthritis, connective tissue disorders, and myopathies.

77.5 Explain the desired outcomes of medical, surgical, and nursing management of the client with rheumatoid arthritis, connective tissue disorders, and myopathies.

77.6 Explain modifications of care for older clients.

UNDERSTANDING PATHOPHYSIOLOGY

1. _____
    is the primary reason for work-related disability and the leading cause of disability in people 65 years old or older.

2. Factors that have been identified by researchers as having a role in the development of autoimmune inflammatory disorders include: (Select all that apply.)
    1. overuse.
    2. injury.
    3. anorexia.
    4. gene defects.
    5. infection.
    6. immunosuppression.
    7. environmental agents.

3. In addition to morning stiffness in joints, other systemic manifestations of rheumatoid arthritis (RA) include: (Select all that apply.).
    1. obesity.
    2. weight loss.
    3. fatigue.
    4. muscle ache.

4. List the three types of deformities that can result from chronic inflammation of joints and synovial involvement:
    a.

    b.

    c.

5. Identify the manifestations that develop with CREST syndrome in clients with systemic sclerosis.
    C:

    R:

    E:

    S:

    T:

6. Describe the physiologic changes that occur during Raynaud's phenomenon.
   WHITE:

   BLUE:

   RED:

7. The rheumatic joint disease _____ _____ can result as sequelae to infection from a tick-borne spirochete.

APPLYING SKILLS

8. When evaluating effectiveness of therapy for clients with arthritis, the American College of Rheumatology has set the standard as _____ _____.

9. The areas most affected by RA include: (Select all that apply.)
   1. wrists.
   2. metacarpophalangeal (MCP) joints.
   3. proximal interphalangeal (PIP) joints.
   4. knees.
   5. feet.

10. A 52-year-old client who has had arthritis for years has undergone a shoulder arthroplasty. Upon returning to the orthopedic unit, the nursing interventions for postoperative care include elevating the HOB to reduce swelling and assessing the operative arm every 4 hours for _____ _____.

11. A 30-year-old bank teller comes to the clinic complaining of fatigue, painful swollen joints, and fever. Upon physical examination, the nurse notes a reddened rash over the bridge of the nose and cheeks. These symptoms may be indicative of the rheumatic disorder _____ _____.

12. Explain why the nurse should evaluate occupation and hobbies when completing a history from a client with complaints of bursitis.

BEST PRACTICES

13. In teaching the client with ankylosing spondylitis (AS) about measures to maintain mobility, the nurse would instruct the client to: (Select all that apply.)
    1. maintain good posture.
    2. engage in exercises that promote stretching/extension of the spine (e.g., swimming).
    3. select ergonomic chairs and work station equipment.
    4. sleep on one side.

14. A client who works in a business office has been diagnosed with RA. Nursing interventions for client education should include all of the following *except*:
    1. use of adaptive equipment to protect joints.
    2. evaluation of work space for ergonomics.
    3. replacement of incandescent lights with fluorescent lights.
    4. medications to reduce inflammation and pain.

15. State the rationale for each type of exercise used to assist the client with RA.
    a. Range of motion:

    b. Strengthening:

16. List four interventions that research has shown to be effective in assisting clients with RA who experience joint pain.

    a.

    b.

    c.

    d.

17. Nursing actions to protect skin integrity for clients with scleroderma include: (Select all that apply.)
    1. use of pressure-reducing beds or air mattresses.
    2. careful removal of dressing.
    3. dressings secured with stretchable gauze.
    4. IM injections/IV therapy at sites free from fibrosis and sclerosis.
    5. use of large amounts of tape.

18. A client with RA complains of fatigue and disrupted sleep. Nursing interventions to assist this client would include: (Select all that apply.)
    1. medication for pain and inflammation.
    2. maintaining a regular sleep schedule.
    3. consumption of one glass of wine before bed.
    4. use of small pillows, lightweight blankets.
    5. engaging in soothing activities.

KEEPING DRUG SKILLS SHARP

19. Common disease modifying anti-rheumatic drugs (DMARDs) used today in the clinical setting include: (Select all that apply.)
    1. methotrexate.
    2. leflunomide.
    3. etanercept.
    4. infliximab.

20. Treatment of systemic lupus erythematosus (SLE) involves use of _____ and _____ to suppress inflammation.

21. Use of NSAIDs to control inflammation in SLE should be closely monitored if there is evidence of _____ _____.

22. To control the symptoms of Raynaud's disease, _____ is used as a calcium channel blocker resulting in vasodilation.

23. In the treatment of scleroderma, _____ _____ is used as an immumodulating agent that interferes with the cross-linking of collagen, reducing the deposits.

24. List the categories of medications used to treat clients with fibromyalgia and the rationale for each.

    a.

    b.

    c.

    d.

    e.

CONCEPT MAP EXERCISES

The following questions are based on the concept map *Understanding Rheumatoid Arthritis and Its Treatment* in the textbook.

25. How does administering intravenous immunoglobulin G treat the manifestations of rheumatoid arthritis?

26. When the synovium of the joint is inflamed, as with RA, how does that result in subsequent destruction of that joint area?

27. What combination of medications is given during the inflammatory phase of RA to decrease pain?

29. What clinical manifestations are treated with direct injection of steroids into the joint space?

28. During the destruction phase of RA, what mechanism *causes* the tissue damage?

30. Which clinical manifestations are permanent without surgical correction?

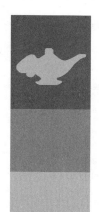

CHAPTER 78

Management of Clients with Acquired Immunodeficiency Syndrome

CHAPTER OBJECTIVES

78.1 Describe the magnitude and the impact of HIV/AIDS in the U.S. and worldwide.
78.2 Describe the etiology and risk factors for HIV transmission.
78.3 Discuss safe sexual practices.
78.4 Relate the magnitude of HIV infections to exposure to contaminated blood.
78.5 Discuss the occupational hazard of HIV for health care workers.
78.6 Describe the pathophysiology of HIV including the mechanism for virus replication.
78.7 Relate laboratory changes in cells to the potential for occurrence of infection.
78.8 Describe clinical manifestations as they relate to the classification system for HIV.
78.9 Discuss the concept of viral load testing.
78.10 Describe medical management goals for the person with HIV infection.
78.11 Identify pharmacologic agents for treatment of HIV including the HAART regimen.
78.12 Identify treatment regimens for infection prevention in HIV clients.
78.13 Describe assessments, outcomes, and interventions for specific nursing diagnoses related to HIV and AIDS.
78.14 Describe education of the client to aid in preventing spread of HIV.
78.15 Discuss compliance related to antiretroviral drug therapy for HIV.
78.16 Describe the AIDS indicator diseases and subsequent treatment.
78.17 Relate stages of AIDS dementia to potential impairment.
78.18 Describe HIV wasting syndrome.

TRENDS AND ISSUES

1. In 2006, there were more than _____ people living with HIV/AIDS.

2. There were more than _____ new HIV infections in 2005.

3. AIDS is the _____ leading cause of death worldwide.

4. Groups at risk for HIV/AIDS include:
    a.

    b.

    c.

    d.

    e.

    f.

5. The cost of treating one person can be more than _____ per year.

6. _____ limits accessibility to appropriate health care in many parts of the world.

UNDERSTANDING PATHOPHYSIOLOGY

7. The genetic subtype of HIV that predominates in North America and Europe is _____.

8. List the three primary modes of HIV transmission:
   a.

   b.

   c.

9. The greatest risk of occupational exposure to HIV for the health care worker is through _____ _____.

10. Place the following steps in the depletion of T helper cells in the order in which they occur.

   _____ The virus is uncoated, and RNA enters the cell.

   _____ HIV attaches to the target cell membrane via its CD4 receptor.

   _____ The cell may function abnormally.

   _____ The newly created DNA moves into the nucleus and the DNA of the cell.

   _____ The enzyme known as *reverse transcriptase* is released, and viral RNA is transcribed into DNA.

   _____ A provirus is created when the viral DNA integrates itself into the cellular DNA or genome of the cell.

   _____ The host cell dies, and viral budding occurs.

   _____ When the provirus is in place, its genetic material is no longer pure cell but is part virus.

11. An individual will likely develop an infection at a CD4 cell count below _____ _____.

12. Differentiate between a long-term nonprogressor and a long-term survivor.

13. Normally antibodies to HIV can be detected _____ weeks after exposure.

14. Which of the following individuals is at risk for having a false-positive test result for HIV?
   1. Person with osteoarthritis
   2. Person with lung cancer
   3. Person with lupus erythematosus
   4. Person with anemia

15. List the four main types of opportunistic infections:
   a.

   b.

   c.

   d.

16. How is the Kaposi's sarcoma in AIDS clients different from that seen in other populations?
   a.

   b.

   c.

17. List one local and one systemic therapy for Kaposi's sarcoma.
   Local:

   Systemic:

18. Clients with invasive cervical cancer often present with _____.

19. The first manifestation of *P. carinii* pneumonia is _____.

20. True or False

   _____ HIV-1 and HIV-2 are two distinct and separate viruses.

   _____ The ability of the HIV virus to change its appearance or mutate is called *genetic promiscuity*.

_____ Sexual preferences versus sexual practices place individuals at greatest risk for HIV.

_____ Most people are infected with *P. carinii* in the early preschool years.

_____ Toxoplasmosis can be acquired through direct handling of contaminated dog feces.

_____ Cervical intraepithelial neoplasia occurs at a high rate in women infected with HIV.

APPLYING SKILLS

21. List two monitoring parameters that are used to follow a client with HIV:

    a.

    b.

22. Which of the following viral load test results poses a high risk for AIDS?
    1.   10,000 copies/ml
    2.   10,000-100,000 copies/ml
    3.   >100,000 copies/ml

23. Prior to initiating teaching for the client with HIV, it is important for the nurse to assess the client's
    _____.

24. List two areas of concern when doing follow-up on a client with AIDS dementia:

    a.

    b.

25. True or False

    _____ Urine tests for detecting HIV infection are as accurate as serologic testing.

    _____ During the assessment of clinical manifestations of HIV-infected clients, it is important to try to quantify the clinical manifestation.

    _____ Clients who manifest an AIDS-defining disease are classified into group B.

BEST PRACTICES

26. Explain how the health care worker can decrease his or her risk of occupational exposure to HIV.

27. List the crisis points at which the nurse can anticipate anxiety, fear, or depression in the client with HIV disease:

    a.

    b.

    c.

    d.

    e.

    f.

28. Which of the following should the nurse include in the teaching plan for an HIV-infected person? (Select all that apply.)
    1.   Interpretation of viral load tests
    2.   The importance of limiting exercise
    3.   Eating a high-calorie, low-protein, low-fat diet
    4.   Routine mouth care
    5.   Proper handwashing
    6.   Skin care

29. List three drugs used to treat HIV wasting syndrome:

    a.

    b.

    c.

30. List the nonpharmacologic nursing interventions for a client with fever:
    a.

    b.

    c.

31. Explain the rationale for avoiding tepid sponge baths for the treatment of fever.

32. The nurse should teach the client with fatigue to avoid consumption of all of the following *except*:
    1. coffee.
    2. tobacco.
    3. sugar.
    4. alcohol.

33. True or False

    _____ Autologous blood programs limit the transmission of HIV through blood product administration.

    _____ Alternative and complementary therapies provide positive benefits and should be encouraged if the client believes they are helpful.

    _____ Aerobic exercise, which increases endurance, can reduce fatigue.

    _____ Cooking with herbs and spices is an appropriate intervention to counter anorexia secondary to hyperosmia.

    _____ Physical therapy modalities such as massage, transcutaneous electrical nerve stimulation (TENS), and application of heat and cold can be helpful in reducing pain.

34. Identify the absolutely, very, and probably safe practices to limit exposure to HIV through injected drug use.
    Absolutely safe:

    Very safe:

    Probably safe:

35. Identify the completely safe and very safe sexual practices to limit exposure to HIV.
    Completely safe:

    Very safe:

KEEPING DRUG SKILLS SHARP

36. The antiretroviral agents that prevent HIV from entering healthy T-cells in the body are:
    1. NRTIs.
    2. PIs.
    3. NNRTIs.
    4. entry inhibitors.

37. The first NRTI was _____ _____.

38. Match each drug with the appropriate reason for administration.

Drug		**Reason for Administration**
_____	a. Trimethoprim-sulfamethoxazole	1. Respiratory infections
_____	b. Clarithromycin	2. Traveler's diarrhea
_____	c. Pyridoxine	3. *P. carinii* pneumonia
_____	d. Ciprofloxacin	4. *M. avium*-intracellulare complex
_____	e. Pneumococcal vaccine	5. Peripheral neuropathy

39. To sustain the durability and efficacy of antiretroviral therapy, clients must maintain compliance _____ of the time.

40. True or False

_____ Most clinicians recommend starting an antiretroviral combination therapy regimen early in the course of the disease.

_____ A potential benefit of antiretroviral therapy is decreased risk for development of HIV resistance to drugs.

_____ A potential risk of antiretroviral therapy is unknown long-term toxicity of antiretroviral therapy.

_____ Amphotericin B is used to treat disseminated disease of *Candida albicans*.

_____ It is unusual for clients to sleep for extended periods during the first few days of a pain control regimen.

_____ Pain therapy regimens increase the diarrhea common in clients with HIV.

41. A client with HIV infection has the nursing diagnosis Risk for ineffective therapeutic regimen management. Which outcome would indicate that goals have been met?
1. No progression to an AIDS-defining illness.
2. The client self reports 100% compliance with drug therapy.
3. Another person reports the client's compliance.
4. The client has a CD4 count drawn every 6 months.

42. List three strategies to improve compliance with the medication regimen.
a.

b.

c.

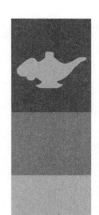

CHAPTER 79

Management of Clients with Leukemia and Lymphoma

CHAPTER OBJECTIVES

79.1 Define *leukemia* and *lymphoma* including Hodgkin's and non-Hodgkin's lymphoma.
79.2 Describe the etiology and risk factors of leukemia and the lymphomas.
79.3 Describe the pathophysiology of leukemia and Hodgkin's and non-Hodgkin's lymphoma.
79.4 Compare and contrast acute and chronic leukemia.
79.5 Differentiate ALL and AML (ANLL), and CML and CLL.
79.6 Identify the similar clinical manifestations as well as the laboratory diagnostic findings of leukemia.
79.7 Identify the goals of medical treatment for acute and chronic leukemia, and the lymphomas.
79.8 Describe the medical treatment to address each goal.
79.9 Identify the nursing management diagnoses and outcomes for the leukemias and lymphomas.
79.10 Describe the staging and classification of Hodgkin's and non-Hodgkin's lymphoma.
79.11 Discuss bone marrow transplants including the indications, harvesting, donor preparation, and nursing management.
79.12 Describe graft-versus-host disease as a complication of transplants.

UNDERSTANDING PATHOPHYSIOLOGY

1. Match each term with the appropriate definition.

Term

_____ a. Hematopoietic cells
_____ b. Lymphoid cells
_____ c. Leukemia
_____ d. Lymphoma

Definition

1. Cancer of the bone marrow
2. Cells that originate in the bone marrow
3. Cancer of the lymphoid tissue
4. Cells that originate in the lymphoid cells

2. List the risk factors for leukemia.
   a.

   b.

   c.

   d.

3. The leukemia most commonly found in children is _____.

4. The leukemia most commonly found in adults is _____.

5. List the three clinical history manifestations commonly associated with leukemia.
   a.

   b.

   c.

6. A complication associated with the rapid destruction of a large number of WBCs is known as
_____.

7. Characteristic clinical manifestations of non-Hodgkin's lymphoma (NHL) include: (Select all that apply.)
   1. ascites.
   2. back pain.
   3. abdominal masses.
   4. painful lymphadenopathy.

8. Identify and explain the three sources of bone marrow.

9. Graft-versus-host disease (GVHD) may occur _____ to _____ days after infusion of viable lymphocytes.

10. True or False
   _____ The client's risk for acquiring chronic lymphocytic leukemia increases with age.
   _____ NHL is 60 times more common in people with AIDS than in the general population of the United States.
   _____ Chronic GVHD resembles systemic lupus erythematosus.

APPLYING SKILLS

11. A client with leukemia reports having an increased sensitivity to sour and sweet tastes. The nurses recognizes this is associated with:
   1. facial nerve involvement.
   2. meningeal irritation.
   3. anorexia.
   4. lymphadenopathy.

12. The primary diagnostic tool for leukemia is _____ _____.

13. A nurse is caring for a client experiencing tumor lysis syndrome. The nurse would expect the electrolytes to reveal:
   1. hyponatremia.
   2. hypercalcemia.
   3. hypokalemia.
   4. hyperkalemia.
   5. hypernatremia.

14. List two criteria the nurse should check for before administering blood to a client receiving treatment for leukemia.
   a.

   b.

15. A nurse is assessing a client with chronic lymphocytic leukemia. Which of the following manifestations would the nurse expect due to the reduced production of RBCs?
   1. Insomnia
   2. Increased appetite
   3. Weight gain
   4. Decreased attention span

16. A manifestation consistent with a decrease in platelet function is:
   1. hard, brown stool.
   2. diminished menstrual flow.
   3. hematuria.
   4. heat intolerance.

17. A client is experiencing altered tissue perfusion related to anemia. The nurse would expect to find all of the following when assessing the vital signs *except*:
   1. increase in respirations.
   2. increase in blood pressure.
   3. increase in pulse.
   4. decrease in blood pressure.

18. True or False
   _____ A complete blood count of a patient with leukemia may reveal a WBC count as normal, low, or high.

Case Study
A client has a nursing diagnosis of Ineffective protection/risk for infection related to neutropenia or leukocytosis secondary to leukemia or treatment.

19. Identify appropriate outcomes for this nursing diagnosis.

20. Calculate the absolute neutrophil count (ANC) for this client with the following values: 1% bands, 42% segs, 1650 WBC.

21. Based on the ANC count of the client described above, would the nurse place the client in protective isolation? Why or why not?

22. The client ordered a fresh fruit salad on the menu but did not receive it when the meal was served. The client noted that the salad had been marked out and was substituted with applesauce. What explanation would the nurse provide to the client?

23. Which of the following orders for this would the nurse question and why?
    a. Notify physician for temperature > 38° C
    b. Frequent oral hygiene with soft-bristle brush
    c. Pericolace, 1 PO, OD
    d. Tylenol suppository for fever > 37.5° C

BEST PRACTICES

24. Explain the rationale for not performing a lumbar puncture during the acute phase of leukemia.

25. What should the nurse teach the client with a nursing diagnosis of Imbalanced nutrition, less than body requirements related to anorexia, pain, or fatigue about his or her diet?

26. A client voices concern about losing his or her hair secondary to chemotherapy. What should the nurse teach the client about this hair loss?

27. Explain the role of the clinical nurse specialist or case manager for the client with a nursing diagnosis of Risk for ineffective therapeutic regimen management and risk for ineffective family therapeutic regimen management.

KEEPING DRUG SKILLS SHARP

28. Which of the following medications is added during stage IV treatment of chronic lymphocytic leukemia?
    1. Prednisone
    2. Leukeran
    3. Fludarabine
    4. Potassium chloride

29. Explain why the client with a nursing diagnosis of Ineffective protection/risk for hemorrhage related to thrombocytopenia secondary to either leukemia or treatment should not receive aspirin or medications containing aspirin.

31. For chronic myelogenous leukemia, Gleevec (imatinib mesylate) inhibits proliferation and induces _____ and targets cells that are positive for the _____

    _____.

30. List the drugs administered in ABVD therapy for Hodgkin's disease and explain why this regimen is preferable to MOPP.

    a.

    b.

    c.

    d.

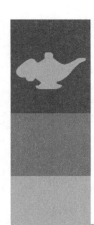

CHAPTER 80

Management of Clients Requiring Transplantation

CHAPTER OBJECTIVES

80.1 Relate the history of transplantation to current transplants for end-stage organ disease.

80.2 Identify the major issues related to organ transplantation.

80.3 Examine the website www.unos.org/data/ for current statistics on organ donors.

80.4 Describe outcome management for the client being selected for and awaiting a donor.

80.5 Discuss organ donation as a "gift of life" and the coordination of donation activities.

80.6 Discuss the role of the nurse in organ donation.

80.7 Describe the preparation of the transplant recipient and the subsequent postoperative immunosuppressive care.

80.8 Identify complications of transplantation.

80.9 Discuss specific organ transplantation.

80.10 Describe self-care necessary to avoid rejection and infection following organ transplantation.

UNDERSTANDING PATHOPHYSIOLOGY

1. There is a significant limitation to organ transplantation due to:
   1. increased use of medications that affect transplant reactions.
   2. shortage of organ donors.
   3. numerous insurance claims which do not cover cost.
   4. clients choosing other options.

2. _____ is the leading cause of morbidity and mortality after transplantation.

3. Acute rejection of organs usually occurs within _____ _____.

4. Chronic rejection of organs usually occurs after _____ _____.

5. Opportunistic infections are very common within the first 6 months after transplantation. These infections include: (Select all that apply.)
   1. *Pneumocystis carinii* pneumonia.
   2. candidiasis.
   3. cytomegalovirus (CMV).
   4. *Staphylococcus aureus*.

APPLYING SKILLS

6. The nurse's role in organ donation and organ recovery includes: (Select all that apply.)
   1. identifying early potential donors.
   2. making referrals to organ procurement organization.
   3. assisting in medical management of organ donors.
   4. acting as a liaison with donor families.

7. The nurse's role in the post-kidney transplant period is to monitor:
   1. fluid and electrolyte balance.
   2. electrocardiograms (ECGs).
   3. overall renal function.
   4. ejection fraction and jugular vein distention.

8. A physiologic alteration seen in the post-cardiac transplantation client is:
   1. absence of angina.
   2. electrolyte imbalances.
   3. severe graft pain.
   4. increased risk of diabetes.

9. Important self-care practices post-transplantation include: (Select all that apply.)
   1. regular dental checkups.
   2. annual ophthalmologic exams.
   3. vigilant monitoring for infection.
   4. influenza vaccine.

BEST PRACTICES

10. The improved success of organ transplantation today is due to: (Select all that apply.)
    1. availability of new immunosuppressive therapies.
    2. advancements in organ preservation.
    3. improved surgical techniques.
    4. risk factor recognition that enhances survival.

11. The _____ (amended 1972) covers the cost of dialysis and transplantation for end-stage renal disease.

12. The criteria used by the Uniform Determination of Death Act state that an individual is considered dead if: (Select all that apply.)
    1. there is irreversible cessation of circulatory and respiratory functions.
    2. there is irreversible cessation of all functions of the entire brain and brain stem.
    3. only respiratory functions remain.
    4. cardiac functions are maintained only due to medication administration.

13. Which act was passed to prohibit the sale of human organs?
    1. Social Security Act of 1972
    2. United Network of Organ Sharing Act
    3. Uniform Determination of Death Act
    4. National Organ Transplant Act 1984

14. _____ is the transplantation of organs, tissues, or cells from one species to another, and has been proposed as one answer to the organ donor shortage.

15. The primary responsibility of an organ transplant team is to:
    1. transplant organs into clients who have the best chance for a long-term successful outcome.
    2. identify donors and maintain a list for future transplants.
    3. maintain a database of successful transplants for future research.
    4. educate other health professionals regarding organ transplant procedures.

16. Successful transplant recipients will have: (Select all that apply.)
    1. improved functional status.
    2. long-term graft function.
    3. improved quality of life.
    4. no need for other medications for life-sustaining purposes.

17. True or False
    _____ The nurse plays an integral role in pre-operative education of potential organ recipients.

    _____ Nurses are encouraged to meet with other health professionals to discuss their feelings and difficult cases, as well as to develop plans of care for their clients.

18. The goal of education of a potential organ recipient is to: (Select all that apply.)
    1. provide the family with factual information regarding waiting time for organs.
    2. explain surgical procedures.
    3. explain post-transplantation regimens (diet, exercise, medications).
    4. explain routine skin grafting procedures.

19. The criteria maintained by the United Network of Organ Sharing (UNOS) for listing a client for organ transplantation is based on: (Select all that apply.)
    1. urgency.
    2. blood type.
    3. recipient weight and height.
    4. medical condition.

20. During the period when clients are waiting for organ transplants, the nurse will: (Select all that apply.)
    1. establish a trusting relationship with the client.
    2. participate in client education.
    3. work with clients so they grasp the realities of life after transplantation.
    4. refer clients to another system of care if needed.

21. Problems that clients with organ transplants may encounter include: (Select all that apply.)
    1. medication side effects.
    2. rejection of organs.
    3. financial limitations.
    4. preservation of other organs.

22. Organ transplantation teams consist of: (Select all that apply.)
    1. transplant surgeon, psychologist, other physicians.
    2. nurse coordinator, nurse practitioner.
    3. social worker.
    4. pharmacist, nutritionist.
    5. clergy.

KEEPING DRUG SKILLS SHARP

23. The goal of immunosuppressive therapy in organ transplantation is to: (Select all that apply.)
    1. suppress immune response to prevent organ rejection.
    2. prolong complications from therapy itself.
    3. give massive doses of medications.
    4. identify graft resources.

24. Excessive immunosuppressive therapy can lead to: (Select all that apply.)
    1. increased risk of infection.
    2. liver or kidney insufficiency.
    3. joint necrosis.
    4. cataracts or malignancies.
    5. rejection of transplanted organ.

USING RESOURCES

25. Log onto the UNOS website at www.unos.org/data/. View the transplant waiting list for your state. How many total individuals are awaiting organ transplantation? Which organ has the longest wait? Why do you think that is? Which organ does not have a long list of people waiting for a long time? Why do you think that is?

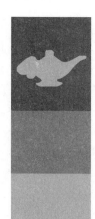

CHAPTER **81**

Management of Clients with Shock and Multisystem Disorders

CHAPTER OBJECTIVES

81.1 Define *shock* and *multiple organ dysfunction syndrome* (MODS).

81.2 Describe the basic etiologies of shock, specific types of shock, and MODS.

81.3 Identify the classifications of shock and MODS.

81.4 Identify similarities and differences among the various types of shock.

81.5 Relate the pathophysiology and clinical manifestations of shock, specific types of shock, and MODS.

81.6 Describe generally recognized stages of shock.

81.7 Explain the systemic effects of shock.

81.8 Identify the diagnostic assessment of client with shock.

81.9 Identify the appropriate outcomes for the nursing and medical interventions for clients with shock and MODS.

81.10 Discuss current medications used to treat shock.

81.11 Discuss the prognosis of the client with MODS.

UNDERSTANDING PATHOPHYSIOLOGY

1. Shock can be defined as:
   1. failure of the circulatory system to maintain adequate perfusion of vital organs.
   2. decreased oxygenation at the cellular level.
   3. anaerobic cellular metabolism.
   4. accumulated waste products in the system.

2. Shock can be categorized into which of following types? (Select all that apply.)
   1. Distributive
   2. Hypovolemic
   3. Cardiogenic
   4. Muscle-related

3. A client admitted to the clinic with burns, hemorrhage, or dehydration may develop:
   1. hypovolemic shock.
   2. distributive shock.
   3. cardiogenic shock.
   4. neurologic shock.

4. Cardiogenic shock is caused by: (Select all that apply.)
   1. inadequate pumping action of the heart.
   2. primary cardiac muscle dysfunction.
   3. mechanical obstruction of blood flow.
   4. valvular insufficiency resulting from disease or trauma.

5. All clients with spinal cord injuries experience some degree of:
   1. septic shock.
   2. neurogenic shock.
   3. distributive shock.
   4. cardiac shock.

6. The primary events that precipitate hypovolemic shock are: (Select all that apply.)
   1. inadequate circulation.
   2. reduction in the circulating blood volume.
   3. metabolic needs of the body not being met.
   4. absence of creatine in the circulation.

7. Clients admitted the clinic with large partial-thickness or full-thickness burns will be prone to: (Select all that apply.)
   1. hypovolemic shock.
   2. distributive shock.
   3. anaphylactic shock.
   4. neurogenic shock.

8. The major pathology behind irreversible or refractory shock is:
   1. renal failure.
   2. intestinal mucosa disturbed.
   3. failure of sympathetic nervous system compensation.
   4. cardiac compromise.

APPLYING SKILLS

9. When mechanical obstructions cause blood flow problems that lead to cardiogenic shock, which of the following may occur? (Select all that apply.)
   1. Large pulmonary embolism
   2. Pericardial tamponade
   3. Tension pneumothorax
   4. Multiple cerebrovascular accidents

10. Clients admitted to the clinic with anaphylactic reactions may be sensitized to which of the following agents? (Select all that apply.)
    1. Penicillin
    2. Bee stings
    3. Chocolate
    4. Snake venom

11. The major cause of death in shock is _____ _____.

12. During shock, the nurse can expect a client's pulse rate to:
    1. usually increase due to increased sympathetic stimulation.
    2. decrease due to vascular collapse.
    3. usually increase with resultant drop in cardiovascular collapse.
    4. undergo no changes.

13. Clients who have a declining diastolic blood pressure can be potential candidates for:
    1. neurogenic collapse.
    2. decreasing systemic vascular resistance.
    3. abnormal pulse pressures.
    4. no significant changes.

14. Clinical manifestations that are expected with hypovolemic shock include which of the following lab data? (Select all that apply.)
    1. Urine osmolarity increases
    2. Specific gravity of urine increases
    3. Sodium and water reabsorption
    4. No change in urine status

15. Confusion, agitation, and restlessness are clinical signs that a client's level of consciousness has changed due to:
    1. decreased circulation to brain tissue.
    2. abnormal output from urinary status.
    3. elevated cardiac enzymes.
    4. constant change in pH values.

16. Clients who have massive thermal burns and are heading toward irreversible shock will show which of the following laboratory findings?
    1. Increased liver enzymes
    2. Decreased cardiac enzymes
    3. Elevated pH levels
    4. Decreased HCO_3 levels

17. When using Ringer's lactate for fluid replacement therapy for clients with shock, the nurse needs to monitor:
    1. serum pH levels.
    2. CPK and LDH levels.
    3. ammonia levels.
    4. serum calcium levels.

18. Arterial blood gas analysis may be done during the shock phase to determine: (Select all that apply.)
    1. if metabolic acidosis that occurs with shock is being effectively combated by hyperventilation.
    2. adequate oxygen levels.
    3. if further respiratory assistance is needed.
    4. a baseline for CO_2 replacement.

19. The primary goals in treating shock are to: (Select all that apply.)
    1. establish vaso-peripheral circulation.
    2. maintain adequate circulating blood volume.
    3. restore vital potassium circulating levels.
    4. increase demands for oxygenation.

BEST PRACTICES

20. The priority in emergency management of shock is to: (Select all that apply.)
    1. provide for emergency intubations.
    2. place client in reverse Trendenlenburg position.
    3. provide fluid resuscitation.
    4. establish intravenous access sites.

KEEPING DRUG SKILLS SHARP

21. The mainstay of hypovolemic shock therapy is: (Select all that apply.)
    1. expansion of circulating blood volume.
    2. IV administration of blood or other appropriate fluids.
    3. increased dilation of heart vessels.
    4. establishment of baseline respiratory status.

22. When large volumes of fluid are given, the nurse must be aware of the client's urinary status. Aggressive fluid replacement should be tapered off when: (Select all that apply.)
    1. urinary output is at least 60 ml/hr.
    2. blood pressure is greater than 100 mm Hg.
    3. heart rate is 60–100 beats per minute.
    4. the client's ability to tolerate foods has been assessed.

23. IV fluids used in shock management may include: (Select all that apply.)
    1. warmed crystalloids.
    2. balanced salt solutions.
    3. colloids.
    4. blood products.

24. When hemorrhage is the primary cause of shock, rapid administration which of the following is indicated? (Select all that apply.)
    1. Large volumes of packed cells
    2. Whole blood
    3. IV fluids of dextrose
    4. Rapid rate extenders of fluids

25. The drug of choice for treating of allergic reactions and anaphylaxis is:
    1. epinephrine.
    2. antibiotics.
    3. urinary stimulants.
    4. glucose inhibitors.

26. Medications that improve myocardial contractions are used in treating types of shock that decrease cardiac output. Examples of these medications include: (Select all that apply.)
    1. digitalis.
    2. amiodarone.
    3. lidocaine.
    4. atropine.

27. Which medication can inhibit coagulation when given to the client in shock?
    1. Drotrecogin Alfa
    2. Naloxone
    3. Epinephrine
    4. Sucralfate

28. When used in a client in shock, naloxone has which action?
    1. Reverses opioid overdose
    2. Reverses hypotension
    3. Improves coagulation
    4. Increases central venous pressure

29. Explain why a nondiabetic client in shock would receive insulin.

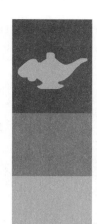

CHAPTER 82

Management of Clients in the Emergency Department

CHAPTER OBJECTIVES

82.1 Describe the scope of emergency care in the United States.
82.2 Identify goals of emergency medical services.
82.3 Describe the focus of emergency nursing.
82.4 Identify important legal and ethical issues that are significant in the emergency department.
82.5 Identify components of care in the emergency department.
82.6 Describe specific emergency conditions, manifestations, and outcomes management.

TRENDS AND THEORIES

1. During the _____, the need for specialized emergency care was recognized as a priority.

2. More than _____ clients use the emergency department (ED) for health services each year.

3. The number of EDs in the United States has decreased/increased (circle one) by _____%.

4. Clients aged _____ to _____ have the most frequent ED visits.

5. The scope of treatment in the emergency department ranges from _____
    _____
    to _____
    _____.

6. Identify the components in the definition of emergency nursing.

UNDERSTANDING PATHOPHYSIOLOGY

7. _____ is the universal blood type that can be infused before cross-matched blood is available if needed.

8. Match the following definitions or descriptions with the correct term.

Definition/Description	Term
_____ a. Chest moves opposite of normal respiratory patterns	1. Pneumothorax
_____ b. Occurs with a sucking chest wound	2. Hemopneumothorax
_____ c. Blood and air in the pleural space	3. Tension pneumothorax
_____ d. Fractures of two or more ribs on the same side	4. Open pneumothorax
_____ e. Blood in the pleural space	5. Flail chest
_____ f. Contents of the mediastinum are pushed toward the unaffected side	6. Mediastinal shift
_____ g. Air enters the pleural space and becomes trapped	7. Paradoxical motion
_____ h. Air in the pleural space	8. Hemothorax

APPLYING SKILLS

9. Which of the following types of incidents seen in the ED must be reported to federal, state, and local authorities? (Select all that apply.)
   1. Suspected child abuse
   2. Suspected domestic violence
   3. Suspected elder abuse
   4. Motor vehicle accidents

10. Match the following definitions or descriptions with the correct term.

Definition/Description	Term
_____ a. Any sudden illness or injury that is perceived to be a crisis that threatens the physical or psychological well-being of a person or group	1. Secondary nursing interventions
_____ b. Interventions may be delayed beyond a few hours	2. Priority nursing interventions
_____ c. Occurs when the ED is called for help with a crisis	3. Emergent
_____ d. A complete focused assessment	4. Emergency
_____ e. Requires interventions within a few hours	5. Urgent
_____ f. Life-threatening: the client may die without immediate interventions	6. Telephone triage
_____ g. Interventions focused on emergency care	7. Nonurgent
_____ h. The process of determining priorities	8. Triage

11. The _____
    obligates ED personnel to follow the client's advance directives.

12. If no written information regarding advance directives is available for a client who requires emergency treatment, ED personnel must: (Select all that apply.)
    1. stabilize the client.
    2. resuscitate any client if necessary.
    3. follow appropriate standard treatment guidelines regardless of a family member's expressed wishes.
    4. not provide any treatment for the client.

13. For any client arriving at the ED with a major traumatic injury, primary assessment includes:
    1. determining when the patient ate last.
    2. overall assessment of vital signs.
    3. evaluation of cervical spine area for any potential injury.
    4. location of relatives in the next state.

14. Before clients can be discharged from the ED, they must receive: (Select all that apply.)
    1. fluid and foods to be eaten at home.
    2. oral and written discharge instructions.
    3. written identification of diagnosed problem.
    4. explanation of treatments, complications, and recheck times.

15. Nursing documentation in the ED must include: (Select all that apply.)
    1. assessment findings.
    2. diagnostic tests and interventions.
    3. responses to treatment.
    4. client education.

16. The first priority of care with any client in the ED is:
    1. maintaining a patent airway.
    2. observing for respiratory distress.
    3. securing medical insurance information.
    4. documenting time of arrival.

BEST PRACTICES

17. The goals of the emergency medical services include: (Select all that apply.)
    1. providing emergency care to a client as quickly as possible.
    2. assuring that the "right client arrives at the right hospital."
    3. maintaining professional relationships with the community.
    4. assisting families in securing appropriate referrals when needed.

18. Minors for whom consent of a parent or legal guardian does not need to be obtained in order to treat them include: (Select all that apply.)
    1. emancipated minors.
    2. minors seeking treatment for communicable diseases.
    3. minor-aged females requesting treatment for pregnancy or pregnancy-related concerns.
    4. children with sore throats and fever.

19. Hospital policies and guidelines must comply with which of the following organizations regarding the use of restraints on clients in the ED? (Select all that apply.)
    1. American Medical Association
    2. Joint Commission on Hospital Accreditation
    3. Centers for Medicare and Medicaid Services
    4. National Alliance of Hospital Organizations

20. The treatment priority for a client with an altered level of consciousness is:
    1. protecting the cervical spine.
    2. establishing and maintaining an airway.
    3. determining the length of time since onset of manifestations.
    4. obtaining a past medical history.

KEEPING DRUG SKILLS SHARP

21. Clients who have received fibrinolytic medications in the ED must be continuously monitored for:
    1. increased intracranial pressure.
    2. active bleeding.
    3. visual disturbances.
    4. beta-blocker corrections.

22. When conscious sedation is used in the ED, nursing responsibilities include: (Select all that apply.)
    1. continually monitoring for airway patency.
    2. maintaining oxygen saturation levels.
    3. monitoring cardiac activity.
    4. determining client response to physical or verbal stimulation.

23. When a client is admitted to the ED for any kind of poisoning, whether accidental or intentional, the nurse must obtain accurate information, including: (Select all that apply.)
    1. amount and time of ingestion.
    2. information about the offending substance.
    3. whether the client has vomited since exposure.
    4. any previous episodes of intentional or accidental poisoning in the past.

24. The drug of choice for clients who present with a narcotic overdose is:
    1. methylpredinosolone.
    2. Narcan.
    3. Valium.
    4. lisinopril.

25. Medications that might be used in the care of a client with a spinal cord injury include: (Select all that apply.)
    1. vasodilators.
    2. high-dose corticosteroids.
    3. vasoconstrictors.
    4. calcium channel blockers.

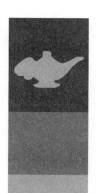

Answer Key

CHAPTER 1

1. a
2. e
3. d
4. f.
5. i
6. c
7. j
8. g
9. h
10. b
11. a. medical or behavior management, such as staying on a healthy diet; b. role management, such as making changes in life roles and adapting to having a chronic disease by modifying behavior such as rehabilitating to optimal functioning; c. affective or emotional, such as learning to accept the illness and managing related emotions.
12. Health literacy, according to WHO, is the cognitive and social skills which determine the motivation and ability of individuals to gain access to, understand, and use information in ways that promote good health. Implications of health literacy include the ability to make effective decisions and to partner with their health care provider in their health care. It has a direct impact on health outcomes.
13. a. 3
    b. 1
    c. 2
14. a. establishing an agenda of client priorities
    b. ask, tell, ask technique of teaching and learning
    c. closing the loop when client restates information
    d. collaborative decision-making or readiness to change
    e. collaborative decision-making or goal-setting and follow-up
    f. adapt teaching to work with older adults
15. a. 2

b. 5
c. 4
d. 3
e. 1
16. 1, 2, 3, 4, 7
17. Heart disease, hypertension, type 2 diabetes, degenerative joint disease, sleep apnea, gallbladder disease, different types of cancer if diet is high in fat.
18. The 3-day dietary log not only identifies what types and amounts of food eaten but when, why, and how the client ate the food. This information helps the client and nurse identify patterns and problem behaviors.
19. 1, 2, 4
20. one
21. Physical activity improves mental functioning, decreases depression, and increases physical endurance.
22. perception, interpretation
23. A broad definition is needed because health can be viewed in many contexts of individual human experience. A broader definition reflects a multidimensional, holistic view.
24. 1, 3, 4
25. a. progression toward a higher level of functioning, b. integration of the whole being, c. an open-ended future with the challenge of fuller potential
26. *Healthy People 2010*
27. True, True, False, False, True, True, True, True
28. fruit, fiber, vegetables
29. 2, 3, 4
30. a. mode, b. intensity, c. duration, d. frequency
31. True, True, True
32. assessment
33. decrease
34. a. Helpful for the worrier. Clients learn to stop obsessive dialogue such as "what if" and replace with positive thought.

b. Based on rational emotive therapy and helps clients recognize irrational thought and replace it with rational self-talk.

c. Clients learn how to imagine a relaxing event or dialogue with self for problem solving.

35. 2, 3, 4, 6
36. 4
37. True, False, True
38. 1, 2, 3, 4
39. *Treating Tobacco Use and Dependence Guidelines*
40. 4
41. 1
42. a. assess lifestyle
    b. assess for risk factors
    c. intervene to modify lifestyle
    d. intervene to reduce modifiable risk factors
43. 4
44. 3
45. 1, 2, 3, 4
46. 4
47. 3
48. 1, 2, 3, 5
49. 4
50. 3
51. 2
52. safety
53. 3
54. 4
55. 3
56. 2
57. 2
58. a. ask all clients if they smoke
    b. ask the client if he/she is willing to quit now
    c. motivation to change
    d. ask what can be done to help
    e. assist the client in problem-solving strategies and skills to assist in stopping smoking
59. Any woman can be a victim of abuse. Identifying abuse using the PVS is a brief and easy to use method and should be used with every woman. Safety is the primary concern.
60. a. keeping immunizations up to date, b. practicing safe sex
61. sigmoid colon, breast
62. 5

CHAPTER 2

1. history of present illness
2. a. 4, b. 2, c. 5, d. 7, e. 3, f. 6, g. 1
3. a. 4, b. 3, c. 1, d. 2
4. a. 2, b. 5, c. 4, d. 1, e. 3

5. A computerized health history assessment provides accurate, legible databases. It can be completed by the client or the nurse and tends to be more complete due to branching programs.
6. These approaches help to identify health issues, deviations from normal, and actual or potential nursing diagnoses in an organized format.
7. See website for chapter 2, Exhaustive Health History Format.
8. See Box 2-5 for answers.
9. 3, 4, 5
10. False, True, False, True, False, False, True, True, True, False, True, True, False, True, True
11. *Long*: also known as exhaustive, uses holistic approach, time-consuming, elicits a wealth of data, may be impractical for an acute care setting
    Short: also known as episodic, used when client presents with an uncomplicated, short-term health problem, proficiency required to perform this type of assessment
12. a. demographic information, b. review of systems, c. family history, d. psychosocial assessment, e. client's health maintenance and health promotion behaviors
13. 2
14. 1, 2, 3, 4
15. 2
16. 1, 2, 3, 4, 5
17. a. 2, b. 3, c. 1
18. anatomy; physiology
19. a. Inspection is a systematic, deliberate visual examination of the entire client. This technique provides information about size, shape, color, texture, symmetry, position, and deformities. It is the first examination technique. b. Palpation is generally the second physical assessment and uses touch. Palpation determines information about masses, pulsation, organ size, tenderness or pain, swelling, tissue firmness and elasticity, vibration, crepitation, temperature, texture, and moisture. Palpation uses the most sensitive parts of the hands to palpate. Palpation uses three levels: light, deep, and bimanual. c. Percussion is used to assess tissue density with sound produced from striking the skin and is usually the third technique. Percussion helps to confirm suspected abnormal findings from palpation and auscultation. There are two methods of percussion: direct and indirect. d. Auscultation is listening to internal body sounds to assess normal sounds and detect abnormal sounds, is the final step in the physical examination, and uses a stethoscope to enhance sounds.
20. inspection
21. True, False

22. 1
23. 4
24. 2
25. 4
26. 3
27. 1
28. 3
29. 1, 3, 4

CHAPTER 3

1. *Thinking* is a special human characteristic that involves organization of new information and the reorganization of previously learned material into forms leading to new responses which can then be generalized to new situations.
Critical thinking is a term used to describe an improved process of thinking by changing the methods of the process of thinking to assure that the conclusion from thinking are self-correctable, reasonable, informed, and precise.
2. See Box 3-1.
3. True, True, True, False
4. Is there anything else you want to tell me about your abdominal pain? Can you give me an example of when your pain was at its worst?
5. The expert nurse has vast experience that allows her to intuitively grasp a situation and zero in on the most important aspect of a problem.
6. outcomes
7. integrating evidence; using one's expertise; considering client preferences
8. self-directed
9. the clinical expertise of the nurse; preferences of the client
10. Clearly identifying clinical problems in practice, searching the literature for relevant research and the best evidence, evaluating and critically appraising the literature using established criteria regarding scientific merit, integrating the evidence from the literature into practice with specific nursing interventions, and evaluating the effect of the change or interventions on client outcomes.
11. a-f
12. Head to toe assessment; immediate priorities would be managing pain, agitation, concern about wife; and psychosocial, emotional, and spiritual concerns. Long-term priorities would concern management for end-of-life care, listening to client and family concerns, perhaps moving him to a facility or back home with care to be with his wife. The client is terminally ill.

CHAPTER 4

1. A group of diverse medical and health care systems, practices, and products that are not presently considered part of conventional medicine
2. Integrative medicine combines mainstream medical therapies and CAM therapies for which there is some high-quality evidence of safety and effectiveness.
3. A placebo effect suggests that the people being treated with the placebo experienced an improvement in their condition as the result of psychological or other factors, rather than because of the inert substance administered. Reiki is based on a Japanese spiritual belief that when spiritual energy is channeled through a practitioner, it heals the client's spirit and consequently their physical body.
4. A redox agent acts in some situations as an antioxidant, whereas in other situations it can act as pro-oxidant.
5. Therapeutic touch is derived from an ancient technique called "laying-on of hands" and is based on a premise that the healing force of the therapist affects the client's recovery. Healing is promoted when the body's energies are in balance. By passing their hands over the client, healers can identify energy imbalances.
6. Complementary medicine is used together with conventional medicine, whereas alternative medicine is used in place of conventional medicine.
7. a. alternative medical systems, b. mind-body interventions, c. biologically based therapies, d. manipulative and body-based methods, e. energy therapies
8. True, False, True, True
9. False
10. The DSHEA ruling of 1994 placed the actual burden of proof on the U.S. federal government to disprove dietary supplement claims.
11. vitamins C, E, and beta-carotene
12. 1
13. 2
14. Create a respectful and open communication environment, ask about CAM at each interaction with the client, educate the client about possible adverse reactions, provide information from NC-CAM, and teach lifestyle modification behavior.

CHAPTER 5

1. Episodic care that is provided by nurses for individuals who seek health care assistance but are able to manage that care by themselves or with the help of significant others outside the institutional setting.

2. Primary health care focuses on the right to basic health care while primary care focuses on the coordinated care by one primary provider.
3. Telehealth nursing practice uses the nursing process to provide care for individual clients or client populations through telecommunications media.
4. 2
5. Primary—health promotion and protection
   Secondary—early diagnosis, prompt treatment, disability limitation
   Tertiary—measures to rehabilitate and maximize remaining capacities
6. a. rapid changes in technology; b. increased emphasis on demonstrated outcomes; c. aging of the population as well as increasing longevity with increasing numbers of chronic diseased; d. reduced revenue to health care organizations from state, federal, and managed care contracts; e. the large number of uninsured people; f. escalating concerns about safety in health care; and g. the growing shortage of nurses.
7. True, False, True, True, True, True, True
8. Because encounters are of short duration, nursing assessment must be clearly focused. Due to the time factor, important assessments may be missed or important questions not asked.
9. physician's offices; hospital outpatient departments; hospital emergency departments
10. Clients are classified by their health status such as acutely ill, chronically ill, or chronically ill with an acute episode. Another classification is by a major illness or body system such as heart failure; diabetes; or ear, nose, and throat. The last type of classification is by the source of reimbursement such as private insurance, Medicare, Medicaid, worker's compensation, or self-pays.
11. During telephone triage, the nurse sorts encounters based on the immediacy of need and type of problem, addresses how the problem should be resolved, and advises the client on whether he/she should be seen in person.
12. cardiac; high-risk obstetric
13. Every encounter should be documented and include assessment data, nursing analysis, recommendations made, client level of understanding of instructions, and requirement for follow-up.
14. Accreditation offers the setting an opportunity to be evaluated by an external group for quality, demonstrates that the setting complies with a uniform set of standards, and allows the organization to be compared with others, thus enhancing a competitive edge.
15. a. Joint Commission of Accreditation of Healthcare Organizations (JCAHO), b. National Committee for Quality Assurance, c. Accreditation Association for Ambulatory Health Care.
16. 2, 3, 4
15. Because the client's family or significant other is responsible for managing the client's care between visits, it is important to understand and respect the client's culture, traditions, and perspectives on health and illness so that care can be provided within this value system.
16. 1, 2, 3, 4
17. Because the client's family or significant other is responsible for managing the client's care between visits, it is important t understand and respect the client's culture, traditions, and perspectives on health and illness so that care can be provided within this value system.
18. 1, 2, 3, 4
19. 2
20. 1
21. 3

CHAPTER 6

1. a. 3, b. 1, c. 2
2. This is a physician who specializes in the care of hospitalized clients.
3. Service lines—care given to groups of clients with similar health problems
4. a. 2, b. 3, c. 1
5. Cross-training is the orientation of nurses to more than one clinical unit so that they can be an effective caregiver on those units.
6. Culturally competent care is knowing, explaining, interpreting, and predicting nursing care within the knowledge of the client's cultural and ethnic beliefs and practices.
7. Risk management is a planned program of loss prevention and liability control.
8. True
9. to determine if the hospital has complied with specific rules and regulations
10. 3
11. diagnosis-related groups (DRGs)
12. client; payer
13. True, True, False, True, False, True, True, False, False, False, False
14. a. government, b. voluntary/not-for-profit, c. for-profit
15. a. promoting self-care, b. upgrading quality of life, c. using resources efficiently
16. To determine if and how a specific job function can be performed more efficiently.
17. quality care is delivered while controlling costs
18. per diem
19. outcome

20. a. Occupational and Safety and Health Act (OSHA), b. Civil Rights Act of 1964, c. Rehabilitation Act of 1973, d. Age Discrimination and Employment Act (ADEA), e. Americans with Disabilities Act

21. a. medication errors, b. complications from diagnostic or treatment procedures, c. falls, d. client or family dissatisfaction, e. refusal of treatment or refusal to sign consent for treatment

22. 1, 2

23. 3

24. Informal education is continuous and includes explanations to clients and/or family members about medications, what to expect during a treatment, or the importance of particular assessments. Informal education is invaluable to client outcomes. Formal education may be provided to individuals or groups of clients and families. More formal methods of teaching are used, including videotapes. The content provided in formal education is consistent among clients.

25. 4

26. 2

27. a. provide excellent nursing care, b. have good medical outcomes, c. provide medical services for complex clients requiring a team of health care providers, d. high retention rate of staff, e. high staff morale, f. good payment systems

28. False, True, True

29. a. budgeting process, b. strategic planning, c. performance improvement plan, d. risk management input, e. utilization review data, f. client satisfaction, g. physician input, h. census data

30. the client's opinion

CHAPTER 7

1. 2
2. 1, 2, 3
3. True, True, False, True, True, False
4. a. These clients often require ventilators to assist with respiration. The equipment requires intensive monitoring and skilled nurses to evaluate the client's response. b. These clients are hemodynamically unstable and require cardiac monitoring—monitoring of the pressures within the heart. These clients require skilled nurses to assess for potential changes and further instability. c. These clients require constant monitoring to assess for changes in the brain's perfusion. d. These clients require constant monitoring to control blood pressure and maintain perfusion of the heart, brain, kidneys, and lungs. In addition, these clients require intensive medication and fluid management. e. These clients require intensive monitoring and medication administration to control and treat the underlying metabolic problems. f. These clients are potentially unstable due to the trauma and loss of blood from major surgery and require intensive hemodynamic monitoring. g. These clients are at risk for cardiac and pulmonary complications due to their previous history and require intensive monitoring to detect any potential change in status.

5. Brain: hemorrhage, stroke, craniotomy, intracranial hypertension, cerebral trauma/edema
   Pulmonary: acute respiratory failure, acute lung injury, pneumonia, pulmonary embolism, status asthmaticus, air leak disorders, thoracic surgery, mechanical ventilation
   Cardiovascular: hypotension, acute coronary syndrome, dysrhythmias, cardiac surgery, vascular surgery, heart failure
   Childbirth/reproductive: premature rupture of membranes, hypertensive crisis, severe hemorrhage, disseminated intravascular coagulation, renal failure
   Endocrine: diabetic ketoacidosis, hyperglycemic hyperosmolar state, diabetes insipidus, syndrome of inappropriate ADH, thyroid storm
   Multisystem: shock, systemic inflammatory response syndrome, multiple organ dysfunction syndrome, burns, organ donation and transplantation, trauma

6. medical/surgical, cardiac, neonatal intensive care, neonatal intermediate care, burn care, other special care, other intensive care

7. Frequent interruptions: plan and group cares, sign on door, have some quiet time when visitors must be quiet to allow sleep
   Personnel and equipment noise: quiet hours, turn alarms down in the room (leave audible at nurses station), phones located away from rooms, keep doors shut
   Constant light: turn lights off or down when client is sleeping, provide periods of light and darkness to mimic day/night, shades on windows
   Lack of privacy: close doors and pull curtains, knock before entering
   Separation from loved ones: allow liberal visitation, allow photos and personal belongings

8. An advocate acts on behalf of another when the other person is not able to do so. The nurse acting as advocate is expected to respect and support the client's values, beliefs, and rights.

9. American Association of Critical Care Nurses, Society of Critical Care Medicine

10. 4

11. These will lead to using best practices. Knowledge in critical care is always expanding and it is imperative to remain current.

CHAPTER 8

1. The skilled services needed to treat an individual's disease and disability in collaboration with his or her family and designated caregivers.
2. 1
3. a. introduce a prospective payment system
   b. initiate a per-client service limit
   c. change billing procedures
   d. mandate the use of Outcome and Assessment Information Set (OASIS)
4. False, True, False, True, True, True
5. The nurse case manager coordinates the delivery and payment of services that target individual client needs.
6. Be prepared. This is important because (1) nurses visiting clients in their homes are on their own, (2) these nurses don't have colleagues readily available for consultation or assistance, and (3) they don't have an endless amount of supplies down the hall. This makes careful preparation and planning essential to make the home visit successful.
7. education; experience; common sense
8. a positive nurse-client relationship
9. a. Domains are four areas that represent groupings of client problems including environmental, psychosocial, physiologic, and health-related behaviors.
   b. Problems is a list of 40 nursing diagnoses that represent matters of concern that adversely affect the client's health status and well-being.
   c. Modifiers are terms used to identify ownership of the problem and degree of severity.
   d. Clinical manifestations are objective and subjective evidence of the client's problem.
10. The Problem Rating Scale for Outcomes provides a framework for measuring a client's problem-specific knowledge, behavior, and status. The scale can be used throughout the time of service to the client and provides a mechanism for documentation. In addition, the scale is used to measure the client's progress and to determine the effectiveness of interventions.
11. True, True, True, True, True, True
12. 1, 2, 4
13. The intervention scheme is an arrangement of nursing actions and activities designed to help the user identify and document plans and interventions. It includes four categories of care such as health teaching, guidance and counseling, targets for nursing interventions, or activities such as dressing change/wound care, and a separate area for identifying client-specific information.
14. Multiple disciplines may be involved in the care of a client at home. It is essential that staff communicate effectively so that services provided by each discipline can be coordinated.
15. Core values include the use and importance of the multidisciplinary team, the provision of care within a seamless health care environment, conducting disease prevention and health promotion activities, respect for the client's rights and responsibilities, recognition that clients must be knowledgeable about their own health and involved in the decision-making process, recognition of the power of the client in that when nurses are in the client's home, it is the client who is in charge, and recognition of the value and contribution of family and other caregivers to the client's health and well-being.
16. The nurse needs to recognize that he/she is a guest in the client's home; the nurse needs to respect the client's cultural, religious, and ethnic beliefs; develop and implement interpersonal skills; enlist the support of the client's family or caregiver; recognize that the nurse's role is to help clients solve their health care problems and to become independent as soon as possible; practice effective communication and collaboration with peer professionals; and maintain a sense of humor.
17. the family or caregiver's beliefs about health care practices and treatment, the extent of their skills, and their availability to care for the client
18. The client's role is to own his/her health care problem and to collaborate with the nurse in order to become as independent as soon as possible.
19. Cell phone: safety, consultation
    Internet: clients view Internet sites to get information; consultation, communication, collaboration
    Telehealth systems: reduce health care barriers by increasing communication, not replace visits

CHAPTER 9

1. 3, 4, 5, 6
2. True, True
3. Hill-Burton Hospital Survey and Construction Act of 1946
4. Omnibus Budget Reconciliation Act of 1987
5. a. an RN must be on duty at least 8 consecutive hours per day, 7 days a week, b. a full-time direc-

tor of nursing must be on staff if the facility has more than 60 beds

6. 14; annually; change in their status
7. Minimum Data Set (MDS)
8. a. assertiveness, b. coaching, c. counseling, d. accurate documentation, e. organizational ability, f. time management, g. effective communication
9. True, True, True, True, False, True, True, True
10. 4
11. 2, 4, 6
12. The MDS does not provide a means of assessing self-concept, spirituality, sense of power, knowledge of health condition and self-care practices, sexuality, patterns of solitude, sense of purpose, immunity, stress management, use of alternative therapies, and attitudes regarding health status and death.
13. a. must be written within 7 days after completion of the assessment, b. the plan is interdisciplinary and nurses coordinate writing of the plan, c. the resident and family should be actively involved in the development, d. the care plan is a working guide to nursing actions, e. nursing assistants must be familiar with the care plan, f. it is the nurse's responsibility to review the care plan with unlicensed caregivers
14. Because of daily contact, nursing assistants may be the first to detect a change in health status; this change must be communicated to the nurse who then performs a further assessment to determine the resident's condition. The nurse must document changes in resident status and communicate these to physicians.
15. a. provide the physician with complete information, b. report symptoms and observations, c. take the order directly from the physician and not office staff, d. repeat the order and when possible ask the physician to fax a copy, e. have the order signed within 24 hours, f. ask the physician for clarification of anything that seems inappropriate and report any continuing concerns to the facility medical director and director of nursing.

CHAPTER 10

1. a. Advances in science and technology have contributed to populations living longer with increased numbers of chronic illnesses.
   b. Changes in health policy and finances have contributed to decreased length of stay in acute care hospitals.
2. The ICF provides a framework for the description of health and health-related states that benefit from rehabilitation services and describes the relationship between body functions and structures, activities and participation, environmental factors, and personal factors.
3. The goal of rehabilitation nursing is "to assist the individual who has a disability and/or chronic illness in restoring, maintaining, and promoting his or her maximal health."
4. altered functional ability and lifestyle
5. 4, 6, 7, 5, 2, 3, 1
6. outpatient, home, day treatment program, subacute, acute
7. client needs and medical stability, services offered in a particular setting, intensity and skill level of needed nursing services, gap between client's current functional ability and realistic, achievable goals of rehabilitation, location of the setting
8. True, True, False, False
9. 3; 2; nursing; medicine
10. a. Client-centered: The client and his unique needs are the focus of care, not the underlying medical diagnosis. Nurses and other team members identify the focus and build a plan of care based on that. In this process, the client's right to make decisions is respected and nurses work to support the client's decision and desired outcomes. The assessment process includes an assessment of the family and the role they will play in the client's rehabilitation.
    b. Goal oriented: Individual goals are determined with the client. Nurses and other team members complete assessments to determine reasonable goals that can be accomplished.
    c. Focus on functional ability: Rehabilitation individualizes an approach to maximize functional ability through training and retraining. Nurses and other team members assess functional ability using the Functional Independence Measures tool and determine areas for improvement.
    d. Team approach: The rehabilitation team is comprised of multiple health care disciplines with the client as a key member. Team members collaborate and cooperate with one another to help the client reach rehabilitation goals.
    e. Quality of life: Successful rehabilitation is dependent upon caregivers understanding what an acceptable quality of life for the client is. Nurses and other team members complete an assessment to determine factors which influence an individual's quality of life that need to be facilitated, maintained, or restored.

f. Wellness: achieving the highest level of wellness for the individual client is the focus. Nurses and other team members maintain, restores, and promote healthy lifestyles for the client within the context of the client's health.

g. Adaptation to change: Coping with change is an innate characteristic of living with a chronic illness or disability. Nurses and other team members help clients recognize the anticipation of change and assist them to learn effective means of coping with change.

h. Coping and adjusting: Clients with a disability or chronic illness will have a psychological reaction to the changes in their lives. Nurses are instrumental in helping clients and their families understand their reactions and providing interventions that will help them cope effectively.

i. Culture: The rehabilitation experience is influenced by the client's culture. Rehabilitation nursing requires cultural competence that will enhance the client's achievement of rehabilitation goals.

j. Client and family education: This is a collaborative process between the client, family, and other team members. Nurses and other team members work together to provide client and family teaching in ways that are accessible and meaningful to the client and family.

11. 1
12. True
13. Because these settings may look physically similar, it may be difficult for clients and family members to understand the differences. By explaining these differences and emphasizing the rehabilitation principles and concepts, the client and family members can make a successful transition from one setting to the other.

CHAPTER 11

1. See Figure U3-1 in the textbook.
2. 7, 2, 1, 6, 3, 4, 5
3. hypo-osmolality
4. vascular, interstitial
5. 1, 5
6. hypertonic, isotonic, hypotonic
7. decreased fluids (or dehydration)
8. 1, 2, 3
9. sugar; caffeine
10. lead to fluid overload
11. See Table 11-5 in the textbook.
12. 135; 145

13. headache; apprehension; increased fluid shifting into the cerebral cells
14. of the competition of Na^+ with Ca^{++} ions for the slow channels in the heart cells
15. 2
16. 1, 2, 3, 4
17. 1, 2, 3, 4
18. 1, 2, 3
19. 1, 2, 3, 4
20. 1, 2, 3
21. 240 ml
22. cerebral edema; pulmonary overload
23. 1
24. 1, 2, 3, 4, 5, 6
25. 1, 2, 3, 4
26. 1, 2, 3
27. 1, 2, 3, 4, 5
28. 2, 3, 4
29. 1, 2, 3, 4
30. D_5W, 0.45% NS
31. NS, LR
32. 3% saline
33. OUTCOMES: The client will have no further losses of fluids and will show improvement in fluid volume.
INTERVENTION #1: Give antiemetics/antidiarrheals/antibiotics as ordered. Rationale: This will prevent further fluid loss.
INTERVENTION #2: Give small amounts of preferred oral fluids hourly; give oral medications one at a time with water or juice. Rationale: small amounts of fluids are better tolerated, giving meds one at a time encourages increased intake.
INTERVENTION #3: Keep water and fluids fresh and within reach. Rationale: Fresh fluids taste better and client is more likely to drink them; client will not have to wait for assistance if he/she can get to fluids without help.
INTERVENTION #4: Administer IV fluids as ordered per IV pump. Rationale: for hydration; IV pump ensures safety.
INTERVENTION #5: Monitor I&O, daily weight, lung sounds. Rationale: to assess fluid balance over time; weight is the best noninvasive indicator of fluid status; lung sounds to monitor for pulmonary overload.
Note: Others are possible.
34. OUTCOMES: The client will show evidence of decreasing body fluid volume and no complications of excess fluid volume or treatment.
INTERVENTION #1: Enforce fluid restriction as ordered and plan fluid distribution with client. Rationale: fluid restriction is to treat excess fluid volume; client is more likely to cooperate if involved in planning.

INTERVENTION #2: Give client cool, not warm, fluids. Rationale: cool fluids are more soothing and decrease sensation of thirst.

INTERVENTION #3: Teach client to hold water in mouth before swallowing. Rationale: this gives sensation of hydrating the tongue and decreases sense of thirst.

INTERVENTION #4: Elevate legs if not severely swollen. Rationale: mobilization of fluids; in severe edema this may cause heart failure.

INTERVENTION #5: Assess skin frequently and provide measures to protect it (elevate heels off bed, turning, keep dry, etc.) Rationale: edematous skin is fragile and prone to breakdown.
Note: Others are possible.

35. a. use large vein
    b. use an IV pump
    c. give slowly

36. OUTCOMES: Client will have no further deterioration in mucous membranes and mouth will remain moist.

INTERVENTION #1: Provide oral care at least every 2 hours. Rationale: promote comfort and moisturizing of tissue.

INTERVENTION #2: Use dilute saline or non-alcoholic mouth rinses. Rationale: alcohol promotes drying.

INTERVENTION #3: Offer cool, nonacidic fluids. Rationale: to improve hydration and comfort without causing increased irritation

INTERVENTION #4: Use a soft toothbrush for oral care. Rationale: to prevent further injury.

INTERVENTION #5: Use a standardized tool to assess oral mucous membranes every 8 hours, or more often as needed. Rationale: a standardized tool makes comparisons from day to day easier and more accurate.
Note: Others are possible.

37. a. importance of taking hourly fluids
    b. avoid excessive caffeinated beverages
    c. fluid intake should reach or exceed 600 ml in 24 hours
    d. keep fresh food and a variety of foods on hand
    e. use community resources such as Meals on Wheels
    f. read food labels and avoid high-sodium foods
    g. consult with physician before using over-the-counter medications or herbal supplements

38. fluid loss; myocardial contractility
39. 1, 2
40. False, True, False, True
41. 4

CHAPTER 12

1. electrolyte deficiency
2. a. Risk for injury
   b. Risk for activity intolerance
   c. Risk for decreased cardiac output
   d. Altered oral mucous membranes
3. dysrhythmias
4. 3.5 mEq/L
5. 1, 2, 3, 4
6. excessive excitability of the myocardial cells
7. decreased
8. carpal spasm when a blood pressure cuff is inflated on the arm for 5 minutes
9. spasm of the facial muscle caused by lightly tapping the facial nerve below the temple region in front of the ear
10. 1, 2, 3
11. 4.5 mEq/L–5.5 mEq/L; 9 mg/dl–11 mg/dl
12. 2.5 mEq/L or 3 mg/dl
13. blocked release of acetylcholine from the myoneural junction; decreases in muscle cell activity
14. a. decreasing the use of magnesium sulfate
    b. saline infusions with a diuretic
    c. IV calcium
    d. albuterol
    e. hemodialysis
15. <1.5 mEq/L or <1.8 mg/dl
16. 1, 2, 3, 4
17. hypokalemia; hypocalcemia
18. a. critical illness
    b. alcoholism
    c. pregnancy and pregnancy-related conditions
    d. diabetes mellitus
    e. infectious diseases
    f. ischemic heart disease
19. impaired absorption or increased loss
20. 1.2 mEq/L–3 mEq/L
21. a. loss of or long-term lack of intake
    b. increased growth or tissue repair
    c. recovery from malnourished states
22. its effect on optimal adenosine triphosphate (ATP) and oxygen supply
23. 3 mEq/L
24. a. limiting high-phosphate foods
    b. limiting carbonated beverages
    c. giving calcium or aluminum products that promote binding and excretion of phosphate
25. 1, 2, 3
26. 1, 2, 4
27. 2, 3, 4, 5
28. 1, 2, 3, 4
29. 1, 2
30. a. agitate the IV bag prior to hanging
    b. dilute to 20–40 mEq/L
    c. do not give IM or IV push

d. may give up to 10–20 mEq/hour
e. use saline as the diluent
f. give through large veins
g. monitor IV site hourly
h. change IV site every 72 hours or earlier if needed
i. use a small IV catheter
j. administer with an IV pump
k. report a urine output of less that 0.5 ml/kg/hour for 2 consecutive hours, a pulse deficit >20/minute, or signs of impaired peripheral tissue perfusion
31. forcing fluids; giving IV saline; giving potassium-wasting diuretics
32. 1, 2, 3, 4, 5
33. 4
34. 1
35. TPN

CHAPTER 13

1. 7.35–7.45
2. 7.35
3. 7.45
4. urine
5. True
6. 2
7. 20:1; pH
8. Acidosis
9. Acidemia
10. Alkalosis
11. Alkalemia
12. chemical, lungs, renal system
13. respiratory
14. respiratory
15. K^+; H^+
16. HCO_3^-
17. treating the underlying cause
18. True, False, True, False, True, False, True
19. 1, 3, 2, 4
20. 1, 2, 3, 2, 3, 4
21. 1, 2, 3, 4, 5, 6
22. oxygen
23. 1

CHAPTER 14

1. Perioperative nursing is using the nursing process to design, plan, and deliver care to meet the identified needs of a client whose protective reflexes or self-care abilities are potentially compromised because of the operative procedure to be performed.

2. increased risk of thrombus formation, decreased oxygen delivery capacity, decreased blood flow to the surgical wound site
3. poor wound healing; wound infection
4. A: airway, B: breathing, C: circulation
5. inadequate ventilation; side effects of anesthetic agents; side effects of preoperative medications; rapid position changes; pain; fluid or blood loss; peripheral pooling of blood after regional anesthesia
6. liver; kidney
7. 2, 4
8. abdominal
9. extremity pain, unilateral edema, warmth in the calf
10. anesthetic agents are fat-soluble and much of the drug dose is deposited from the blood into fatty tissue; therefore, excretion of these agents is slower in obese clients
11. True, False, True, True, False, True, False
12. Allergies, Bleeding tendencies or use of medications that might alter coagulation, Cortisone or steroid use, history of Diabetes mellitus, previous Embolic events
13. 3
14. CXR: to identify abnormalities and possible respiratory infections; pulse oximeter: to obtain baseline oxygen saturation information
15. a. BUN
    b. creatinine
    c. urinalysis
16. a. albumin
    b. hemoglobin and hematocrit
    c. BUN
    d. creatinine
17. 2
18. identify the right client, position the client properly, prevent wrong site surgery, check equipment for safety, count supplies, maintain surgical asepsis
19. a. heads the surgical team and makes decisions about surgical procedures
    b. alleviates pain, provides relaxation, maintains the airway, ensures adequate gas exchange, monitors vital signs, estimates fluid and blood loss, administers blood or fluids, administers medications to maintain hemodynamic stability, provides anesthesia
    c. coordinates all team members, advocates for the client
    d. organizes surgical equipment, handles surgical instruments
20. 1, 2, 5
21. a. recovery from anesthesia
    b. discharge from PACU until first day or so

c. time to complete healing
22. a. general
    b. regional
23. 96.8° F or 36° C
24. color, type, amount
25. coughing and deep breathing
26. 3
27. 4
28. 1, 2, 3, 4
29. 3
30. put bed in lowest position, put side rails up, instruct the client not to get up without assistance
31. 3
32. operative site, age/size of client, anesthetic used, client's complaints of pain
33. 4
34. 2, 3, 4, 5
35. airway patency; lateral Sims'
36. 4
37. ventilation with a bag-valve-mask
38. 2
39. return the client to bed if necessary, cover the wound with sterile dressings moistened with normal saline, monitor the vital signs, keep the client calm, notify the surgeon immediately, and prepare the client for emergency surgery
40. wound care, drain and tube care if any, medications, what to report to the health care provider, when to return for follow-up care
41. True, True, False
42. 2, 4, 5
43. 2, 1, 4, 5, 3
44. 4
45. a. spinal
    b. epidural
    c. caudal
    d. topical
    e. local infiltration
    f. field block
    g. peripheral nerve block
    h. IV regional block
46. 4
47. 2, 3
48. 2, 3, 4
49. a. respiratory status
    b. circulatory status
    c. neurologic status
    d. wound/dressing condition
    e. IV lines—patency, what is infusing, correct rate
    f. drainage tubes—patency; amount, type of drainage
    g. presence of pain
    h. presence of nausea and vomiting
50. See Table 14-4 for various answers.

CHAPTER 15

1. a. potential application of pharmacogenomics to predict individual responsiveness to drugs
   b. carrier screening for selected genetic disorders
   c. prenatal diagnosis
   d. diagnostic genetic testing for adult-onset disorders
   e. genetic testing for complex trait disorders
   f. predisposition testing for complex trait disorders
   g. genetic-based therapeutics
   h. gene therapy
2. genes
3. 23
4. autosomes
5. two X; one X and one Y
6. False, True, False, False, True, True, False, False
7. a. autosomal recessive: disorders are caused by the inheritance of two copies of an altered or nonfunctioning gene. Both parents are carriers. Each child has a 25% chance of inheriting two copies of the mutated gene and being affected, a 50% chance of being a carrier and unaffected, and a 25% chance of neither having the disorder nor being a carrier.
   b. autosomal dominant: only one mutated gene needs to be present in order to be affected. The mutated gene dominates the normal gene. Each child of a parent who has an autosomal dominant condition has a 50% chance of inheriting the gene and being affected and a 50% chance of inheriting the wild-type gene (normal) and not being affected.
   c. X-linked inheritance: caused by an alteration on the X chromosome. Girls have two X chromosomes, but boys only have one X; the other is a Y. A mutation on the X chromosome will always be expressed in boys because they do not have a normal copy of the gene. Each son of a female carrier has a 50% chance of inheriting the mutated gene and a 50% chance of inheriting the normal one. Each daughter of a female carrier has a 50% chance of inheriting the abnormal gene and being a carrier and 50% chance of inheriting the normal gene. All daughters of men affected by an X-linked disorder will be carriers. All sons of affected men are neither carriers nor are they affected by the disorder.
8. autosomal dominant
9. random mutations
10. 1, 2, 3
11. 1
12. True, True

13. 1, 2, 3, 4
14. 1, 2, 3, 4, 5
15. to provide at-risk families with information so they can make informed choices during pregnancy
16. The role will vary depending on expertise and practice area. In all settings, nurses are responsible for providing legally and ethically sound care. Nurses should be able to provide a basic assessment of the client and family, construct a pedigree, identify potential genetic concerns, and provide basic genetic education. The nurse should also assess psychosocial aspects like coping and adaptation, support systems, and health beliefs and practices.
17. Privacy and confidentiality, informed consent, stigmatization, potential for discrimination, and disruption of family and social relationships

CHAPTER 16

1. lump
2. mass of tissue
3. spread of cancer to distant organs
4. 1
5. Medical oncologist
6. Epidemiology
7. a. 2, b. 1, c. 3
8. a. 2, b. 1, c. 5, d. 3, e. 4, f. 6, g. 7
9. a. carcinogenesis
   b. initiation—when a carcinogen causes cell changes at the genetic level
   c. promotion—further genetic damage from additional assaults to cells
   d. malignant conversion—when genetic events cause the cells to change to malignant cells
   e. progression—when cells become increasingly malignant
10. Stage 1—the progressive alteration of malignant cells with additional genetic changes results in a heterogeneous population of malignant cells with varying degrees of metastatic potential.
    Stage 2—Cancer cell migrate via the lymph or blood circulation or by direct extension.
    Stage 3—Cancer cells are established at the secondary site.
11. immune system
12. True
13. Smoking

14. True
15. 1, 2, 3, 4
16. 1
17. 1, 2, 3, 4
18. 1, 2, 3, 4
19. It means they are more like the cells from which they arose and are less likely to metastasize.

CHAPTER 17

1. 1, 2, 3
2. 20
3. True, True, True, False
4. destroy malignant tumor cells without excessive destruction of normal cells
5. 1, 2, 3, 4, 5
6. TNM; T = characteristics of the primary tumor; N = involvement of lymph nodes; M = evidence of metastasis
7. 1, 2, 3, 4
8. True
9. 1, 2, 3, 4, 5
10. Pain
11. True, True
12. 1, 2, 3
13. time, distance, and shielding
14. erythropoietin
15. early aggressive interventions usually offer the best hope of cure
16. from tumors that tend to shed cells from their surface
17. chemotherapy; RT to shrink the tumor mass and decrease the likelihood of micrometastasis
18. 1, 2, 3, 4, 5
19. 1, 2, 3, 4
20. 1, 2, 3, 4
21. infection; catheter occlusion
22. 1, 2, 3, 4
23. surgery
24. 1, 2, 3
25. extravasation
26. True

CHAPTER 18

1. 1
2.

Phase	Activity
Vascular	Blood vessels constrict Clotting process begins Platelets release factors to stimulate healing Capillaries dilate: wound area is red and warm
Inflammation	Occurs whenever cells are injured Limits harmful effects of bacteria Inflammatory response: destroy organism "Walling off" effect: fibrin clot blocks lymph WBCs clean up wound and initiate further healing
Proliferative	Collagen deposition Angiogenesis (new vessels) Granulation tissue development Wound contraction
Maturation	Remodeling of scar: collagen synthesis and lysis Capillaries disappear Scar regains 2/3 original strength

3. 2, 4
4. bands
5. matrix mealloproteases
6. True, False, True, False, True, True, True, False, True, False, False, False, True, True, True, True
7. a. tertiary, b. primary, c. secondary (See Figure 18-3 in textbook.)
8.

Factor	Effect
Diabetes mellitus	Accelerated atherosclerosis: impairs blood supply to wound
Lack of vitamin C	Impaired collagen synthesis
Neuropathy	Unregulated blood flow to wound Possible unintentional injury to area
Foreign bodies	Increases risk of infection
Protein malnutrition	Reduced collagen deposits Decreased WBC function
Smoking	Reduces blood flow; vasoconstriction CO reduces tissue oxygen levels

9. dilutes toxins released by bacteria, brings nutrients to wound, and carries phagocytes to wound for defense
10. prealbumin level
11. infection
12. Mark the area to be measured on the client's leg with a pen and a matching area on the noninjured leg.
13. pain level
14. True, True, False, True, True, True, False
15.

Appearance	Clinical Significance
Edges approximated	Normal healing with collagen synthesis
Open wound, edges apart	Possible infection in wound, opening to drain nonhealing wound
Healing ridge under skin	Normal finding in 5–7 days
Serous exudates	Normal finding
Purulent exudates	Infection, infiltration by WBC, macrophages
Eschar	Necrotic tissue, needs to be removed
Granuloma	Chronic infection, "walled off" area

16. Cold compresses cause vasoconstriction to reduce the effects of edema. Application of heat will dilate the blood vessels and increase blood flow and removal of waste products.
17. 3

18.

Method	Procedure
Sharp	Surgical removal of eschar
	Used for large wounds with thick eschar
	Eschar removed down to level of bleeding tissues
	Done under sterile conditions
	May need anesthesia or sedation
	Pain medications needed after
Mechanical	Use of irrigation or dressings
	Removes debris, bacteria, necrotic tissue
	Wet-to-dry dressings
	"Nonselective" debridement
	Used only until wound is clean and has granulating tissue
Enzymatic	Proteolytic enzymes applied to necrotic tissue
	Used when client cannot tolerate surgical excision
	Slow process
	Should not be used with infected wounds
	Medicate prior to use: burning pain
	Wound needs to be moist, not dry
	Do not place on viable tissue
Autolytic	Use of body's own digestive enzymes to break down necrotic tissue
	Occlusive dressing over wound
	Slow process
	For clients who cannot tolerate other types of procedures
	Contraindicated for infected wounds

19. normal saline
20. The eschar can be scored with small cuts to enhance penetration.
21. Steroids cause a depression of the immune system by blocking prostaglandin production and decreasing the inflammatory response.
22. True, False, True, False, True
23. The increased capillary permeability and blood flow causes edema. Rest, Ice, Compression, and Elevation reduce that edema.
24. by blocking the production of prostaglandins which cause inflammation
25. histamine

CHAPTER 19

1. 1, 2, 3, 5
2. 1, 2, 3
3. a. person, b. plant, c. soil, d. food, e. other organic substance, f. combination of substances
4. A carrier may be asymptomatic and can be shedding organisms, spreading the infection unknowingly.
5. 1, 3, 4, 5
6. Cultural practices involving food or hygiene may increase the risk of exposure (bathing in contaminated water, eating uncooked foods).
7. 2
8. colonization
9. latent period
10. incubation period
11. 1, 2, 4
12. False, True
13. 1, 2, 3, 4, 5, 6
14.

Category	Etiology
Postoperative	Immobility, decreased cough, pain with deep breathing
Diminished consciousness	High risk for aspiration
Impaired gag reflex	High risk for aspiration
Intubation	High risk for aspiration
Tracheostomy	High risk for aspiration
Old age	Decreased immune response, poor nutritional status, decreased activity level
Chronic lung disease	Reduced defenses, fatigue
Cardiac disease	Reduced defenses, respiratory congestion
Renal insufficiency	Decreased immune response
Malignancies	Decreased immune response, medications, malnutrition

15. True, True, False, True, True, False, True, True
16. Clients are asymptomatic but can still transmit pathogens to health care workers or other clients.
17. It damages the epithelium and impairs the skin's defense mechanism; increases risk of infection.
18. semi-permeable
19. Handwashing; alcohol-based
20. a. gloves, b. gowns, c. masks, d. protective eyewear
21. a. contact precautions, b. droplet precautions, c. airborne precautions

22. 1, 2, 3
23. 3
24. 1, 2, 3, 4, 5
25. True, False, True, True, False, True, True, True

CHAPTER 20

1. Pain serves as a warning about potential physical harm and alerts us to problems.
2. Nociception is a measurable physiologic event that carries information to the brain about body tissue damage. Although pain may not accompany nociception, it is a critical component of the body's defense system and may have pain that accompanies it.
3.

Type	Characteristics
Acute pain	Short duration: less than 6 months Identifiable, immediate onset Limited and predictable duration Described as shooting, stabbing, sharp Motivates the person to obtain relief Person can return to pre-pain state
Chronic pain	Lasts months and years Constant, continuous May originally have been acute pain Many causes remain unknown Multiple treatment approaches may fail

4. a. nonmalignant: nociceptive or neuropathic problem, myofascial pain, regional pain syndrome, rest-reinjury cycle
   b. intermittent: migraine headaches, sickle cell crisis
   c. malignant: due to cancerous growths
5. a. superficial/cutaneous: skin and subcutaneous tissues
   b. somatic: muscle, bone, ligaments, joints, blood vessels, and nerves
   c. visceral: organs and their capsules
6. False, True, False, True, True
7. Referred pain
8. a. tolerance to pain, b. age of client (coping mechanisms, previous experiences), c. gender (cultural expectations of gender), d. degree of anxiety, e. past experiences (positive or negative), f. meaning of pain (childbirth pain vs. surgical pain), g. culture and ethnicity, h. expectation and the placebo effect.
9. Pain threshold is the lowest intensity of painful stimulus perceived as pain. Tolerance is the amount of pain a person is willing to endure.
10. 1, 3, 4
11. Transcutaneous electrical nerve stimulation (TENS) unit
12. All pain is real even if the nurse cannot ascertain it or its cause.
13. 1, 2, 3, 4
14. 1, 2, 3, 6, 7
15. a. recognize and treat pain promptly
    b. make information about analgesics readily available to clients
    c. promise attentive analgesic care
    d. define explicit policies
    e. examine processes and outcomes with goal of continuous improvement
16. the client's report
17. Wong-Baker
18. 1, 2, 3, 4
19. Nurses are the primary advocates for the client, assessing pain and providing pain relief measures.
20. a. educate clients about pain and pain control measures, b. obtain accurate pain history and assessment
21. False, True, True, True
22. a. quiet, clean, soothing environment
    b. position changes
    b. back massage
    c. teach client self-management strategies such as guided imagery and deep breathing
23. chronic intractable
24. comfort measures, cognitive behavioral interventions
25. a. Step 1: nonopioids, such as NSAIDs or acetaminophen
    b. Step 2: mild opioids, such as codeine PLUS nonopioids
    c. Step 3: strong opioids, such as morphine with/without nonopioids
26. terminally ill cancer client
27. NSAIDs
28. none (there is no ceiling dosage for morphine)

29.

Agent	Characteristics
Lidocaine	Local anesthetic Acts within 5–10 minutes Lasts 2 hours
Bupivacaine	Local anesthetic Long acting; 4–8 hours 4 times more potent than lidocaine 4–6 times more toxic Blocks sensory nerves over motor nerves

30. EMLA cream
31. True
32. high-fiber diet, fluids, senna-based medications
33. IV: 15 minutes
    IM: 30 minutes
    SC: 90 minutes
    Epidural: 4–12 hours
34.

Medication	Category	Indication
Tegretol	antidepressant	neuropathic pain
Dilantin	anticonvulsant	neuropathic pain
Neurontin	anticonvulsant	muscle spasms from pain
Decadron	corticosteroid	bone pain
Lioresal	muscle relaxant	muscle spasms from pain

35. a. transdermal patch, b. "lollipop"
36. PCAs deliver medication intravenously and are controlled by the client at a preset rate ordered by the physician. The client receives pain medication without delay, reducing anxiety and increasing the client's independence and control over situation.
37. 3
38. Peak effect is the maximum effect of a drug at a certain time after its administration. Client activities are best planned at the peak effect of pain medication administration.
39. a.   medication allergies
    b.   time of last dose and response to it
    c.   other medications being taken
    d.   individual pain experience
    e.   CNS status
40. True, True, True

CHAPTER 21

1. a. denial, b. anger, c. bargaining, d. depression, e. acceptance
2. Alleviation of symptoms and maximizing quality of life. Palliative care does not emphasize cure.
3. 1, 2, 3, 4, 5
4. a. socioeconomic status, b. physical health, c. relationships with friends and family, d. satisfaction with self
5. 1, 2, 3, 4, 5, 6, 7
6.

Problem	Example
Disease/treatment-related	Surgery Radiation Chemotherapy Infection/anemia Malnutrition/cachexia
Physiologic	Overexertion Immobility Poor sleep Pain/discomfort
Psycho-emotional	Stress Anxiety Grief/depression
Spiritual	Fear Distress

7. disease trajectory
8. Mini-Mental Status Exam (MMSE)
9. 1, 2, 3, 4, 5, 6, 7
10. hearing
11. Assessment of sleep disturbances includes review of sleep schedule and the intake of stimulants that interfere with proper rest, evaluation of activity level, and daytime napping. Once treatable causes of sleep disturbance are addressed, the client will have proper rest and can be medicated for pain relief without increasing drowsiness.
12. Disturbed thought processes including acute confusion or delirium, decreased urinary elimination, reduced peripheral tissue perfusion with mottling of the skin, ineffective breathing patterns (Cheyne-Stokes respirations), congested breathing, periods of apnea
13. 1, 2, 3, 4, 7, 8
14. 3
15. a. nonjudgmental and nonthreatening attitude; b. listening skills that encourage client to talk; c. use of therapeutic silence, paraphrases, reflections; d. offering structure to conversation
16. a. accepting the reality of the loss, b. experiencing the pain of loss, c. adjusting to the environment where the deceased is missing, d. finding

a way to remember the deceased while moving forward with life

17. 1, 3, 4
18. none (no ceiling amount; titrate to effect to relieve discomfort and achieve satisfactory analgesia)
19.

Medication	Action	Indication
NSAIDs	Antiinflam-matory	When inflammation is causing pain (i.e., metastatic bone disease)
Tricyclic antidepressants Anticonvulsants	Analgesic effect	Pain syndromes with neurologic component (i.e., pain described as "burning," "shooting pains," or "shock-like")
Anticholinergics	Relieve smooth muscle spasm	"Colicky pain"
Benzodiazepines	Relieve anxiety	Physical, emotional, and spiritual concerns with terminal illness

20. True, True, False, True, True, False, True
21. haloperidol (Haldol)
22. 4
23. anticholinergics
24. tricyclic antidepressant
25. corticosteroids
26. equianalgesic

CHAPTER 22

1. True, True, False, True, False
2. 2, 3
3. 3
4. stress
5. 4
6. elevated blood pressure, risk for stroke and heart attack, and psychological disorders
7. a. Time-zone-change syndrome is experienced by individuals who cross several time zones. b. Shift-work sleep disorder may be experienced by those who have a history of long-term shift work where the usual sleep-wake cycle is altered to accommodate work schedules. c. Irregular sleep-wake patterns are seen in older adults and the chronically ill. Erratic schedules or ignoring external cues contributes to erratic periods of sleeping and wakefulness.

8. a. In Parkinson's, 70% of those diagnosed report sleep disorders characterized initially by insomnia followed by disturbances in the sleep-wake schedule and visual hallucinations. b. 90% of people with depression suffer from a sleep disturbance. It is most often characterized by sleep-onset insomnia. c. Alzheimer's and other dementias are often accompanied by frequent awakenings, with agitation that progresses to loss of sleep-wake consolidation.
9. a. 4, b. 5, c. 2, d. 1, e. 6, f. 3
10. 3
11. noise level, 24-hour lighting, frequency of care-giving interruptions
12. 1, 2, 5
13. True
14. 4
15. The nurse needs to be aware that older adults take longer to fall asleep and are more easily awakened, that REM sleep decreases, and that it takes longer for the older adult to get back to sleep once wakened.
16. depression
17. polysomnography
18. circles under the eyes, lack of coordination, drowsiness, irritability
19. weight; gender; history of snoring; short, thick neck
20. feeling tired upon waking, erectile dysfunction, snoring getting progressively worse
21. Taking benzodiazepine. This is a hypnotic sedative which can increase clinical manifestations because of its selective effect in relaxing muscles of the upper airway and depression of arousal.
22. Alcohol is a depressant and can contribute to relaxation of muscles in the upper airway.
23. Teach the client that this is the treatment of choice. Continuous positive airway pressure (CPAP) is applied through a face mask. The increased pressure keeps the airway open. The CPAP mask should be applied over the nose and secured in place and should be worn when the client is ready to go to sleep. Inform the client that the machine is portable and can be battery-operated. Inform the client he may experience nasal congestion, air leaks, and pressure marks on the face and that if these occur to call the nurse for assistance or referral.
24. 90
25. 4
26. 1, 4, 5
27. The nurse should explain that conventional indoor lighting is not strong enough to have a therapeutic effect. The light being prescribed is very intense and should only be applied for the

specific amount of time. During light application, the client should protect her eyes from overexposure.

28. If a male client with an indwelling catheter has REM-associated erections, the nurse must use caution when securing the indwelling catheter. A sufficient amount of slack in the tubing must be present to accommodate the erection.

29. a. mimic usual sleep activities if possible, b. reduce noise and interruptions, c. provide relaxation measures such as a back rub, d. if prescribed, administer a hypnotic agent.

30. These clients are at risk for having symptoms worsen or for having a prolonged relapse with overexertion.

31. evening

32. Narcolepsy causes significant disruptions to social and occupational roles and subsequently may affect a client's self-esteem. Decreased self-esteem contributes to depression as does the impaired release of neurotransmitters such as dopamine.

33. They often diminish the limb movements associated with this disorder and thus decrease the frequency of sleep arousals.

34. 3

CHAPTER 23

1. 1, 2, 3, 4
2. a. anxiety, b. stress, c. coping mechanisms, d. self-esteem. Related factors include culture and family background, exposure to similar stressors, and repeated exposure to stressors.
3. 1
4. Emotion-focused coping behaviors alter a client's response to stress through actions to make him or her feel better such as talking or crying. On the other hand, problem-focused coping behaviors are aimed at altering the stressor such as getting more information or making a plan to relieve the stress.
5. a. 2, b. 1
6. One cause is biology. There is some evidence of a genetic influence as well as evidence of abnormalities in brain structure and neurotransmitters. Additionally, the limbic system is altered with mood disorders and the frontal and temporal lobes and brain stem are altered with anxiety disorders. The second cause is psychological. Alterations in defenses, thinking, and learning processes can distort a person's view of reality.
7. 3
8. a. 1, b. 1, c. 1, d. 1, e. 2, f. 1, g. 2, h. 2
9. 4

10. 1, 3, 4
11. False, False, True, True
12. Denial
13. 3
14. False
15. 4
16. a. definition of the illness, b. medication options, c. treatment options, d. relapse prevention
17. family member
18. 4
19. True
20. a. 3, b. 1, c. 2, d. 3, e. 2, f. 1

CHAPTER 24

1. 1
2. psychoanalytic: person is fixed at the oral stage of development, seeking gratification of needs through drinking; psychodynamic: person experiences interpersonal and intrapersonal difficulties that provide foundation for addiction; behavioral: addiction is a learned behavior that can be unlearned; family systems: emphasizes that relationships and roles and unhealthy communication patterns among family members contribute to addiction
3. a. 4, b. 6, c. 5, d. 7, e. 8, f. 1, g. 3, h. 2
4. 1, 3, 4
5. acute intoxication
6. 1, 3, 4
7. 3
8. cardiovascular; central nervous system
9. 1, 3, 4
10. endorphin
11. 3
12. 1, 4, 6
13. headache
14. marijuana (cannabis)
15. False, True, False, True, True, True, False, True, False
16. 1, 3, 4
17. Respiratory depression places the client at risk for respiratory arrest.
18. brain; 0.08
19. 4
20. 4; 6
21. 1, 4, 5, 6
22. False
23. self-awareness
24. 2
25. buprenorphine hydrochloride and buprenorphine hydrochloride with naloxone dehydrate
26. a. maintain adequate respiratory status, b. maintain adequate circulatory status, c. provide hydration

27. 2
28. a. education, b. outpatient services, c. impatient or outpatient detoxification and rehabilitation
29. 1, 3, 4, 5
30. True, True, True
31. These drugs cause less respiratory depression and hypertension, and they help prevent delirium tremens (DTs).
32. 1, 2
33. a. providing rest, b. orienting the client as necessary, c. intervening to prevent complications, d. monitoring for both physical and mental changes.
34. 2, 3, 4

CHAPTER 25

1. See Figure U6-1 in textbook.
2. See Figure U6-3 in textbook.
3. 1, 2, 3, 4
4. a. pain
   b. swelling
   c. tenderness
   d. joint stiffness
   e. cramps, muscle spasms
   f. deformity
   g. reduced movement or range of motion
5. 9, 8, 6, 7, 4, 5, 2, 3, 1
6. 2
7. a. pain
   b. pallor
   c. temperature
   d. pulses
   e. capillary refill
   f. paresthesia
   g. mobility of affected joints
8. circulatory compromise
9. 2
10. a. ANA
    b. CRP
    c. ESR
    d. RA
    e. CBC
    f. calcium
    g. phosphorus
    h. alkaline phosphatase
    i. creatinine kinase
    j. lactate dehydrogenases
    k. aldolase
11. aches: muscle strain
    sharp pain: fracture or infection
    throbbing: bone-related
12. a. glucosamine: pain relief
    b. chondroitin: pain relief
    c. fish oil: anti-inflammatory, relieves morning stiffness

d. avocado/soybean: persistent pain
e. topical capsaicin: persistent pain
f. devil's claw: persistent pain

CHAPTER 26

1. True, True, True, False, True, True
2. large weight-bearing joints
3. knee
4. 4, 1, 7, 1, 7, 2, 6, 2, 5, 3, 3, 2, 2, 4, 5, 6
5. 1, 3, 4
6. 1, 2, 3, 4
7. 1
8. 2
9. 2
10. 1, 3, 4
11. 3
12. 3
13. 2
14. 1, 2, 3
15. 3
16. 1, 2, 3, 4
17. 5
18. 2
19. 2, 3
20. 1
21. 3
22. 1, 2, 3
23. 2

CHAPTER 27

1. False, True, True, True, False, False, True
2. 1
3. 1, 2, 3, 4
4. 6, 1, 9, 2, 5, 7, 4, 10, 3, 8, 16, 14, 15, 12, 13, 11
5. 1
6. fat embolus
7. True, True, False, True, True, False, True
8. 24; 48
9. Paralysis
10. 1
11. 2
12. 1
13. 1, 2, 3, 4, 5
14. 1
15. 1, 2, 3, 4
16. higher than the client's heart
17. 1, 2
18. Bivalving
19. dislocation
20. are in partial contact but their relationship is abnormal
21. 1, 2, 3, 4, 5
22. 1, 2

CHAPTER 28

1. See Figure U7-2 in textbook.
2. cellular
3. a. decreased protein
   b. decreased fat
   c. restricted carbohydrates
4. a. increased caloric intake
   b. sedentary lifestyle
5. Primary starvation is when inadequate nutrients are delivered to the GI tract over an extended period of time; secondary starvation is when the upper GI tract fails to absorb, metabolize, or use delivered nutrients.
6. 1, 2, 3, 4, 5, 6
7. ulcerative colitis, Crohn's disease, ulcers, cancer, diabetes, alcoholism
8. a 24-hour diet recall
9. 3
10. Albumin has a long half-life and is a general indicator of nutritional status. Prealbumin has a short half-life and reflects acute nutritional changes.
11. height, weight, BMI, frame size, circumferential measurements
12. BMI
13. False, True, False, True, True
14. refer to a specialist to rule out cancer; oral cancers are often asymptomatic
15. McBurney's point
16. True, False, True, True
17. bruit
18. to assess for dysphagia which would put the client at high risk for aspiration
19. a. flat plate
    b. upper GI series
    c. modified barium swallow
    d. computed tomography
    e. ultrasound
20. direct visualization of the GI system by means of a lighted flexible tube or scope
21. a. dysphagia
    b. esophageal reflux
    c. esophageal spasm
    d. motility disorders
    e. hiatal hernia
22. Nutrition screening is a method of categorizing clients as high or low risk for nutritional disorders. It is quicker and includes generalized questions about nutritional status and GI health. It should be done on all clients. Nutritional assessment is an in-depth history and physical examination along with diagnostic testing to determine actual or potential problems involving the upper GI tract or nutrition.
23. 1, 2, 3, 4
24. a. abdominal pain
    b. nausea and vomiting
    c. indigestion
    d. diarrhea
    e. changes in weight or appetite
25. 1, 2, 3, 4
26. The nurse should specifically ask about the relationship between diarrhea and food/fluid intake.
27. a. types of foods eaten in the past 2–3 days
    b. how this food was prepared
    c. if anyone else who ate the food got ill
28. a. bleeding
    b. liver disease
    c. peptic ulcers
    d. vomiting blood
    e. anemia
    f. gallbladder disease
    g. pancreatitis
    h. change in bowel habits/characteristics
    i. weight changes
    j. results of any diagnostic tests
29. Food allergies typically have systemic manifestations, whereas food intolerances usually manifest with GI symptoms.
30. 1, 2, 3, 4
31. drug-nutrient interactions, interference with nutrition and the absorption, processing and excretion of nutrients
32. a. aspirin/aspirin-containing products
    b. NSAIDs
    c. antacids
    d. laxatives
33. There is wide variation in content and they can have potential side effects and interactions with nutrients.
34. anticholinergic

CHAPTER 29

1. Malnutrition can describe undernutrition or overnutrition related to deficient or excess energy or nitrogen stores, possibly due to altered dietary intake. Protein energy malnutrition results when the body's needs for protein or energy are not adequately supplied.
2. a. increased needs for growth and development
   b. increased needs to sustain pregnancy and to produce milk
   c. medical or socioeconomic status may limit their ability to obtain and ingest nutritionally adequate diets
3. 4
4. 1, 2, 3, 4, 5
5. True, False, True, False

6. a. environment
   b. genetic tendencies
   c. socioeconomics
   d. ethnic disparity
7. 1
8. False, True, True, True, True, False
9. Nurses are there as the client enters the health care system, have constant contact during the hospitalization, and are the last contact as the client leaves the hospital. Early identification of nutritional problems and constant monitoring of progress can help prevent further problems.
10. a. Parkinson's disease
    b. Alzheimer's disease
    c. CVA
    d. side effect of medications
11.

Protein Intake	Caloric Intake	Appearance
Marasmus	Inadequate	Inadequate Thin, cachectic
Kwashiorkor	Inadequate	Adequate Body weight within the normal range

12. 1, 2, 3, 4, 5, 6
13. a. activities to support a client's knowledge of normal nutrition; example: diet information related to decreasing risk for cancer
    b. targeting specialized diet therapy for a clients with an illness; example: Crohn's disease
    c. activities to assist the client to return to normal nutritional behaviors; example: retraining a client to swallow after a stroke
14. 1, 2, 4
15. 1, 2, 3, 4, 5
16. 2, 3, 4
17. Suction
18. False
19. a. raise head of bed to 45 degrees for 1 hour before, during, and for 1 hour after the feeding
    b. continuous tube feedings require the client's head of bed to be raised at all times
    c. check gastric residuals every 4 hours
    d. avoid adding blue dye to the formula
20. 1, 2, 3, 4
21. 2
22. a. anorexiant: Meredia (sibutramine)
    b. thermogenic: phentermine
    c. peripheral lipase inhibitor: Xenical (Orlistat)

23.

Classification	Sample Product
Semi-elemental, predigested	Vivonex TEN, Peptamen, Reabilan, Criticare HN
Standard protein	Isocal, Osmolite, Resource
Fiber supplemented	Jevity, Ultracal, Fibersource
High protein	Traumacal, Alitra Q, Impact, Replete, Promote
Calorie dense	Isocal HN, Nutren 2.0
Diabetes	Glucerna
Renal failure	Nepro

CHAPTER 30

1. The buildup of plaque and bacteria around the tooth causes inflammation of the tissue. The supporting structures of the tooth are damaged, causing the tooth to fall out or to require extraction due to severity of the periodontal disease.
2. a. mechanical trauma—injury from jagged teeth, cheek biting
   b. chemical trauma—drugs from chemotherapy, chemicals in mouthwashes
3.

Classification	Etiology	Examples
Primary	Direct infection of tissues	Canker sore Herpes simplex Vincent's angina
Secondary	Opportunistic infection (immunosuppression)	Candidiasis

4. 1, 2, 3, 4
5. biopsy
6. odynophagia
7. The pain from heartburn usually means substernal, midline burning that radiates in waves upward toward the neck. Clients often describe it as "cramping" or "knotting." In contrast, angina pectoris tends to be a heavy, crushing, or tightening sensation in the chest that tends to radiate toward the left arm.
8. Achalasia

9.

Name	Procedure	Result
Nissen fundo-plication	Suturing fundus around the esophagus	Creates valve-like sphincter, prevents reflux
Hill operation	Narrows esophageal opening	Reinforces sphincter, anchors stomach and distal esophagus, recreates gastroesophageal valve
Belsey (Mark IV) repair	Suturing the stomach onto the distal esophagus	Creates esophagogastric angle without opening esophagus or diaphragm

10. The extensive lymphatic supply to the mucosa allows the cancer to spread widely and quickly. By the time the client develops swallowing problems, the cancer has invaded the esophagus and spread to other adjacent structures.

11. Leukoplakia is a potentially precancerous, yellow-white lesion that occurs in any region of the mouth. The lesions are usually elevated and have a roughened or leathery surface and clearly defined borders. Leukoplakia is common. Erythoplakia is a red, velvety-appearing patch that often indicates early squamous cell carcinoma.

12. Hiatal hernia: client experiences heartburn 30–60 minutes after a meal; may have substernal pain. Rolling hernia: client may complain of fullness after a meal or complain of difficulty breathing; may experience chest pain similar to angina; pain is worse when client lies down

13. venous drainage causes darker coloration of the skin

14. True, False, True, False

15. a. maintain pressure over extraction site to reduce bleeding
    b. decrease blood flow to area of extraction and reduce edema
    c. small amount of bleeding expected, call physician if bleeding lasts more than 1 hour
    d. extraction site is sensitive to temperature extremes
    e. prevent recurrence of bleeding at extraction site
    f. patient comfort, encourage oral intake
    g. prevent dehydration

16. 1, 2, 3

17. 1, 3, 4, 5
18. False, False, False
19. 1
20. a. Imbalanced nutrition, less than body requirements
    b. Impaired swallowing
    c. Risk for injury
    d. Risk for ineffective coping
21. a. wound healing
    b. wound care
    c. nutrition
    d. respiratory care
    e. medications
    f. what manifestations to report
    g. contact information
    h. date/time of follow-up appointment
22. antimicrobial
23. 1, 2, 3
24. 1, 2, 5, 6

CHAPTER 31

1. a. chemical irritation of nerve endings from stomach acid
   b. stretching and contracting of stomach caused by muscle tension as in obstruction
2. esophageal varices
3. potassium
4. 1, 2, 3, 4, 5
5. gastric cancer
6. pernicious anemia
7. High gastric acid secretion and rapid emptying of food from the stomach into the duodenum characterizes duodenal ulcers. Gastric ulcers are caused by a break in the mucosal barrier exposing the stomach to hydrochloric acid.
8. upper GI bleeding
9. vagotomy: eliminates acid-secreting stimulus to gastric cells
   vagotomy with pyloroplasty: prevents gastric stasis and enhances emptying
   gastroenterostomy: permits regurgitation of alkaline duodenal contents which neutralize gastric acid; drains acid away from ulcerative areas, promoting healing
   antrectomy: reduces acid-producing portions of the stomach
   subtotal gastrectomy: treatment of duodenal ulcers
   total gastrectomy: treatment of extensive cancer
10. alkalosis
11. 1, 3, 4, 6, 7
12. 1, 2, 3, 4, 5, 6, 7, 8
13. indicates GI tract bleeding

14. assess for clinical manifestations, review laboratory test reports, report any sign of electrolyte abnormality to the physician
15. True, False, True, True
16. 3
17. Manifestations appear 5–30 minutes after eating and involve vasomotor disturbances such as vertigo, tachycardia, syncope, sweating, palpitations, diarrhea, and nausea
18. a. decompression
    b. lavage
    c. gastric analysis
    d. tube feeding
19. 4, 1, 5, 2, 6, 3
20. 1, 3, 4
21. right
22. False
23. The nurse should report this finding and take vital signs.
24. The important concept here is that of accurate I&O. The irrigation solution IS added to the intake if the same amount is NOT subtracted from the output. If it is added to the intake, it should be separated from the remains of the intake as a separate source. If the irrigation solution is subtracted from the output, there is no need to add it to the intake. As long as the measurements are done accurately and consistently, it doesn't matter which way the nurse does it, unless the physician has a preference.
25. Room-temperature saline is cooler than body temperature and promotes mild vasoconstriction.
26. Maintaining adequate perfusion to the kidneys is vital to client stability; urine output should be monitored hourly with a Foley catheter in place.
27. The tube could be positioned over a suture line and moving it might cause trauma.
28. a. Imbalanced nutrition, less than body requirements
    b. Acute pain
    c. Ineffective therapeutic regimen management (individual)
    d. Fear
    e. Risk for injury
29. Compazine
30. Loss of prostaglandins exposes the gastric mucosa to acid secretions, resulting in ulcers
31. False
32. because many of these contain aspirin or NSAIDs
33. Enteric-coated aspirin: protects against irritation from lost mucosa
    Cytotec: same as above
    Histamine receptor antagonists: decrease gastric acidity

Proton pump inhibitors: block gastric acid secretion

CHAPTER 32

1. weight loss, accessory organ symptoms such as jaundice, postsurgical diarrhea
2. current complaints, GI complaints, fluid intake changes, congenital problems
3. 2, 3, 4, 5, 6, 8
4.

	Urine Output	Associated Conditions
Anuria	Less than 100 ml per 24 hours	Acute or chronic renal failure
Oliguria	100–600 ml per 24 hours	Acute or chronic renal failure, shock, dehydration, reduced cardiac output, renal injury or obstruction with stones
Polyuria	Unusually large daily amounts	Systemic diseases such as diabetes mellitus, diabetes insipidus, diuretic medications, chronic renal disease

5. a. Etiology: postoperatively or postpartum, use of certain medications
   b. Manifestations: sudden inability to void, severe suprapubic pain and urgency
   c. Treatment: medical emergency; requires immediate urethral or suprapubic catheterization
6. Urinary incontinence is the involuntary loss of urine. Causes include urge, reflex, stress, mixed, overflow, and functional.
7. a. abdominal pain—depends on location, maybe emergent such as appendicitis, bowel obstruction
   b. dyspepsia—may indicate ulcer pain
   c. blood in the stool—if visible, diverticulosis, hemorrhoids, ischemic colitis
   d. diarrhea—inflammatory bowel disease
   e. fecal incontinence—impaired neurologic sensation
   f. infection—possible hepatitis, pancreatic disease
8. True, False, True, True, True, True, True, True, False
9. glomerular
10. all
11. False, True, True, True
12. 5–10

13. 2; 1
14. 1, 2, 3, 4, 5
15. 1, 2, 4, 6, 7, 8
16. 1, 2, 3, 4, 5, 6
17. 2
18. a. Computed tomography: useful alternative for clients who cannot retain barium; can identify masses
    b. Ultrasonography: used to identify pathology in pancreas, liver, gallbladder, spleen, and retroperitoneal tissue; abdominal gas can interfere with ultrasound waves
    c. Proctosigmoidoscopy: examination of distal sigmoid colon, rectum, and anal canal; not as thorough as colonoscopy but safer
    d. Colonoscopy: visual exam of entire colon with flexible fiberoptic endoscope; used to screen clients at high risk for colon cancer
    e. Flat plate of abdomen—x-ray of abdominal organs, used to identify tumors, obstructions, etc.
    f. Occult blood—home-based test on three consecutive stools, for lower GI bleeding, source unknown
    g. Video capsule endoscopy—capsule swallowed by client to transmit digital images of small intestine, used for GI bleeding or lesions
19. True, False, True, True
20. True, True, False, True
21. a. KUB-screening or preliminary test for lithiasis, shows calcifications and large soft tissue masses in the abdomen
    b. IVP—visualize the renal pelvis, collecting system, and ureter, gold standard to find filling defects
    c. CT—well-tolerated imaging method for renal and retroperitoneal pathology, used to stage malignancies
    d. cystourethroscopy—direct visualization of urinary tract, used to find calculi, infection, reflux, obstruction, cancer
    e. urinalysis—can quantify red and white blood cells, used for UTI
    f. creatinine clearance—determines glomerular filtration rate and tubular excretion ability of kidney, may be diminished in renal disorders, used to make this determination
    g. serum creatinine—blood test not affected by fluid status, used to diagnose glomerulonephritis through renal failure
    h. BUN—measure of renal function looking at urea as an end product of protein metabolism that is excreted by kidneys, used to support findings of renal insufficiency, starvation, dehydration, etc.
22. 1–5
23. True

CHAPTER 33

1.

Disorder	Etiology
Hemorrhage	Trauma, ulcerations, or inflammation
Pain	
Visceral	Mechanical factors causing stretching/distending
Somatic	Inflammation of specific area, more intense
Referred	Pain felt at a distance from affected organ
Nausea/vomiting	Distention of the duodenum
Distention	Excessive gas in the intestines; blockage
Diarrhea	Infections, malabsorption syndromes, medications
Constipation	Inadequate fluid or bulk, mechanical blockage

2. 1–5
3. True, False, True, True, True
4. 1, 2, 3, 5
5. 1, 3, 4, 5

6.

	Crohn's Disease	**Ulcerative Colitis**
Area affected	Entire GI tract All layers of bowel	Entire colon Mucosa/submucosa
Age of client	15–30 yrs of age	15–30 yrs. of age
Amount of diarrhea	Urgency at night	10–20 stools/day
Appearance of stool	Liquid, no blood	Bloody, mucus
Systemic symptoms	Fever, fatigue, weight loss, pallor	Fever, fatigue, weight loss, pallor
Nutritional deficiencies	Malabsorption	Malabsorption
Medical treatment		
Medications	Antidiarrheals Anti-inflammatory Corticosteroids Salicylates Mesalamine, Flagyl/antibiotics	Antidiarrheals Corticosteroids Salicylates
Surgical intervention	Not curative, only if complications	Remove colon, cure
Prognosis	Chronic; recur	Chronic; recur

7. Polyps
8. Diverticulosis is the presence of noninflamed diverticula. Diverticulitis is inflammation of the diverticula.
9. 5
10.

	Cause	**Injuries**	**Treatment**
Blunt trauma	Steering wheel Pedestrian accidents	Shearing Crushing Compressing Rupture of bowel	Observation
Penetrating injury	Gunshot wounds Stabbings	Damage all structures Perforations Peritonitis/sepsis	Surgery IV antibiotics

11. 3
12. False
13. a. Temperature: increases signify complications
    b. Blood pressure: decrease can signify shock
    c. Respiratory rate: monitor for adult respiratory distress syndrome
    d. Bowel sounds: monitor return of normal functioning
    e. Urine output: evaluate fluid status of client
    f. Skin turgor/mucous membranes: assess hydration status
    g. Laboratory tests (CBC, electrolytes): prevent complications, return levels to baseline
14. 4
15. 3
16. a. Rest: reduce energy demands on patient
    b. NPO status: rest the bowel, reduce diarrhea
    c. Fluids: replace losses from diarrhea and vomiting
    d. Electrolytes in fluids/IV: return balance to vascular system
    e. Perineal/skin care: remove irritating fluids; prevent breakdown
17. 1, 2, 4
18. a. Acute pain related to inflammation
    OUTCOME: The client describes decreased postoperative pain.
    INTERVENTION #1: Medicate as ordered and evaluate effectiveness.
    INTERVENTION #2: Teach the client splinting of the abdomen .
    b. Risk for infection related to rupture of appendix
    OUTCOME: Infection will not develop/rupture will be diagnosed early.
    INTERVENTION #1: Monitor vital signs closely.

INTERVENTION #2: Monitor pain closely for rigid, board-like abdomen.

19. a. Diet high in calories, protein, and carbohydrates: To provide the nutrients necessary to assist patient cope with stress of surgery and ensure proper wound healing postoperatively.
    b. Diet low in residue/liquid diet: To reduce peristalsis, rest bowel.
    c. Cathartics, such as GoLYTELY or Fleet Prep Kit: Clean out the bowel and minimize bacterial growth in the bowel.
    d. Administration of antibiotics: Reduce bacterial growth and prevent postoperative infections.

    e. Administration of enemas: To clean the lumen (inside) of the bowel; remove bacteria.
    f. Blood transfusions (if needed): Correct severe anemia and enhance wound healing.
    g. Enterostomal nurse consult: Provide emotional support and information before the surgery.

20. a. Insertion of a nasogastric tube: Decompress; remove fluids/gas
    b. NPO status: Rest the bowel
    c. IV fluids with electrolytes: Replace losses; maintain balance
    d. Monitor vital signs frequently: Signifies complications; infection

21. gastroenteritis
22. it has been shown to cause spasms of the colon

23.

Medication	Indication for Use	Action
5-ASA Azulfidine Asacol/Rowasa Dipentum	Ulcerative colitis (UC) and Crohn's	Block production of prostaglandins/leukotrienes decrease inflammatory process
Steroids	UC and Crohn's Inflammatory bowel disease (IBD) fails to respond to salicylates	Reduce inflammation
Antacids Antihistamines	Steroid use for UC/Crohn's	Prevent gastric ulceration
Budesenide	Crohn's	New, nonsystemic steroid
Purinethol	UC and Crohn's	Immunosuppression
Methotrexate Imuran Sandimmune	IBD fails to respond to salicylates/ steroids	Immunoregulatory
Remicade	Crohn's	Block action of tumor necrosis factor
Antegren	IBD	Immune modulator Attach to immune cells and prevent them from leaving bloodstream to go to site of inflammation
Anticholinergics	UC and Crohn's	Relieve abdominal cramps
Antidiarrheals	UC and Crohn's	Relieve diarrhea
Antispasmodics	UC and Crohn's	Reduce spasms, rest the colon
Flagyl	UC and Crohn's	Prevent/control infection
Cipro	Infection	Treat anal fistulas/perianal disease

CHAPTER 34

1. microorganisms; 100,000
2. a. length of the male urethra
   b. antibacterial properties of prostatic fluid
3. 1, 2, 3, 5, 6, 7
4. urine culture

5. pyelonephritis
6. urethritis
7. a. urinary stasis, b. supersaturation of the urine with poorly soluble crystals

8.

Type of Calculi	Etiology
Calcium	Paget's disease Hyperparathyroidism Impaired renal absorption Increased intestinal absorption
Oxalate	Inflammatory bowel disease Postileal resection of bowel Overdose of ascorbic acid Concurrent fat malabsorption
Struvite	Certain bacteria, Proteus "urea-splitter"
Uric Acid	Increased urate excretion Fluid depletion Low urinary pH Increased uric acid production
Cystine	Congenital metabolic error
Xanthine	Rare, hereditary condition Xanthine oxidase deficiency

9. True, True
10. benign prostatic hypertrophy (BPH)
11. 6
12. 1, 2, 4, 6, 7, 8
13. 1, 2, 3, 4, 5
14. 1, 2, 3, 4, 5, 6
15. 1, 2, 4
16. False, True, True, True, True, True
17. 4
18. a. Encourage fluid intake of at least 3 liters per day: flush bladder
    b. Avoid caffeinated beverages/alcohol: irritates lining of bladder
    c. Learn risks associated with spermicides: alters pH, irritates
    d. Remind client to void every 2–3 hours: mechanical clearing
    e. Instruct female clients to void before and after coitus: prevent bacterial infection
19. OUTCOME: Client will have return of normal voiding habits within 3 days of starting antibiotic treatment
    INTERVENTION #1: provide instructions about antibiotic therapy
    INTERVENTION #2: instruct on dietary changes/fluid intake
20. OUTCOME: Complications will not develop or will be minimized
    INTERVENTION #1: Administer antispasmodics
    INTERVENTION #2: Increase fluid intake
    INTERVENTION #3: Administer urinary tract antiseptics/analgesics
21. irrigation
22. 1, 2, 3, 4, 6
23. Phenazopyridine (Pyridium)
24. a. Renal and hepatic function: ability to clear medications
    b. Cardiovascular status: ability to handle fluid intake
25. clean catch urine collection
26. BCG is instilled into the bladder through a urethral catheter. The catheter is clamped or removed, client retains the fluid for 2 hours moving side to side or supine to prone changes in position. After 2 hours, the client voids in a sitting position or catheter is unclamped.
27. a. Maintain adequate fluid intake, b. perform Kegel exercises, c. develop a voiding schedule

CHAPTER 35

1. 1, 2, 3, 4, 5, 6, 7
2. hypertension
3.

	Acute	Chronic
Etiology	Bacterial contamination of urethra	Chronic obstruction with reflux
Manifestations	Enlarged kidneys, abscesses, fever/chills, flank pain/CVA tenderness, cloudy or foul-smelling urine	Hypertension, azotemia, pyuria, anemia, proteinuria
Testing	UA with C&S, KUB x-ray, cystourethrogram, MRI/CT	UA with C&S, blood pressure
Medical treatment	Antibiotics, sulfonamides for 10–14 days, analgesics	Control hypertension, increase fluid intake, antibiotics

4. Removing the obstruction causes sudden release of pressure and diuresis which can lead to dehydration.
5. True, True, False, False, True, False, True, True, True, True
6. a. hematuria, b. flank pain, c. palpable abdominal or flank mass

7.

	Acute	Chronic
Cause	Allergic reaction	Progressive fibrosis
Onset	Rapid	Slowly progressive
Manifestations	Fever, rash, oliguric renal failure, hematuria	Chronic inflammatory cell infiltration with atrophy, interstitial edema, altered renal vasculature, interstitial fibrosis
Prognosis	Complete recovery or rapid progression to renal failure and death or change to chronic form	Similar to chronic pyelonephritis

8.

	Acute	Chronic
Onset	Sudden	Insidious
Manifestations	Hematuria, proteinuria, fever/chills, weakness, pleural effusions, ascites, pallor, generalized edema	Malaise, weight loss, edema, irritability/mental cloudiness, metallic taste in mouth, polyuria, nocturia, headache, dizziness, GI disturbances, respiratory difficulty, angina

9. a. contusion, b. minor laceration, c. major laceration, d. "fractured" kidney (shattered), e. vascular injury
10. Hematuria
11. a. renal agenesis—unilateral may be normal function; bilateral agensis is fatal
    b. supernumerary—usually asymptomatic
    c. ectopic—no renal problems, but may cause respiratory difficulty, pain, and difficulty in childbirth
    d. aplasia—small, contracted kidneys have no functioning renal tissue

    e. hypoplastic—miniature kidneys have some functioning renal tissue and may be asymptomatic or may cause hypertension and recurrent UTI
    f. horseshoe—may be asymptomatic but susceptible to hydronephrosis, infections, and calculus formation
12. Heavy metals: lead, mercury, bismuth, arsenic, copper, cadmium, gold, lithium
    Poisons: mushrooms, insecticides, herbicides, snake venom
    Solvents: ethylene glycol, gasoline, kerosene, turpentine, tetracholoroethylene, carbon tetrachloride, tricholoroethyline, chlorinated hydrocarbons
    Other agents: anesthetics, contrast dyes
    See Box 35-1 for comprehensive list.
13. 1, 2, 4
14. Spontaneous pneumothorax
15. Damage caused by streptococcal infections may lead to glomerulonephritis.
16. Measures to prevent recurrent pyelonephritis are similar to those for cystitis: see chapter 34, but includes adequate fluid intake, good perineal hygiene, voiding before and after sexual intercourse for female clients, and voiding on a regular basis. The client also needs to know the manifestations of UTI and get quick medical attention.
17. Rhabdomyolysis: maintain adequate perfusion through kidneys and decrease muscle metabolism, prevent further damage to the kidneys
    Hypertension: decrease BP and stop damage to aterioles/arteries
18. 3
19. OUTCOME: The client will have balanced I&O, maintain adequate hydration, and will have no manifestations of dehydration.
    INTERVENTION #1: Prepare the client for diagnostic tests and probably antibiotic therapy.
    INTERVENTION #2: Maintain IV hydration.
20. OUTCOME: The client will report no pain or will report that pain is controlled.
    INTERVENTION #1: Administer analgesics as ordered and evaluate their effectiveness.
    INTERVENTION #2: Force fluids to 3–4 L/day.
21. a. decrease pain so client can participate in coughing and deep breathing exercises or spirometry; allow client to become mobilized as soon as possible
    b. decrease pain so client can participate in coughing and deep breathing exercises or spirometry
    c. identify problems with renal function early
    d. assess for paralytic ileus which is common

22.

Plan		Intervention(s)
a.	Maintain fluid and electrolyte balance	Daily weight, I&O, administer loop diuretics and/or plasma volume expanders, dietary restriction of Na$^+$, water, and possibly protein
b.	Decrease inflammation	Administer steroids
c.	Prevent thrombosis	Administer anticoagulants, teach client to monitor for hemorrhage or thrombotic events
d.	Minimize protein loss	Increase dietary protein to 1–1.5g/kg/day, 24-hour UA to monitor loss, treat inflammation to decrease losses

23. decrease
24. 2, 3, 4
25. Excessive fluid loss can cause hypotension. Hypotension leads to decreased renal perfusion.
26. a.   Older adults vary in sensitivity and response to medications.
    b.   Older adults typically have decreased renal perfusion and therefore decreased ability to excrete drugs.
27. 1, 3, 4, 5, 7, 8
28. sulfonamides; sulfamethoxazole with trimethoprim
29. corticosteroids; immunosuppressants
30. ACE inhibitor
31. streptokinase

CHAPTER 36

1. 1, 3, 4
2. prerenal: dehydration
   intrarenal: nephrotoxic agents
   postrenal: prostatic hypertrophy
3. True, False, True, False, True, True, True, True, True

4.

	Nonoliguric Renal Failure	Oliguric Renal Failure
Urine output	2000 ml/day	<400–600 ml/day
Urine	Dilute Low specific gravity	Concentrated High specific gravity Proteinuria
Clinical signs	Tachycardia Dry mucous membranes Poor skin turgor Hypotension Orthostatic hypotension	Precipitating event Edema Weight gain Weakness Anemia
Prognosis	Less morbidity/mortality	Mortality as high as 50%

5. 1
6. Ultrafiltration is the removal of fluid from the blood; it uses either osmotic or hydrostatic pressure. Diffusion is that passage of particles from an area of higher concentration to an area of lower concentration.
7. Rapid solute removal from the blood changes the osmotic pressure gradient; the cerebral tissues now absorb more fluids which leads to cerebral edema and increased intracranial pressure.
8. a.   decreased seizure threshold
   b.   anemia
   c.   bleeding problems
9. Hematologic: anemia, bleeding tendencies, platelet abnormalities
   Immunologic: depression of humoral antibody formation, suppression of delayed hypersensitivity, decreased function of leukocytes
   Musculoskeletal: osteodystrophy, osteomalacia, osteoporosis, osteosclerosis, impaired conversion of vitamin D to active form, reduced absorption of calcium from intestines, increased phosphate retention
   Changes to medication metabolism: high risk for medication toxicity; changes in absorption, distribution, metabolism, excretion
   Psychosocial: powerlessness, lack of control, restrictions imposed by regimens, changes to body image, changes to sexuality, role reversal, loss of work/financial strain, scheduling problems
10. 1, 3, 4, 5
11. Palpate the site for a thrill and auscultate for a bruit to ensure adequate blood flow through the graft
12. 1

13.

	Advantages & Disadvantages	Contraindications	Specific Nursing Care
Hemodialysis	Can be accomplished quickly, temporarily Requires venous access	Cardiovascular disease	Assess access site Strict aseptic technique; dressing changes No BP in arm with access device
Peritoneal	Relative ease allows it to be used in the community or at home A possible disadvantage for each type of peritoneal dialysis is the need for a well-trained and compliant client	Hypercatabolism Poor condition of peritoneal membrane Several relative contraindications exist Peritonitis is a major concern Client unwilling or unable to perform treatment	Assess effluent for infection Monitor catheter insertion site Monitor patency of catheter Review knowledge at every opportunity
CAPD	No need for machinery or water source during the day; normal activities possible Body better maintains homeostasis: may need fewer dietary restrictions		
Continuous cyclic peritoneal dialysis	Reduced risk of infection Longer daytime dwell means no exchanges at work or school		
Intermittent peritoneal dialysis	May dialyze a client for up to 48 hours in a row if needed		
Nightly intermittent peritoneal dialysis	No daytime dwells		

14. a. prevent fluid overload and reduce workload of the kidneys
   b. must account for insensible losses to balance overall fluid level
   c. kidneys not functioning properly, avoid dehydration
   d. kidney's inability to excrete potassium and regulate other electrolytes is impaired
   e. check for effects of hyperkalemia or hyponatremia
   f. avoid foods that contain magnesium which cannot be excreted in renal failure, protein and fluid restrictions to avoid overworking kidneys

15. a. reverse process of gluconeogensis
   b. reduce workload of kidneys when trying to excrete nitrogenous waste
   c. impaired excretion
   d. if oral intake is not sufficient to meet needs

   e. impaired renal excretion

16. OUTCOME: The client will regain/maintain balanced intake and output
   INTERVENTIONS: Accurate I&O, fluid restriction, monitor vital signs, assess skin turgor and mucus membranes, daily weight, obtain urine specific gravity

17. OUTCOME: The client will maintain adequate nutrition as evidenced by sufficient intake to prevent protein catabolism and maintain lab values within safe limits
   INTERVENTIONS: Work with client to establish preferences, provide a pleasant environment at meals, medications to alleviate the discomfort of stomatitis/nausea, provide enteral or parenteral feedings

18. magnesium

19. a. remove end products of protein metabolism from the blood

b.   maintain a safe concentration of serum electrolytes
c.   correct acidosis and restore bicarbonate level
d.   remove excess fluid from the blood
20. potassium chloride
21. increased quality of life
22. 1, 2
23. 1
24. decreased incidence of infection
25. noncompliance with medication regimen
26. Lasix
27. Due to decreased kidney function they are at higher risk of nephrotoxicity and alterations in pharmacokinetics
28. 1, 2, 5, 7, 8
29. erythropoetin
30. increased BUN and creatinine levels
31. The urine will be very dilute, with large quantities produced. In addition, there will be a loss of sodium in the urine resulting in hyponatremia.
32. edema, hypertension, heart failure
33. Decreased excretion of nitrogenous waste accumulates in the CNS.

CHAPTER 37

1.   See Figure U9-1 in textbook.
2.   See Figure U9-2 in textbook.
3.   See Figure U9-4 in textbook.
4.   4
5.   pelvic exams; Pap smears
6.   soft tissue radiographic breast examination; tumors and benign lesions
7.   3
8.   2, 4, 7, 5, 6, 3, 1
9.   1, 2, 3, 4, 5, 6, 7
10. 1, 2, 4
11. 3
12. 1, 2
13. gynomastia
14. many women go to an OB/GYN physician for all their health care needs
15. tail of Spence
16. 1, 2, 3, 4
17. a.   pelvic pain
     b.   breast pain
     c.   abnormal uterine bleeding
     d.   infertility
     e.   infection
18. a.   pain
     b.   testicular or scrotal problems
     c.   sexual function issues
     d.   lower urinary tract symptoms/complaints
     e.   infertility
     f.   infection

19. 1, 2, 3, 4, 5
20. 1, 2, 3, 4
21. 1, 2, 3, 4, 5
22. general questions as to whether the woman is satisfied and comfortable with her current sexual activity
23. urinary; gastrointestinal
24. weight—both obesity and anorexia—can affect menstruation and fertility and can contribute to general health problems
25. so the client is more comfortable and the nurse has had the chance to establish rapport
26. 20
27. abnormal Pap smears
28. True, False, False, False, False, True, False
29. reassure him that this is a normal occurrence and has no sexual meaning
30. 1, 2
31. a.   caffeine
    b.   alcohol
    c.   tobacco
    d.   recreational drugs
32. antihypertensive medications (methyldopa, clonidine, guanethidine, hydralazine), antidepressive medications, medications to treat prostate cancer

CHAPTER 38

1.   they regard such problems as a potential threat to their sexuality or identity as a man
2.   a.   sensitivity to fear and embarrassment
     b.   respect for privacy and confidentiality
     c.   careful history-taking
     d.   addressing information needs
3.   reproductive and genital disorders affect relationships
4.   50
5.   219,000
6.   threats to individual self-concept, gender roles, relationships, and sexual interaction
7.   embarrassment
8.   2
9.   3
10. 1, 2, 7, 8, 5, 6, 4, 3
11. 3, 4
12. 1
13. 1, 2, 3, 4, 5
14. 1, 2, 3, 4
15. 3
16. 4
17. 2
18. 3
19. 1, 2, 3, 4, 5
20. inflatable; semi-rigid
21. 2

22. 2, 3, 4
23. 1, 2, 3, 4
24. bladder
25. True, True
26. sildenafil (Viagra)

CHAPTER 39

1. 3
2. 1, 3, 7, 4, 6, 5, 2
3. 2
4. 3
5. uterus; cervix
6. tubes; ovaries
7. 1, 3, 4
8. 1
9. hot flashes, night sweats, palpitations, dizziness
10. 1, 2, 3, 4
11. 1, 2, 3
12. 4
13. 2
14. 1, 2, 3, 4, 5
15. 2
16. 1, 2
17. 1, 2, 3
18. 1
19. 4
20. 2
21. 2
22. Some Hispanic cultures discourage menstruating women to walk barefooted, wash their hair, or take showers or baths.

    In some cultures, menstruating women may be subject to restrictions on work and physical activities.

    In some cultures, women have to abide by rules related to disposal of menstrual fluid and sanitary products.

    Many cultures do not permit intercourse during menstruation.

    Some religions require women to engage in certain practices during and after menstruation.

    Some religions are strictly against contraceptives, sterilization, and abortion.

    Some cultures practice female genital mutilation.
23. 2, 4, 3, 6, 1, 5

CHAPTER 40

1. age
2. 1
3. 4
4. True, False, True, True, False
5. 4
6. 1, 2, 3, 4

7. 1
8. 2
9. 3, 2, 4, 5, 1
10. 1, 2, 3
11. 3
12. cyst
13. nonpalpable lesions
14. modified radical mastectomy
15. 1, 2 , 3
16. True
17. 2
18. 1, 2, 3
19. 1, 2
20. 1, 2, 3
21. 1, 3, 4
22. 2

CHAPTER 41

1. Compare: Both terms are used to described infections that are transmitted by sexual activity. Contrast: *Venereal disease* was used to describe diseases transmitted only by sexual intercourse. *Sexually transmitted infection* is used to describe any infection transmitted by any sexual activity or contact.
2. *Sexarchy* means the beginning of sexual activity.
3. 1, 2, 3, 4, 5
4. Chancroid
5. *Chlamydia trachomatis*
6. 1, 2, 3
7. 2
8. 4
9. 3
10. 1
11. 3
12. 1
13. 1, 3, 4
14. 1, 2
15. 1
16. 4
17. 2, 3
18. 2
19. 3, 4
20. Answers will vary.
21. 1, 2, 3, 4
22. job training sites, any site where teens gather such as concert venues
23. Belief that the older adult does not engage in sexual activities.
24. 1, 2, 4
25. Partners of clients who have STIs deserve to know their status and to receive examination and treatment if needed. If left untreated, the consequences of many STIs can be devastating (infer-

tility, life-long infection, possible involvement of other organs). One argument against requiring clients to report names of contacts is that clients who are embarrassed might not get care themselves.

CHAPTER 42

1. See Figure U10-2 in textbook.
2. True, True, True
3. 12, 11, 10, 9, 4, 7, 8, 1, 3, 2, 6, 5
4. 1, 2, 3, 4
5. 1, 2
6. 4
7. liver, pancreas, biliary tract
8. True, True, False, True, False
9. Biopsy
10. Paracentesis
11. 1
12. 1, 2, 3
13. because manifestations can be vague and because these disorders can affect multiple body systems
14. thyroid gland
15. having blood tests, receiving a blood transfusion, body piercing, tattoos, dental procedures, or intravenous injection with a potentially contaminated needle
16. liver or pancreas
17. color, pigmentation, striae, ecchymoses, mottling
18. color, texture, brittleness, presence of ridges, peeling
19. blood glucose
20. primary hypothyroidism
21. 1, 2, 3, 4
22. False, True, True, False, False, True

CHAPTER 43

1. euthyroid
2. 1, 2, 3, 4
3. 1, 2, 3, 4
4. 1
5. 2
6. 1, 2, 3
7. myxedema
8. 1
9. 2, 3, 4
10. Graves' Disease
11. 2
12. 1, 2
13. 1, 3, 4, 5
14. 1, 4
15. 1, 3, 4
16. 1, 2

17. 1, 2, 3, 4, 5
18. 1, 2, 3, 4, 5
19. 1, 2
20. 1, 2, 3, 4, 5
21. 1
22. musculoskeletal, GI, renal, neurologic
23. manifestations are often vague; manifestations may be attributed to something else
24. hypocalcemia
25. 1, 2
26. cancer
27. hyperthyroidism
28. 1, 2, 3, 4
29. 1, 2, 3
30. a.   normal urine output
    b.   no stones
31. 3
32. 1, 2
33. 1, 2, 3
34. 1
35. 1, 2, 3, 4
36. potassium iodine
37. 1, 2, 3
38. hypothyroidism
39. 1, 2, 3, 4
40. 4
41. vitamin D
42. 1, 2, 3, 5

CHAPTER 44

1. 1, 2, 3, 4
2. Autoimmunity
3. 1, 2
4. 1, 2, 3, 4
5. 1, 2
6. Primary aldosteronism
7. Secondary aldosteronism
8. Hyperpituitarism
9. Hypopituitarism
10. 3
11. True, True
12. 1, 2, 4
13. 1, 2, 3
14. 3
15. 4
16. 1
17. 3
18. angiotensin II, plasma renin activity
19. decreased renal perfusion
20. Cushing's syndrome, acromegaly, amenorrhea, galactorrhea, hyperthyroidism, rare hypergonadism in males
21. 1, 4
22. 3

23. 1, 2, 3, 4
24. 1
25. 1, 2
26. osteoporosis
27. 1
28. True
29. 1, 2, 3
30. 1, 4

CHAPTER 45

1. 21 million; 7
2. 6 million
3. 6th, $132 billion
4. Islet cell transplant
5. insulin deficiency (defect); insulin resistance; obesity
6. 1, 3
7. 1, 2
8. type 2
9. 3
10. insulin dependent diabetes mellitus (IDDM)
11. 1, 2, 3
12. glycosuria
13. ketones
14. 4
15. 1
16. hemoglobin A1C, or glycosylated hemoglobin
17. ketones
18. glucose
19. microalbuminuria or proteinuria
20. self-monitoring of blood glucose (SMBG)
21. 1
22. 1, 2, 3
23. 1
24. 2 hours after eating
25. 3
26. 2
27. 4
28. 2
29. 3
30. 1
31. 2
32. when starting a new diabetic agent; when starting another medication that can affect blood glucose; when sick/stressed; when you think your blood sugar is too high or too low; when you lose or gain weight; when you have a change in your medical regimen, diet plan, or activity plan
33. To help the diabetic client become responsible for, and competent to, make informed decisions regarding diabetes care
34. True, True, False, False, False
35. 1, 1, 2, 2, 1, 2

36. Macrovascular: coronary artery disease, cerebrovascular disease, hypertension, peripheral vascular disease, infections
    Microvascular: diabetic retinopathy, nephropathy, neuropathy
    Macrovascular (especially coronary artery disease)
37. elevated triglyceride levels
38. Health promotion: managing obesity and maintaining ideal body weight, exercising, not smoking, achieving normal blood lipid levels
    Health maintenance: prompt recognition and treatment of hyperglycemia, aggressive management of hypertension, screening high-risk clients
39. urinary tract infections
40. nonproliferative, preproliferative, proliferative
41. 2
42. 2
43. 1
44. 1, 2, 4, 5

CHAPTER 46

1. digestion; utilization of glucose
2. True, True
3. 1, 2, 3
4. a. cholecystitis, b. cholelithiasis, c. hyperlipidemia, d. hypercalcemia, e. pancreatic tumor, f. pancreatic ischemia, g. certain medications and alcohol abuse
5. removal of the gallbladder
6. jaundice
7. a. cholesterol—most common type, increases with age, prevalent in women, stones smooth and whitish-yellow to tan
   b. pigment—present in 30% of people with cholelithiasis in the U.S., stones are black or earthy calcium bilirubinate
   c. mixed—combination of cholesterol and pigment stones or either with some other substance, calcium carbonate, phosphates, bile salts, and palmitate are the other constituents
8. autodigestion
9. bluish discoloration of the left flank
10. bluish discoloration of the periumbilical area
11. 1, 2
12. 1, 2
13. 3, 4
14. 4
15. 1, 4
16. pain or biliary colic
17. coronary heart disease
18. 1, 2, 3
19. 1, 2, 3, 4

20. 1
21. 1, 2, 3, 4
22. False, True, True
23. Morphine
24. 2
25. calcium gluconate
26. 2

CHAPTER 47

1. 1
2. 1, 2
3. 1, 2, 3, 4
4. 1, 2
5. a. 2, 5, 9; b. 2, 3, 6, 8; c. 2; d. 1; e. 10; f. 7
6. hemorrhage
7. 1, 2, 3, 4
8. 1, 2, 3, 4
9. 1
10. 1, 2, 3
11. 1, 2, 3, 4
12. 1, 2, 3, 4
13. 1, 2, 3
14. 1
15. 2
16. 1
17. 1, 2, 3

CHAPTER 48

1. See Figure U11-1 in the textbook.
2. persistent itching or pruritus
3. An allergy is an immunologic response that happens consistently with exposure. An irritation is unpredictable.
4. alopecia, ichthyosis, atopic dermatitis, psoriasis
5. scabies
6. hirsutism
7. nutrition; respiratory
8. anemia
9. A callus is a flat painless thickening of a circumscribed area of skin. A corn is a horny induration and thickening of the skin caused by friction and pressure and is often painful.
10. Linear lesions appear in a straight line. Satellite lesions appear as small peripheral lesions around a larger central lesion.
11. False, False, False, True, True
12. A: asymmetry; one half in unlike the other half
    B: border; irregular, scalloped, or poorly circumscribed
    C: color: varied from one area to another, shades of two colors, or changing color
    D: diameter; larger than 6 mm as a general rule

13. this may explain unusual lesions or their location
14. A large number of skin disorders are caused or worsened by exposure to irritants and chemicals in the home or workplace.
15. 6, 7, 8, 11, 1, 4, 9, 10, 5, 2, 3
16. well-lit: to better visualize the skin and other structures
    private room: so client feels comfortable getting undressed and wearing a gown
    moderate temperature: overly warm temperatures cause vasodilation and redness; overly cool temperatures can cause vasoconstriction and possible blue or pale tint to skin
    neutral wall colors: painted walls affect the hue of the skin tone
17. buccal mucosa; nail beds, lips, or palms; white of sclera; hard palate
18. dorsum of hand
19. location, distribution, size, arrangement, color, configuration, secondary changes, presence of drainage
20. palpate
21. True
22. See Figure 48-3 in the textbook.
23. A culture is indicated for an infection that does not respond to the usual treatment.
24. A patch test is used to identify substances that produce an allergic reaction.
25. Contraindications include presence of dermatitis, taking oral steroids, or if the allergen would worsen a dermatitis
26. Aspirin products can cause prolonged bleeding
27. Place a small amount of antibiotic ointment on the site and cover with a clean, dry dressing, make sure client understands any wound care instructions and when to return for follow-up.
28. cutaneous
29. sunburn-like rash in areas of sun exposure
30. 2, 3, 4, 1
31. aloe vera

CHAPTER 49

1. 3, 5, 2, 1, 6, 4
2. pruritus
3. body fluids such as urine
4. one month, 3–4 days
5. scalp, elbows, knees, genital area, sacral area
6. 30; 50; women; men
7. First-degree sunburn is mild, tender erythema followed by desquamation and healing. Second-degree sunburn is more extreme erythema and edema. Blistering results from damage to the epidermal cells.

8. basal cell, squamous cell, malignant melanoma
9. 3
10. fair complexion, excessive childhood sun exposure with blistering burns, increased number of dysplastic moles, family history of melanoma, presence of a changing mole on the skin
11. asymmetry, border notching, color variegation, diameter >6 mm
12. depth
13. cutaneous T cell lymphoma
14. itching, post-herpetic neuralgia
15. aesthetic, reconstructive
16. thrombosis
17. False, False, True, True, True, True, True, False, False, True, True, False, False, True
18. all pressure ulcers are contaminated with surface bacteria and a surface swab only grows this surface bacteria
19. 12
20. excessive swallowing
21. False
22. Application of moisturizers is more frequent if bathing can't be done often; assistive personnel may be needed to apply topical treatments, oral antihistamines are administered in small doses due to possible decreased tolerance
23. 2, 5, 6, 1, 3, 4
24. limits skins destruction, prevents edema, and possible decreases blistering
25. 1
26. 3, 4, 5, 1, 2
27. protect the blood supply to the flap
28. control of hemorrhage through application of direct pressure
29. True, False, False, False, False, True
30. age, size of affected region, condition of stratum corneum, cutaneous blood supply, molecular weight of drug, medication vehicle
31. 2, 4
32. Tacrolimus ointment (Protopic), pimecrolimus cream (Elidel)
33. taper the dose as the drug is discontinued
34. 4

CHAPTER 50

1. 8, 4, 6, 5, 2, 3
2. ability to maintain normal body temperature, risk of infection secondary to loss of skin barrier, evaporative water loss
3. 3, 4, 5, 6, 1, 2
4. 15%
5. higher
6. wound contracture; hypertrophic scarring
7. True, True, True, False, False

8. Thermal: exposure to or contact with a flame, hot liquid or semi-liquid, or hot objects.
   Chemical: tissue contact with strong acids, alkalis, or organic compounds
   Electrical: heat that is generated by the electrical energy as it passes through the body
   Radiation: exposure to a radioactive source
9. 44.77, or 48 ml/hour
10. 3
11. 24; 48
12. 2
13. 4
14. Background pain: experienced when the client is at rest or engages in nonprocedure-related activities. It is described as continuous in nature and low in intensity.
    Procedural pain: experience during the performance of therapeutic measures and is described as acute and high intensity.
15. 1; 2
16. pulses, capillary refill, color, movement, sensation
17. 3099 Kcals
18. 8672.4 ml/24 hours (2ml/kg/TBSA) – 17,334 ml/24 hours (4ml/kg/TBSA)
19. upper extremities: 18%, ½ of face: 4.5%, hand-sized burns 4% (1% x 4) = 26.5% TBSA (22.5% are second degree)
20. visible
21. not visible; large; irregularly shaped
22. 3, 2, 1
23. elevate the head of the bed
24. 75; 100
25. The tissue serves as a medium for bacteria growth
26. strict handwashing
27. 3
28. therapeutic positioning, ROM exercises, splinting, client and family education
29. hip extension
30. 3
31. calories; protein
32. Because the cases are considered contaminated and are done last to prevent cross-infection of other clients.
33. False
34. 5, 2, 7, 3, 11, 1, 6, 8, 4, 10, 9 (During the acute phase, the burn is not closed, making Risk for infection a higher priority than it would be normally for a "risk for" diagnosis. Also Impaired physical mobility, although a physical and actual diagnosis, is not as critical in the acute phase. The three psychosocial diagnoses could themselves be in any order, except that physical diagnoses always take priority over psychosocial)

35. 4
36. 1, 2, 3, 5
37. 1, 2, 4
38. Resuscitative phase: fear and anxiety are most common

    Acute phase: anxiety, fear, grief, perceived role/identity changes, depression, withdrawal, regression, other signs of poor coping, nightmares, need to discuss accident, acting out

    Rehabilitative: self-image concerns, problems with reintegration into society, need for vocational rehabilitation and related role changes, fear and anxiety continue, acting out, poor self-confidence
39. morphine sulfate
40. gastric ulcers (GI bleeding)
41. False, False, True, False, True

CHAPTER 51

1. See Figure U12-2 in textbook.
2. Any of the following: predictable, reproducible, goes away with rest
3. 1, 3, 4
4. Lipodermatosclerosis
5. True, False
6. Age: incidence of atherosclerosis and vascular problems increases with age

    Occupation: work involving heavy physical labor, long periods of standing in one place, or sedentary activities increase risk
7. baseline
8. True, True
9. contralateral
10. Allen's test
11. Doppler
12. 1, 2, 3, 4, 5
13. 2; some diagnostic studies use iodine-based contrast dye
14. 1. a
    2. c, d
    3. a
    4. c
    5. a
15. Air plethysmography and/or impedence plethysmography
16. intermittent claudication; lifestyle
17. 1
18. 2
19. 1, 2, 3, 4

CHAPTER 52

1. 2
2. 50 million
3. 25
4. lack of client compliance; providers' ignorance of the need to prescribe and manage complex holistic treatment protocols
5. heart attack
6. increase in peripheral arterial resistance
7.

Type	Characteristics
Primary	90% of all known cases unknown etiology Usually appears between the ages of 30 and 50
Secondary	Due to an identifiable cause Glomerulonephritis and renal failure most common causes

8. a. renin is an enzyme produced in the kidneys
    b. renin converts angiotensin I to angiotensin II
    c. angiotensin II causes vasoconstriction and stimulates the release of aldosterone
    d. aldosterone causes sodium and water retention
    e. the increase in volume and the vasoconstriction both lead to hypertension
9. cortisol
10. 1, 3, 4
11. syncope (orthostatic hypotension or postural hypotension)
12. damage to target organs
13. 140 mm Hg; 90 mm Hg
14. a. the desired target BP is reached and maintained
    b. treatment choices are tolerated and safe
    c. the client is willing to commit to the regimen over the long term
15. True, False, True, True, True
16. 1, 2, 3
17.

Risk Factor	Action
Stress	Identify coping mechanisms Learn and use relaxation techniques Identify stress triggers
Obesity	Lose weight; 10% reduction is helpful Maintain BMI at <27 Increase exercise: 30–45 minutes on most days Aerobic exercise best; light weight-lifting OK Moderate intensity exercise is fine Low saturated fat, low cholesterol, increase polyunsaturated fats
Nutrients	Low sodium (less than 2.3–6 grams per day) Increase calcium, magnesium, potassium through natural sources Adequate water intake
Substance abuse	Stop smoking, no tobacco or nicotine Caffeine is OK Moderate use of alcohol (1.0 ounces/day/men; 0.5 ounces/day/women)

18. Allow the client to sit quietly and rest for 5 minutes before taking the blood pressure.
19. a. weight reduction
    b. sodium restriction
20. compliance
21. a. have clients move slowly when changing position
    b. have clients breathe deeply and keep eyes open
22. Any of the following: to prevent the rise of blood pressure with age, to decrease the existing prevalence of hypertension, to increase hypertension awareness and detection, to improve control of hypertension, to reduce cardiovascular risks, to increase recognition of the importance of controlled isolated systolic hypertension, to improve recognition of the importance of persistent damage from high-normal blood pressures, to reduce ethnic, socioeconomic, and regional variations in hypertension, to improve opportunities for treatment, to enhance community programs
23. Community blood pressure screenings are usually nurse-driven and help assess the approximately 20% of Americans not in regular contact with any part of the health care system. Most people learn of their hypertension via incidental blood pressure readings.
24. OUTCOME: any of the following: the client will

actively participate in creating a treatment plan, the client will describe the underlying causes of hypertension and self-care strategies, the client will adhere to scheduled follow-up appointments, the client will describe the action and side effects of medications, the client will express commitment to and self-responsibility for controlling hypertension

INTERVENTIONS/RATIONALE:
a. Explain the asymptomatic nature of the disease—will help client not minimize the problem
b. Assist clients to incorporate needed changes into lifestyle—changes are often difficult and a source of noncompliance; client being in control helps facilitate compliance
c. Educate client on action of needed medications, side effects, and encourage client to report annoying side effects that may cause him/her to stop taking the drug—clients may consider the treatment worse than the disease and stop taking the drugs
d. Provide follow-up appointments and discuss progress—communication with the client and continued education helps improve compliance
e. Provide education on the disease and potential complications—allows client to understand importance of compliance even though the client may be asymptomatic now

25. a. diuretics
    b. beta blockers
26. 1 year
27. Client will demonstrate knowledge of hypertension and its risk factors, client will list all medications including dosage, possible side effects, and indications for use, client will demonstrate proper technique for measuring BP with home BP machine.
28. Older clients are more likely to experience adverse reactions to antihypertensives. Too rapid a reduction in blood pressure can affect cerebral perfusion and result in changes in mental status, dizziness, or weakness. Medications are started at low doses and changes made over longer amounts of time.
29. By blocking the increased aldosterone secretion that causes fluid retention; the reduced fluid volume will result in a decreased cardiac volume and lower blood pressure.
30. Calcium channel blockers relax the blood vessels and decrease heart rate which will cause a decrease in blood pressure.
31. stimulation of the sympathetic nervous system

which increases heart rate and blood pressure

32. after identification of high blood pressure readings, treatment is aimed at the cause and at the high blood pressure in order to prevent complications from the hypertension

CHAPTER 53

1. atherosclerosis
2. diabetes, smoking, increased blood lipid levels
3. primary: caused by lymphatic vessels that are missing or impaired
   secondary: caused by lymphatic vessels that are damaged or have been removed
4. 2, 3, 5, 6, 7, 8
5. the client's own saphenous vein
6. infection
7. pain, pallor, pulselessness, poikilothermy, paresthesias, paralysis
8. atherosclerosis, hypertension
9. 6 cm
10. Pallor: stimuli leads to spasm of digital arteries, blood flow is decreased
    Cyanotic: resulting tissue hypoxia and venous congestion
    Rubor: spasm resolves and blood flow returns
11. Venous stasis: immobilization, lack of use of the calf muscle pump
    Hypercoagulability: dehydration, blood dyscrasias
    Injury to vessel wall: IV injections, fractures, dislocations
12. True, False, True, True, False, True, True, True, True, False
13. constant, reproducible, not positional
14. Mr. Thomas has limb-threatening disease with a poor prognosis
15. Doppler ultrasound
16. dorsalis pedis, posterior tibial, popliteal, femoral
17. 1, 2, 3, 4
18. documenting character of pedal pulses, comparing one side with the other, marking the pulses that can be felt with an ink pen
19. myoglobin release secondary to muscle ischemia (compartment syndrome)
20. True
21.

Goal	Specific Teaching Area
Reduce risk	Stop smoking; meticulous skin care; moderate program of exercise; decrease body weight if needed; low-fat, low-cholesterol diet
Promote arterial flow	Medications: Trental, cilostazol, aspirin, clopidogrel, reverse Trendelenberg position, fleece boots to keep feet warm and protected
Save the limb	Arterial bypass surgery to restore blood flow

22. reverse Trendelenberg
23. preventing injury to the extremities, especially the feet
24. 1, 2, 3, 4
25. 2, 3
26. 24 hours
27. A traumatic amputation can sometimes be replanted as the client and the limb were healthy up to the time of the injury, depending on the severity of the injury. However, the client has not had time prior to surgery to grieve the loss of the limb and adjust to perceived alterations in body image. Clients with PVD have been chronically ill for some time and have other medical conditions, which would affect the outcome. If planned, clients can start to adapt to their new body image preoperatively.
28. a. ambulate as tolerated, including stairs and outside
    b. no lifting >15 pounds for 6–12 weeks
    c. no activities requiring pushing, pulling, or straining
    d. driving is restricted
29. True, False, True, True, False, False
30. Age-related changes and impairments of physiologic functions along with arterial disease may increase Activity intolerance, altered, Peripheral tissue perfusion, and Pain
    Physical or cognitive impairments, ongoing drug therapy, and psychosocial factors may limit pain recognition.
    Sight reduction and flexibility limitations may prevent or decrease self-care
    Sight reduction may increase the risk for falls or other injury
31. disruption in the suture line, pseudoaneurysm formation, slipped ligature, reclotting of the graft
32.

Medication	Indication	Route	Nursing Considerations
Coumadin	Thrombus DVT	PO	Given after acute DVT has been treated with injectable heparin; long half-life. Must be stopped 3 days before any invasive procedure; prescribed based on INR 2.0–3.5; administer in the evening for a hospitalized client; antidote: vitamin K. Teaching: avoid other anticoagulants, don't change the amount of green leafy vegetables you eat, bleeding precautions: electric vs. standard razor, gentle tooth brushing, monitor for bleeding/bruising.
Heparin	Acute DVT	IV, SQ	Continuous IV infusion dosed according to PTT at or above 60 seconds; therapeutic level 1.5–2.5 times normal or baseline. Infused at the rate of 700–1400 units/hour. Bleeding precautions; short half-life. Reversed with protamine injection, increased effects when given with other anticoagulants.
LMWH	Acute or postacute conditions	SQ	Longer acting; more reliable; no monitoring needed. Expensive. High bio-availability. Same bleeding precautions and drug-drug interactions as with heparin.

33. nifedipine (Procardia)

34. True, True

CHAPTER 54

1. See Figure U13-2 in textbook.
2. 1; 37.3
3. $403.1 billion
4. individuals in their peak, midlife years
5. the prevalence, incidence, and mortality varies among differing races and by gender
6. True, True, True
7. coronary artery disease, hypertension
8. 1, 2, 3
9. 1, 2, 3, 4, 5
10. 1, 2
11. childhood and infectious diseases; immunizations; hospitalizations; OB history; major illnesses; prior history of rheumatic fever, scarlet fever, severe strep infections, enlarged heart or murmurs; congenital abnormalities; renal and neurologic manifestations
12. 1, 2, 3, 4, 5
13. True, True, True, True, True, True, True, True, True
14.

S_1	Patho: closure of mitral, tricuspid valves; marks the onset of systole Heard best: at the apex and left lower sternal border with the diaphragm Sounds like: "lub"
S_2	Patho: closure of pulmonic and aortic valves; signifies onset of diastole Heard best: at the aortic area with the diaphragm Sounds like: "dup"
Gallop	Patho: sudden changes of inflow volume causing vibration of the valves and ventricular supporting structures. S_3: passive, rapid filling of the ventricle in early diastole. Benign except in adults over 30. S_4: increased stiffness of the ventricles Heard best: S_3: at the apex with the bell while client is in left lateral recumbent position S_4: at the apex with the bell, client in the supine, left lateral recumbent position Sounds like: S_3: dull, low pitched, follows S_2 immediately S_4: heard immediately before S_1

Friction rub:	Patho: inflamed layers of the pericardial sac rubbing against each other Heard best: with the diaphragm at the apex and along the left sternal border Sounds like: scratching, rubbing sound; heard throughout the respiratory cycle
Murmurs:	Patho: turbulent blood flow through valves and great vessels Heard best: with the bell, client in left lateral recumbent position Sounds like: blowing or swooshing

15. bruits, ascites, hepatojugular reflex
16. color, temperature, capillary refill, edema, turgor
17. a. Hematocrit: decreased oxygen-carrying capacity in anemia can cause angina
    b. WBC: often elevated after acute myocardial infarction
    c. Myoglobin: cardiac enzyme, released quickly after infarction
    d. CK-MB: enzyme specific to myocardial tissue released within 2 hours of damage
    e. Troponin: most specific cardiac enzyme but long half-life makes it impossible to use to diagnose second injury within a week
    f. PT/PTT: coagulation factors are increased after myocardial infarction and puts client at greater risk for new clotting phenomena or extension of MI
    g. LDL: increased risk of cardiovascular disease with increased levels
    h. HDL: decreased risk of cardiovascular disease with increased levels
    i. Sodium: reflects water balance; low sodium might indicate hypervolemia which stresses the heart or could indicate heart is not pumping well
    j. Potassium: abnormalities affect cardiac electrical instability
    k. BUN/creatinine: increased values may indicate heart is not pumping well enough to perfuse kidneys; also IV contrast dye is excreted through the kidneys
    l. Glucose: elevated after MI; also may indicate uncontrolled/undiagnosed diabetes
18. occupation, hobbies, family history of cardiovascular disease, substance abuse, lifestyle, household members, marital status, children, relationships, religious beliefs, support systems, home safety, location/accessibility of resources
19. 20
20. Primary prevention efforts are aimed at people who do not have a diagnosis of cardiovascular disease; secondary prevention efforts are aimed at people who do have a diagnosis of cardiovascular disease. Actual activities may be the same.

Modifiable Risk Factors
Smoking: don't start or quit (secondary: be aware that nicotine products, such as patches, still produce vasoconstriction; if the client can stop smoking without using these products it is better)
Diet: lose weight; low-sodium, low-fat diet
Alcohol intake: alcohol in moderation
Inactivity: begin structured exercise program (secondary: obtain physician OK prior to starting)

Metabolic Risk Factors
Dyslipidemia: low-fat diet, increase exercise, medication
Hypertension: keep BP under control with lifestyle modification, medication (secondary: add medications earlier in the presence of cardiovascular risk factors)
Obesity: lose weight (secondary: physician-approved diet regimen planned in consultation with registered dietitian)
Diabetes: maintain strict glycemic control
Metabolic syndrome: control disorder through weight loss, lifestyle modifications

21. 1, 2, 3
22. 1, 2
23. influenza
24. thrombophlebitis
25. 1, 2, 3, 4
26. dysrhythmias
27. angelica, astragalus, canola, ginkgo, motherwort, khela, cinchone

CHAPTER 55

1. 2201
2. the lack of donor hearts
3. 10–20%
4. in the first 30 days after transplant
5. cardiomyopathy
6. 1, 2, 3, 4
7. rheumatic fever
8. 1, 2
9. 1
10. 2
11. 1, 2, 3
12. 1, 2, 3
13. Acute pericarditis
14. a. 7, 8, 9
    b. 4, 5, 6
    c. 1, 2, 3

15. murmur
16. 2
17. 1, 2, 3, 4, 5
18. True, False, True, True, False, True, True
19. 1, 2, 3
20. Aschoff's bodies
21. 3
22. 1, 2, 3
23. 1, 2, 3, 4
24. 1, 2, 3, 4
25. 1, 2, 3, 4
26. 1, 2, 3, 4
27. 1, 2, 3, 4
28. pericardiocentesis
29. 2
30. 3
31. 1
32. 2
33. atrial fibrillation
34. Anticoagulants
35. 1, 2, 3
36. Aspirin
37. infection

CHAPTER 56

1. True, False, True, True
2. True, True, True, True, True
3. smoking, hypertension, obesity, elevated serum lipids, physical inactivity, diabetes
4. 1, 2, 3
5. menopause
6. intima; arterial wall
7. collateral circulation
8. Conditions that cause increased preload: mitral or tricuspid valve regurgitation, hypervolemia, congenital defects, ventricular septal defect, atrial septal defect, patent ductus arteriosus
   Conditions that cause increased afterload: hypertension (pulmonary or systemic), myocardial infarction, aortic or pulmonic stenosis, high peripheral vascular resistance, myocarditis, cardiomyopathy, ventricular aneurysm, long-term alcohol consumption, coronary heart disease, metabolic heart disease, endocrine heart disease, mitral or tricuspid stenosis, cardiac tamponade, constrictive pericarditis, hypertrophic obstructive cardiomyopathy
   Conditions that precipitate heart failure: dysrhythmias, systemic infections, anemia, thyroid disorders, pulmonary embolism, thiamine deficiency, chronic pulmonary diseases, medication dose changes, physical or emotional stress, endocarditis, myocarditis, or pericarditis, fluid reten-

tion from medication or salt intake, a new cardiac condition

9.

Right-Sided Failure	Left-Sided Failure
"R" is for the "rest" of the body Peripheral edema Anorexia Abdominal pain Nausea JVD Anasarca Cachexia	"L" is for "lungs" Dyspnea Orthopnea Paroxysmal nocturnal dyspnea Cough S_3, S_4 heart sounds Signs of cerebral hypoxia Fatigue, muscular weakness

10. True, True
11. 1, 2, 3, 4
12. True, True
13. 1, 2, 3, 4
14. 1, 2, 3, 4
15. 1, 2, 3
16. a. Decreased cardiac output
    b. Excess fluid volume
    c. Impaired gas exchange
    d. Ineffective tissue perfusion
    e. Risk for activity intolerance
    f. Risk for impaired skin integrity
    g. Risk for anxiety
17. The client will have an increase in cardiac output as evidenced by regular cardiac rhythm, heart rate, blood pressure, respirations, and urine output within normal limits.
18. assess BP, RR every hour, assess heart rate and rhythm every hour, document and analyze rhythm strips every 4–8 hours or per protocol, report dysrhythmias and/or treat per protocol, monitor appropriate lab work (see Care Plan), auscultate heart sounds every 1–2 hours, monitor lung sounds every hour, assess for changes in mental status, assess peripheral pulses every 2–4 hours, administer medications as ordered, encourage both physical and psychological rest, avoid rectal temperature or medication administration, serve small meals (sodium-restricted), and have client rest after eating
19. See Box 56-2 in textbook.
20. 1, 2, 3
21. 1, 2, 3, 4
22. sympathetic nervous system
23. 1, 2, 3
24. True
25. 1, 2, 3, 4
26. morphine sulfate

CHAPTER 57

1. 1, 2
2. 1, 2
3. 1
4. sudden death
5. 1, 2, 3
6. 1
7. accelerated
8. reentry
9. sinus exit block
10. 1, 2, 3, 4, 5
11. 1, 2, 3, 4
12. first-degree AV block
13. 1, 2, 3
14. 1, 2, 3, 4
15. 1, 2, 3, 4
16. 1, 2, 3, 4
17. coarse, fine
18. 1, 2, 3, 4
19. 1, 2, 3
20. atrial flutter, saw tooth
21. 1, 2, 3
22. 1, 2, 3
23. 1, 2
24. 1
25. 1, 2, 3, 4
26. 1, 2
27. normal sinus rhythm
28. ventricular tachycardia
29. atrial fibrillation
30. sinus rhythm with PAC
31. sinus rhythm with unifocal PVC
32. atrial flutter
33. sinus tachycardia
34. sinus bradycardia
35. 1, 2, 3, 4
36. 1, 2, 3, 4
37. 1
38. 1, 2, 3
39. 3
40. warfarin sodium (Coumadin)
41. 1, 2, 5
42. magnesium sulfate

CHAPTER 58

1. 1 million
2. 250,000
3. 6,400,000
4. a. adjust activity to a level below that which causes angina
   b. encourage frequent, brief rest periods
   c. have an earlier bedtime
   d. take longer or more frequent vacations

   e. seek counseling
   f. learn and practice relaxation techniques
5. a. dysrhythmias
   b. heart failure
   c. pulmonary edema
   d. cardiogenic shock
   e. pulmonary edema
   f. complications from myocardial necrosis
   g. pericarditis
   h. Dressler's syndrome
   i. recurrent MI
6. atherosclerotic lesions OR atherosclerosis
7. 1, 2
8. stable angina
9. unstable angina
10. variant angina
11. anterior wall of the left ventricle near the apex
12. 1, 2, 3, 4
13. 1, 2, 3, 4
14. chest pain OR angina pectoris
15. 1, 2, 3, 4
16. 1, 2, 3, 4
17. 1, 2, 3
18. True, True, False, True, True, False
19. dysrhythmias
20. 1, 2, 3
21. Morphine
    Oxygen
    Nitroglycerin
    Aspirin
22. A: aspirin and antianginal therapy
    B: beta blockers and blood pressure control
    C: cigarettes and cholesterol
    D: diabetes and diet
    E: education and exercise
23. 1, 2, 3, 4
24. 1
25. 1, 2, 3
26. 1, 2, 3
27. 1
28. 1, 2
29. Stop the activity and sit down. Take nitroglycerin, one pill sublingually, every 5 minutes up to three doses if the pain continues. After the third pill, if the pain continues or worsens, take an aspirin and have some one call 911. Family members should not drive the client to the hospital.

CHAPTER 59

1. 2, 3, 5, 6
2. 3
3. Noncardiac chest pain may be related to a cardiac or GI problem. Cardiac chest pain is usually described as an aching, heavy, squeezing sensation

with pressure or tightness in the substernal area and can radiate into the neck or arms.

4. 1, 2
5. True, True, False, False
6. the Visual Analogue Scale, Modified Borg Category Ratio Scale for Assessment of Dyspnea
7. sinusitis
8. stridor
9.

Factor	Area to Be Assessed
Occupation	Exposure to respiratory irritants; hobbies may involve chemicals, dust, airborne particles
Geographic location	Recent travel to areas where respiratory diseases are prevalent Air pollution
Environment	Living conditions Crowded household Air conditioning Climb stairs at home?
Habits	Smoking Smokeless tobacco Drug use Alcohol use
Exercise	Onset of wheezing with exercise Change in activities due to respiratory problems Typical activities during the day
Nutrition	Decreased nutrition due to fatigue

10. viral infections; normal aging; head injuries; local obstruction, emphysema
11. compare one side of the chest to the other side to note abnormalities.
12. say 99; check for symmetry on both sides
13. True, False, True, True, False
14. Fine crackles—discontinuous, high-pitched, short, crackling, popping sounds heard during inspiration, late = restrictive disease, pneumonia; early = COPD, asthma
Pleural friction rub—superficial sound that is coarse and low-pitched, has a grating quality like two pieces of leather rubbing together; pleuritis with pain on breathing
High-pitched wheezing—high-pitched musical squeaking sound that is mostly in expiration but can be in both; asthma or emphysema
15. inhaled; metered dose inhaler
16. moderately hypoxemic
17. vital capacity; expiratory volume; FRC; TLC; RV
18. Paco$_2$
19. less invasive

20. no physical symptoms are present
21. infectious; cancerous

CHAPTER 60

1. a. use of sedatives or anesthetic agents, b. deteriorating level of consciousness, c. any other condition potentially affecting ventilatory efficiency
2. cigarette smoking
3. 1, 2, 4
4. 1, 3
5. edema; suture line healing; swallow secretions
6. 2
7. beta-hemolytic streptococci
8. 4
9. topical nasal decongestant sprays; intranasal cocaine
10. gastric acid
11. hoarseness
12. True, False, False, False, False, True, True, True, False, True, True, True, True
13. 1, 2
14. 2
15. a. abnormal respiratory rate and pattern, b. use of accessory muscles to assist breathing, c. abnormal pulse and blood pressure, d. abnormal skin and mucous membrane color, e. abnormal ABG levels or oxygen saturation
16. 2, 3, 4
17. Mild bleeding
18. a. presence of bowel sounds, b. passage of flatus, c. complaints of hunger
19. a. coughing upon swallowing, b. ineffective cough, c. decreased breath sounds, d. crackles, rhonchi, or wheezes
20. False, False
21. 4, 3, 5, 1, 2
22. ability to speak; ability to eat
23. greater than 45 degrees
24. ice
25. True, True, False, False, True, True
26. 1, 2, 3, 4
27. epinephrine 1:1000

CHAPTER 61

1. 4
2. 1, 3, 5, 6
3. 3
4. 1, 2
5. 2
6. 4
7. ventilation-perfusion mismatch
8. 2, 3, 4, 5

9. 25 mm Hg
10. pulmonary vasoconstriction from chronic hypoxia
11. 1, 2, 3, 4, 5
12. False
13. 4
14 spiral CT scan
15. 1
16. An indication of approaching acute respiratory failure is an inability to auscultate wheezing during exhalation. The airways are too narrow to allow airflow.
17. 4
18. 3, 4
19. 2
20. 2
21. 3
22. 1, 2, 3, 4, 6
23. pursed-lip breathing
24. a. Severity of dyspnea is one measure to determine effectiveness of therapy.
    b. Spirometry is an effective tool to determine effectiveness of therapy and to anticipate exacerbations. Accuracy of assessment is important if it is to be used to plan therapy.
    c. Medication delivery is dependent on accuracy of use.
    d. Allergens may be a trigger for asthma attacks.
    e. Some clients may be taking medications which can cause bronchospasms, such as Inderal.
    f. History of triggers is needed to prepare a plan for prevention and control.
    g. Need to know abilities so that guidance can be provided to the client on disease management.
    h. Chronic disease management may be overwhelming. Family support helps decrease anxiety and the burden of self-care. Unsupportive family can increase stress.
    i. This assessment helps identify the presence of possible environmental triggers which can be modified.
25. 3
26. a. early ambulation, b. leg exercises, c. sequential compression stockings, d. low-dose heparin prophylaxis
27. When elevating the legs, flexure of the hips occurs which can contribute to stasis of the lower extremities and thus increase the risk for further clot formation.
28. 2
29. a. 2, i; b. 1, ii; c. 2, ii; d. 1, iv; e. 1, iv; f. 2, vi; g. 2, v
30. 1
31. 1
32. 2
33. 1, 3, 4, 5
34. 3

CHAPTER 62

1. a. fever, b. myalgias, c. cough
2. a. advanced age, b. history of smoking, c. upper respiratory infection, d. tracheal intubation, e. prolonged immobility, f. immunosuppressive therapy, g. nonfunctional immune system, h. malnutrition, i. dehydration, j. chronic disease states, k. homelessness
3. 1, 2
4. a. 6, b. 1, c. 5, d. 3, e. 2, f. 4, g. 7
5. atelectasis; chest x-ray
6. Ghon complex
7. a. advanced age, b. HIV infection, c. immunosuppression, d. prolonged corticosteroid therapy, e. malabsorption syndromes, f. low body weight, g. substance abuse, h. presence of other diseases, i. genetic predisposition.
8. True, False, False, False, True
9. a. small-cell carcinoma, b. non-small–cell that includes squamous cell carcinoma and adenocarcinoma, c. large cell, d. metastatic
10. cigarette smoking
11. False, False, True
12. a. 3, b. 4, c. 1, d. 2
13. distal; large
14. interstitial
15. True, True
16. empyema; drainage
17. diagnosis
18. True, False, False, False, True, True, True, True, True, True, True, False, True
19. areas of consolidation
20. a. assess rate and character of respirations, b. auscultate the breath sounds, c. assess skin and nail beds to determine the severity of hypoxia
21. Induration
22. AFB smear; culture
23. a. if the pulse rate becomes rapid, b. the blood pressure drops
24. Intermittent bubbling is normal and indicates that the system is accomplishing one of its functions. Continuous bubbling during inspiration and expiration indicates that air is leaking into the drainage system or pleural cavity.
25. Rapid bubbling in the absence of an air leak indicates considerable loss of air from an incision or tear in the pulmonary pleura.
26. True, True, True
27. side-lying
28. 1, 2, 3, 4

29. increased ability to perform ADLs; increase in physical activity with less dyspnea and fatigue
30. Coughing and deep-breathing promote lung expansion and the expulsion of air and fluid from the pleural space by increasing intrapulmonary and intrapleural pressures.
31. a. promote adequate oxygenation, b. maintain a patent airway, c. achieve the highest possible functional level
32. a. adequate hydration, b. bronchodilators and mucolytic aerosols, c. effective coughing techniques, d. twice daily inhalation of hypertonic saline solution, e. Synthetic DNase
33. False, True, False, False, True, True, True
34. prior to
35. two
36. amphotericin B
37. Corticosteroids
38. Cyclosporin A

CHAPTER 63

1. oxygen, carbon dioxide
2.

Hypoxemic	Ventilatory
Severe arterial hypoxemia	Client unable to support adequate gas exchange
Minimally responsive to oxygen	Results from CNS depression, inadequate neuromuscular ability to sustain breathing, respiratory system overload
Caused by diffuse problems such as pulmonary edema, near-drowning, ARDS, localized problems	

3. True, True, True
4. 3
5. carbon dioxide
6. pulsus paradoxus
7. decreased cardiac output
8. 4
9. 2, 3, 4
10. 1, 2, 3, 4
11. inflammatory response; increases permeability of the alveolar membrane; interstitial; alveolar; leads to; noncardiogenic; decreases lung compliance; oxygen transport
12. alveolar; surfactant
13. fibrin
14. increased respiratory rate; profound dyspnea
15. internal bleeding; punctured organs
16. a. atelectasis, b. hemopneumothorax, c. flail chest, d. aspiration, e. pulmonary contusion

17. 3, 4
18. air; pleural
19. spontaneous; traumatic
20. 4
21. 2
22. 1
23. 3
24. 1
25. True, True, True, False, True, False, True
26. 3, 4
27. 20
28. 1
29. a. airway patency, b. adequacy of breathing, c. circulatory sufficiency
30. absent; decreased
31. 2
32. 3
33. Raising edematous legs increases venous return and will stress the overtaxed left ventricle. Keeping the legs dependent decreases preload.
34. a. 4, b. 3, c. 1, d. 2
35. a. 4, b. 3, c. 2, d. 1
36. CPAP is applied to a client with spontaneous respirations, whereas PEEP is applied during mechanical ventilation. Both are used to apply positive pressure to keep the alveoli open and reduce shunting.
37. High-pressure alarms are triggered when there is increased airway resistance or decreased lung compliance such as secretions in the tube or kinking or dislodging of tube. Low-pressure alarms occur when the tubing is disconnected, ET cuff leak, or apnea.
38. Placing the client in a prone position creates a change in the dependent portions of the lung resulting in increased perfusion to the less damaged portions of the lungs and decreases pulmonary shunting.
39. clear communication; frequent updates
40. a. decreased, b. decreased, c. decreased, d. decreased
41. False, True, True, False
42. 4
43. vecuronium (Norcuron); pancuronium (Pavulon)
44. 1, 3
45. 1
46. 4
47. False, False
48. 2
49. 3
50. 4

CHAPTER 64

1. 1–8

2. True, False, False, False
3. 2, 4, 5, 7
4. False, False, True, False, True
5. vision, appearance, pain and comfort
6.

Complaint	Possible Cause
Hearing loss	Conductive from damage to middle ear or otosclerosis Sensorineural from disease of the inner ear, nerve pathways, from loss of hair cells CNS disorder
Pain	Related problems with nose, sinuses Oral cavity, pharynx, or TMJ
Ear drainage	Bleeding Infection
Tinnitus	In absence of sound waves

7. True, True, True
8. Photophobia
9. 1, 3, 4, 5
10. deeper internal aching
11. asymptomatic
12. HTN: can affect blood flow to eyes; retinopathy
Headache: can signal a brain tumor if visual changes present
13. normal (The position properly protects the sclera of the eye.)
14. corneal reflex
15. normal
16. light up; have consistent color
17. black; round; smooth borders; equal
18. image edema; areas of demyelinization; vascular lesions
19. Tonometry
20. 8; 21
21. a. hearing acuity, b. balance, c. equilibrium
22. 2
23.

Test	Purpose
Weber test	To assess conduction of sound through bone
Rinne test	Distinguishes conductive loss from sensorineural hearing loss
Romberg test	Assess the inner ear for balance

24. The cornea of the eye must be anesthetized with topical anesthetic drops.
25. Fruits, vegetables, fish, vitamins C and E, and beta carotene have potential to reduce the incidence of visual problems like macular degeneration.

26. identify; quantify; localize the source
27. Presence of clear drainage may be due to infection, fistulas, or leakage of CSF. The physician should be notified and a specimen collected for analysis.
28. 1, 2, 3, 4, 5
29. Over-the-counter preparations may contain antihistamines and decongestants which can dry the ocular surface of the eye.

CHAPTER 65

1. 4
2.

Type	Cause	Manifestations
Primary open angle	Aqueous humor flow is obstructed by trabecular meshwork	No early signs Later: increased intraocular pressure (IOP) Bilateral
Angle closure	Anatomically narrow anterior chamber angle Sudden blockage of anterior angle by base of iris	Unilateral, develops suddenly Severe pain, blurred vision/vision loss
Normal tension	Normal-high IOP	Optic nerve is damaged IOP not high Resembles primary open-angle
Secondary	Edema, eye injury, inflammation, tumor, cataracts, diabetes block outflow of aqueous humor	unilateral/bilateral

3. a. hypertension, b. diabetes, c. cardiovascular disease, d. obesity
4. 1, 2, 4, 5, 6, 7, 8, 10
5. False
6. central

7.

Type	Etiology	Manifestations
Dry	Atrophy and degeneration of retina	Thinning of macula deposits into retina
Wet	Bleeding within and beneath the retina	"Metamorphopsia," distorted lines in vision Opaque deposits Central vision more distorted Scar tissue formation Dark, blurry area in center of vision or "white out" Color perception changes

8. burning, itching, sensation of something in the eye

9.

Type	Etiology	Manifestation
Myopia	Light rays focus in front of the retina	Difficulty seeing things far away (nearsighted)
Hyperopia	Eye is deficient in focusing light rays Image that falls on the retina is blurred	Difficulty seeing things near (farsighted)
Astigmatism	Rays of light are not equally bent in all directions	Poor vision for both distant and near objects

10. 12; 22
11. awakening
12. True, False, True, True, True
13. retinal detachment
14. a. Graves' disease: exophthalmos
    b. Rheumatoid arthritis/connective tissue disorder: Sjögren's syndrome
    c. SLE (lupus): retinopathy of SLE—cotton wool spots, optic neuropathy, discoid lesions of eyelids
    d. Myasthenia gravis: ptosis of eyelids, diplopia, nystagmus, ocular myopathy, cranial nerve palsy
    e. Multiple sclerosis: optic neuritis
    f. Hypertension: vasoconstriction, leakage, arteriosclerosis of ocular vessels, hypertensive retinopathy, retinal vein occlusion

g. AIDS: cytomegalovirus retinitis, bacterial corneal ulcers, fungal corneal ulcers, protozoan/viral infections, HIV retinopathy, Kaposi's sarcoma, non-Hodgkins' lymphoma

h. Lyme disease: optic neuropathy, keratitis, choroiditis, exudative retinal detachment

15. 1, 3, 4, 5
16. blood pressure
17. 3
18. Prolonged vomiting can result in increased IOP and wound dehiscence.
19. a. observe the eye patch for any drainage (only serous drainage is expected), and b. assess the level of pain and presence of nausea.
20. 1, 2, 3
21. True, False, True, True, True, True
22. Miotics
23. Topical beta-blockers
24. False, True, True
25. 4

CHAPTER 66

1. Hearing impairment
2.

Type	Cause	Results
Conductive	Anything that blocks external ear—thickening, scarring, retraction, or perforation of tympanic membrane Any pathophysiologic change in middle ear that affects the ossicles	Interference with sound transmission through external and middle ear
Sensorineural	Congenital/hereditary, noise injury, aging Meniere's disease, ototoxicity	Impairment of the function of the inner ear, eighth cranial nerve, or brain
Mixed hearing loss	Combined	Both components present (sensorineural and conductive)

3. buildup of matter
4. Otitis media
5. 1, 2, 3, 4
6. Presbycusis
7. 1

8. 1, 2, 3, 4, 5
9. 1, 2, 3, 4, 5, 6
10. True, False, True, False, True, True
11.

Disorder	Cause	Manifestations
Benign paroxysmal positional vertigo	Follows head injury or viral infection of inner ear Calcium crystals deposited on otoliths	Slow responses to head movement Brief attacks of vertigo Rapid head tilt to affected ear Self-limited, resolves over weeks to months
Labyrinthitis	Infection or inflammation of cochlear or vestibular portion of inner ear Syndrome occurs in spring or early summer Preceded by URI	Vertigo Nausea Vomiting No hearing changes Resolves in 1–2 weeks
Meniere's disease	Excess endolymph in vestibular and semicircular canals	Hearing changes episodic; waxes and wanes Paroxysmal whirling vertigo Fluctuating hearing loss Tinnitus Aural fullness

12. a. vestibular system (labyrinth or inner ear), b. visual system, c. proprioceptive system (joints and muscles), d. cerebellar system
13. a. Rinne's test: hearing loss results in greater conduction by bone
    b. Weber test: sound will lateralize to the more affected ear
14. Gently pulling on the pinna causes pain when the infection is in the outer ear because the area is inflamed. Touching the ear does not cause pain when the infection is in the middle ear.
15. 6
16. transient ischemic attack
17. 1, 2, 3, 4

18. OUTCOME: Client will develop effective methods to communicate needs and will be included in conversation
    INTERVENTIONS: writing requests, visual aids (pictures, diagrams), use of an expert interpreter
19. 3
20. 1, 2, 4, 6
21. a. meticulous cleaning of ear canal, b. warming of irrigation solution
22. complete
23. 2, 3, 4
24. corticosteroids
25. boric acid and alcohol
26. 1, 3, 4

CHAPTER 67

1. 1, 2, 4, 5
2. family, friends, ambulance team
3. pyramidal tract disorders
4. 5
5.

Area	Clinical Significance
Growth and development	Was neurologic dysfunction present at early age? Prenatal exposure to disease Full term vs. preterm Did client accomplish major developmental tasks?
Family health history	Presence of genetic risk factors Epilepsy Huntington's disease ALS Muscular dystrophy HTN/stroke Psychiatric disorders
Psychosocial history	Educational background Level of performance Changes in sleep patterns Perceived stressors Exposure to toxic substances at work

6. Level of consciousness
7. 1, 2, 3, 4
8. 7s; 3s
9. a. inspection, b. palpation, c. percussion, d. auscultation
10. Raccoon eyes
11. nuchal rigidity

12.

Cranial Nerve	Function	Testing Method	Indication of Dysfunction
I	Smell	Ask client to identify aromatic odor (coffee, vanilla)	Anosmia
II	Visual acuity	Snellen chart; visual fields	Amorosis (blindness): decreased or absent central vision Vision loss in one or more direction or in a portion of the visual field (half of visual field, middle portion, or both sides). Diabetic retinopathy, loss of venous pulsation Papilledema: optic disc swelling
III, IV, VI	Eyes; eye movement	Test direct/consensual response Test accommodation Pupillary light reflex Check six cardinal directions of gaze	CN III: ptosis: upper eyelid droop; Inability of an eye to move nasally, up and nasally, up and temporally, or downward. Irregularly shaped pupils Aniscoria: unequal pupils; no or sluggish response to light or accommodation Nystagmus (involuntary eye movements): seen as fine, rhythmic eye movements that can be vertical, horizontal, or rotational Inability to look down or to walk down steps due to visual disturbance Inability of an eye to move laterally outward; diplopia
V	Muscles of mastication	Clamp jaws shut, open mouth against resistance Open mouth widely test corneal reflex	Weakness (rare), aching, or spasm of masseter or temporal muscles Facial pain, paresthesias
VII	Facial expression	Ask client to frown, smile Raise eyebrows, tightly close eyes Show teeth, puff out cheeks	Central deficits: affects the lower half of the face only; due to CNS defect Peripheral deficit: deficit involving both upper face and lower face; due to CN VII lesion Facial asymmetry, loss of nasolabial fold, inability to close the eye and blink reflexively, drooling, difficulty swallowing secretions, loss of tearing Loss of taste on the anterior two-thirds of the tongue
VIII	Hearing; bone and air conduction; equilibrium	Listen to whispered voice Tuning forks Romberg test	Whispered words, fingers rubbing not heard correctly or equally Sound lateralized to one side (negative Weber): Sound lateralizes toward side with hearing loss (conductive); sound lateralizes toward side w/o hearing loss (sensorineural) Bone conduction equal to or longer than air conduction (negative Rinne) Swaying, wide-based stance to maintain balance (positive Rhomberg) No response

IX, X	Pharynx	Open mouth wide and say "Ah" Test gag reflex Ask client to cough and speak	Uvula deviates, palate fails to rise Hoarse voice Nasal voice No gag Weak cough Loss of taste, tachycardia, ileus
XI	Sternocleido-mastoid; trapezius muscles	Elevate shoulders with/without resis-tance, turn head to one side, then other Resist attempt to pull chin back to midline push head forward against resistance	Drooping of a shoulder, muscle atrophy, weak shoulder shrug, or weak turn of the head
XII	Tongue	Open mouth wide, stick out tongue; check to see if midline	Deviation of tongue to weak side, atrophy, fas-ciculations, slurred speech (dysarthria)

13. Ask the client to stand quietly with feet together; assess balance and sense of body position.
14.

Type	Method of testing
Stereognosis	Place three small familiar ob-jects into client's hands; ask cli-ent to identify with eyes closed
Graphesthesia	Trace different, separate letters and numbers on client's palm; ask client to identify with eyes closed
Extinction phe-nomenon	Simultaneously prick client's skin at same point on two sides of the body at same time; ask client whether they felt one or two pricks
Two-point simulation	Simultaneously prick the skin with two pins at varying dis-tances; identify the smallest distance which the client can perceive two pricks

15. Babinski
16. False, True, True, False, True
17. blood flow
18. brain death
19. Pain—focus on location of pain such as head, back, sudden or gradual onset, frequency, dura-tion, character (if throbbing, achy, dull sharp). Also ask what factors accompany the pain.
    Dizziness—ask how the client defines dizziness. Is it related to postural changes, head movement changes, vision problems? What helps it or makes it worse?

Sensory complaints—ask client to describe the sensation if they can't see, taste, hear, smell, or feel. Ask what kind of sensation it is, whether shooting, dull, stabbing, sharp. Ask when it hap-pens and how long it lasts.
Motor complaints—ask the client about weak-ness or coordination problems, involuntary movements. Inquire about the site, onset, fre-quency, and duration of any manifestations. What starts them and what makes them better?
Loss of consciousness/alterations in mental sta-tus—ask family or friends when the problem began, how long it lasts. Was there any trauma or other injury that started the problem? Are there other symptoms that accompany it? Ask if there are other illnesses that might contribute to this problem.
20. True, True, False, True, True, True
21. Many over-the-counter medications contain ingredients that affect the CNS and can alter functioning. Many herbal remedies, which are advertised as "natural," have active chemical components that alter CNS function too.

CHAPTER 68

1. Structural lesions
2. Metabolic disorders
3. True
4. metabolic
5. contractures
6. a. aphasia, b. apraxia, c. agnosia

7.

Manifestation	Example of Client Behavior
Disorder of attention	Patient may fear they are "going crazy" May appear preoccupied
Fluctuations in cognition	Totally irrational one moment, then lucid More disoriented at night Unfamiliar surroundings Unfamiliar noises Unfamiliar people Lack of window in room: disoriented
Loss of memory for recent events	Hallmark of metabolic disorders Difficulty with immediate recall and abstract thought Quickly lose orientation to time
Perceptual errors	Mistaking the nurse for daughter Hallucinations, illusions, delusions
Hallucinations	Client hears, sees, feels, smells, or tastes something that is not present
Illusions	Misinterpretation of something actually in the environment; e.g., mistaking shadows for a real person
Delusions	Thoughts or beliefs with no basis in fact; e.g., believing they have been robbed or poisoned when no basis exists for the belief

8. The client cannot actively participate in care/decisions; therefore the family serves as the client in these circumstances.
9. impaction
10. 1, 2, 3, 4, 5
11. doll's eye
12. 1, 2, 3, 4, 5, 6, 7, 8
13. mortality or significant morbidity
14. Glasgow Coma
15. 3
16. Reposition the patient often and tape the eyes closed if needed
17. False, True, True, True, False
18. high Fowler's
19. Turn off tube feedings several hours before the meal to stimulate appetite.
20. Resume the tube feeding. Volumes under 100 ml do not require delaying tube feeding.
21. 1, 2, 3, 4, 6

22.

Task	Responsibility	Can RN Delegate?
Verification of physician order	RN	no
Verification of placement of feeding tube	RN	no
Reconstitution of feeding	RN/licensed	yes*
Preparation of feeding	RN/licensed	yes*
Priming the feeding pump	RN/licensed	yes*
Irrigation of feeding tube	RN	no
Tube site care	RN/licensed	yes*
Monitoring fluid/ nutritional balance	RN	no

*RN is responsible for the care of the patient. If tasks are delegated, the RN retains the responsibility for ensuring proper instructions were given and verifying competence in performing.

23. professional; compassionate; cope; support; talk
24. diazepam
25. Empty the catheter bag to assist with clear assessment of diuretic effect per urine volume obtained.

CHAPTER 69

1. seizure
2. Epilepsy
3. During continued seizure activity, the brain requires increased oxygen and glucose to meet the energy demands. If the seizures continue, as in status epilepticus, the supplies are exhausted and result in anaerobic metabolism.

4.

Area of Brain	Manifestations
Motor cortex	Motor manifestations, upper extremity with spreading of movements centrally to entire limb, one side of face and lower extremity (Jacksonian)
Parietal region	Sensory phenomena; numbness or tingling
Occipital region	Bright, flashing lights in field of vision opposite the side of the focus
Posterior temporal area	Difficulty speaking or aphasia
Anterior temporal lobe	Begin with psychic manifestations; "aura"

5. 3, 4, 1, 5, 2
6. True, False, True, True, False, True
7.

Area of Brain	Manifestations
Frontal lobe	Inappropriate behavior Speech disturbance Bowel/bladder incontinence Gait disturbances
Temporal lobe	Receptive aphasia Visual field changes Tinnitus Headache
Parietal lobe	Sensory deficits Right/left disorientation Psychomotor seizures
Occipital lobe	Headache Homonymous hemianopsia
Cerebellar	Unsteady gait Falling/incoordination Tremors Nystagmus
Brain stem	Vertigo/dizziness Vomiting Sudden death from cardiac/respiratory failure
Pituitary/hypothalamus	Hormonal dysfunction Sleep disturbance Temperature fluctuations Cushing's syndrome
Ventricle	Obstruction of CSF circulation Hydrocephalus Rapid rise in ICP Postural headache

8. 1

9.

Type	Etiology	Manifestation
Tension	Muscle contraction, fatigue and stress	Tight, band-like, posterior neck
Cluster	Form of migraine triggered by alcohol	Cyclical pattern, boring, intense pain, constricted pupils
Migraine	Vascular headache	Vasospasm, unilateral, throbbing/pulsatile, photophobia, anorexia, nausea and vomiting, aura

10. EEG
11. Details about the seizure, its starting point, and progression can aid in diagnosing cause.
12. The nurse should look at the stereotypical movements and paroxysmal nature of seizures. Clients exhibiting pseudoseizures make different movements with each seizure.
13. Absence—in children or adolescents
Myoclonic—sudden uncontrollable jerking movements in single or multiple muscle groups; client sometimes falls, loses consciousness, and then confused postictally; seizures occur often in the morning
Clonic—rhythmic muscular contraction and relaxation lasting several minutes, no distinct phases
Tonic—abrupt increase in muscular tone and muscular contraction, loss of consciousness and autonomic manifestations, last 30 seconds to several minutes
14. aneurysm
15. blood
16. a. Nuchal rigidity: stiffness of the neck, pain upon movement
    b. Brudzinski's sign: forward neck flexion of a supine client results in flexion of both thighs at the hips and flexion of ankles
    c. Kernig's sign: with client recumbent, thigh flexed at right angle to abdomen, knee flexed 90 degrees; extending the leg causes pain, spasm of hamstring, and resistance to further extension
17. a. prevent injury during seizures
    b. eliminate factors that precipitate seizures
    c. diagnose and treat cause of seizures
    d. control seizures to allow desired lifestyle
18. 1, 2, 3, 5

19. Do not attempt to use an oral airway or open the client's mouth with your fingers
20. 1, 2, 3, 5
21. Complete history and physical assessment with documentation of LOC, orientation, neurologic checks, cranial nerve function, limb strength and movement, mental status
22. Immediate notification of observation to physician to evaluate for presence of CSF fluid.
23. 1, 3, 4, 5, 6, 7
24. LOC; blood pressure
25. Monitor dosage and side effects carefully due to decreased elimination and increased half-life resulting in higher plasma levels of medications.
26. immediately
27. Alcohol lowers the seizure threshold and is detoxified by the liver. Most anticonvulsant drugs are also metabolized by the liver; this would place an increased strain on the metabolizing functions of the liver.
28. diazepam
29. vasopressin
30. The osmotic diuretic mannitol disrupts the barrier, allowing greater concentration of the chemotherapy agents.
31. Corticosteroids
32. Temozolamide
33. gastrointestinal motility

CHAPTER 70

1. a. Ischemic: caused by a thrombotic or embolic blockage of blood to the brain
    b. Hemorrhagic: bleeding into the brain tissue; may be due to aneurysm
2. ischemic
3. oxygen
4. Atherosclerosis causes a narrowing of the blood vessel with deposits; turbulent blood flow causes platelets to adhere to the plaque.
5. diabetes
6. hypertension
7. a. hyperlipidemia, b. cigarette smoking, c. heavy alcohol consumption, d. cocaine use, e. obesity
8. 50
9. bifurcation of the common carotid
10. The speech center for most right-handed clients is in the left cerebral hemisphere. The nerve fibers cross over in the pyramidal tract as they pass from the brain to the spinal cord. Therefore, a stroke to the left side of the brain results in loss of speech control and right-sided hemiplegia.
11. With dysarthria, the client understands language but has difficulty pronouncing words and may slur them. Aphasia may involve deficits in speaking, reading, and writing.
12. TIAs are brief episodes of neurologic dysfunction, lasting less than 24 hours, and recovery is complete. TIAs serve as a warning sign of an impending stroke, the effect of which may be permanent. The pathophysiology of a TIA is similar to that of a stroke. Differences are in duration of ischemia and the lack of permanent deficits.
13.

Type	Characteristics
Wernicke's	Receptive aphasia clients can speak but do not understand spoken words
Broca's	Expressive aphasic clients can understand spoken words but cannot speak clearly
Global	Affects both speech comprehension and speech production

14.

Type of Stroke	Warning Manifestations
Ischemic	Transient hemiparesis, loss of speech, hemisensory loss
Thrombotic	Develops over minutes to hours to days. First partial and then complete occlusion of the affected vessel.
Embolic	Occurs suddenly, without warning.
Hemorrhagic	Occurs rapidly Severe occipital headache Vertigo/syncope Paresthesias Transient paralysis Epistaxis Retinal hemorrhage

15. 1, 2, 4
16. a. level of consciousness, b. pupillary response to light, c. visual fields, d. movement of extremities, e. speech, f. sensation, g. reflexes, h. vital signs
17. a. acoustic aphasia: Clients can hear the sounds of speech but the parts of the brain that give meaning to these sounds are damaged. They do not understand. b. visual aphasia: Clients cannot read words but can see them. They do not understand the symbols.
18. 1, 2, 3, 4
19. 2
20. maintaining a patent airway

21. Elevated temperatures require increased metabolic needs, which in turn will cause cerebral edema and increased risk of ischemia.
22. a. prevents joint immobility, contractures, and muscle atrophy, b. stimulates circulation, c. helps to reestablish neuromuscular pathways
23. Assist client to lie prone for 15–30 minutes several times a day and place a pillow under the pelvis to hyperextend the hip joints. When positioning the client on his or her side, do not flex the hip acutely.
24. 1, 2, 3, 4, 6
25. Neurologic status
26. To rule out hemorrhagic stroke as the cause of acute neurologic changes. Hemorrhage would contraindicate using thrombolytics.
27. 1, 3, 4, 5, 7
28. 6 hours
29. 24
30. 1.5–2.5

CHAPTER 71

1.

Cause	Example
Biomechanical and destructive	Compression of disks, herniation of disks, torsion injuries
Destructive origins	Infections, tumors, rheumatoid disorders
Degenerative	Osteoporosis, spinal stenosis
Other	Depression, unhappy in work setting, involved in litigation

2. Changes in cartilage and elasticity of the disk cause the disk to prolapse.
3. True, True, False
4. a. Lordosis: excessive backward concavity of lumbar spine; results in swayback and kyphosis, back pain
   b. Spondylothesis: forward slipping of vertebra; occurs at L4–L5; loss of spinal alignment
   c. Spondylosis: defect of lamina; vertebral arch slips forward; lumbar area most common
   d. Spinal stenosis: ligamentous infolding and hypertrophy of the bone; produces pressure on entire spinal cord, weakness or paralysis
5. contralateral paralysis
6. Neurofibromas; meningiomas
7. fifth
8. seventh; unilateral paralysis

9.

Type	Manifestation
Motor nerves	Muscle weakness Cramps Spasms Loss of balance/coordination
Sensory nerves	Tingling Numbness Pain: burning, freezing, or electric-like sensations, sensation of wearing an invisible "glove" or "sock," sensitivity to touch
Autonomic nerves	Orthostatic hypotension, bradycardia Reduced ability to perspire Constipation Bladder dysfunction Sexual dysfunction

10. carpal tunnel
11. True, False, True, True,
12. To identify workplace causes for back strain and correct them
13. bone graft donor
14. swelling
15. See Figure 71-11 in the textbook.
16. Surgeons frequently inject local anesthetic into surgical site. Assessment of sensation can be done after the effects have worn off.
17. progressive weakness or paralysis of the lower extremities; loss of sphincter control; anal numbness; urinary retention
18. Place the client in a lateral position with knees flexed.
19. 1, 2, 4
20. strengthening of back and abdominal muscles through daily exercises
21. logrolling
22. Pillows should not be placed under the popliteal space as this increases risk of DVT
23. 8
24. 1, 2, 3, 5
25. 2
26. opioids
27. The chemical in the hot pepper extract added to the cream is useful in relieving neuropathic pain by blocking pain impulses.
28. The discomfort is an indicator of the need to make adjustments in lifestyle to preserve function. Medicating will mask the need for changes.
29. Tegretol

CHAPTER 72

1.

Type	Characteristics
Alzheimer's disease	Progressive decline in two or more areas of cognition Most common form of dementia in people 65+ years of age Cause is unknown Presence of neurologic plaques/tangles widely distributed throughout brain
Multi-infarct disease	Second most common cause of irreversible dementia Blood clots block small vessels in brain Men Over 50 years old Progressive decline in cognition
Lewy body dementia	Similar to Alzheimer's Progresses more rapidly Abnormal brain cells, "Lewy bodies"
Pick's disease	Form of dementia, different from Alzheimer's "Pick's bodies" within neuron cells sharply confined to front parts of brain

2.

Stage	Manifestations
Preclinical	Disease begins near hippocampus (essential for short- and long-term memory); affected regions begin to shrink Memory loss begins Period can last 10–20 years
Mild Alzheimer's	Cerebral cortex begins to shrink memory disturbances noticed by family or coworkers before client does May have poor judgment or problem-solving skills May become careless in work habits Confused where they are/get lost easily Client may become irritable, agitated
Moderate Alzheimer's	Language disturbances: circumlocution Paraphrasias Palilalia Echolalia Motor disturbances: apraxia Forgetfulness: safety concerns Depression and irritability worsen Delusions/psychosis may appear Wandering at night is common Occasional incontinence
Severe Alzheimer's	Clients cannot recognize family/friends; do not communicate in any way; voluntary movement is minimal, limbs are rigid; urinary/fecal incontinence frequent; high risk for aspiration

3. 50
4. 2
5. 1, 3, 4, 5, 6, 7
6. descending
7. ACh receptors
8. cognition
9. respiratory failure and death from pneumonia
10. Myasthenic crisis: precipitated by infection or sudden withdrawal of anticholinesterase drugs; difficulty swallowing or breathing
    Cholinergic crisis: result of overmedication; abdominal cramps, diarrhea, excessive pulmonary secretions
11. 1, 2, 3, 4, 5
12. a. bradykinesia; b. rigidity; c. tremor at rest; d. flexed posture of the neck, trunk, and limbs; e. loss of postural reflexes; f. freezing movement
13. muscle weakness and fatigue that worsens with exercise and improves with rest
14. ptosis
15. improvement
16. a. identification of potential safety hazards (loose rugs, hot tap water, inadequate lighting, unlocked doors); b. teach family members how to safeguard home; c. place identification badge on clients in case they become lost; d. place dangerous items out of reach; e. supervise potentially dangerous activities
17. a. stretch spastic muscles at least twice a day through full range of motion, b. assess muscle spasticity, c. administer medications to relieve muscle spasms, d. avoid intense aerobic activity, e. use ambulation aids such as cane or walker
18. 1
19. 1, 2, 3, 5
20. 1, 2, 3
21. 1, 3, 4, 5

22. They are used to help retain ACh in the neuro-junctions in clients with Alzheimer's disease. Clients will experience improvements in thinking abilities and are less likely to demonstrate manifestations of wandering, agitation, or socially inappropriate behavior.
23. Levodopa is a precursor to dopamine, a necessary neurotransmitter, which is deficient in Parkinson's disease.
24. Haloperidol
25. IV corticosteroids (methylprednisolone)

CHAPTER 73

1. 20
2. a. space-occupying tumors, b. cerebral infarction, c. obstruction of the outflow of CSF, d. ingested or accumulated toxins, e. impaired blood flow to or from the brain, f. systemic hypertension
3. a. movement of CSF out of the cranium, b. reduction of blood flow to the brain, c. displacement of brain tissue (herniation)
4. a. any alteration in level of consciousness, b. decrease in the Glasgow Coma Scale
5. increased systolic blood pressure; widened pulse pressure; bradycardia
6. motor vehicle accidents
7.

Injury	Characteristics
Concussion	No break in the skull No visible damage on CT or MRI
Open head injury	Penetrates the skull
Closed head injury	Blunt trauma
Contusions	More extensive damage Brain is damaged
Subdural hematoma	Collection of blood in the subdural space Brain or blood vessel laceration

8. a. Transcalvarial—brain tissue is extruded through an unstable skull fracture, variable manifestations depending on location
   b. Central—result of downward displacement of the brain tissue through the tentorial notch, rapid change in the LOC, changes in respiratory patterns, pupils go from small and reactive to dilated and fixed
   c. Lateral transtentorial—occurs from displacement by masses in or along the temporal lobe, called *uncal herniation*, pupils sluggish then unresponsive, first ipsilateral, then contralateral, decreasing LOC, abnormal respirations, posturing
   d. Cingulate—frontal lobes are compressed, ischemia, congestion, edema, IICP
   e. Infratentorial—when cerebellar tonsil shifts through the foramen magnum compressing the medulla, rapid progression of blood pressure changes, pulse and breathing, decreased LOC, arched stiff neck, quadriparesis
9. males; 16; 30
10. Flexion injuries
11. 1, 2, 3, 4
12. quadriplegia
13. paraplegia
14. 1, 2, 3, 4, 5, 6, 7
15. 3
16. 1, 2, 3, 4, 5, 6
17. basilar skull fracture of the frontal and temporal bones
18. It helps to determine the extent of the injury, client's activity, and LOC before and after the injury.
19. 2
20. dermatomes
21. a. intubation followed by hyperventilation, b. osmotic diuretics: Mannitol, c. elevation of the head: to promote venous drainage
22. 1, 2, 4
23. a. elevate the head of the bed to a sitting position immediately, b. check blood pressure, c. check for possible sources of irritation, d. remove stimulus if possible, e. administer antihypertensives if needed
24. logrolling
25. 2, 3, 4
26. a. proper fitting of wheelchair to meet client's ability
    b. ROM exercises, oral antispasmodic medications
    c. intermittent catheterization, suprapubic catheters
    d. use of suppositories or digital stimulation every day
    e. frequent turning, pressure-relieving devices; thorough skin assessment
    f. incentive spirometry, diaphragmatic breathing
    g. nonopioid analgesics, TENS units
    h. peer group counseling sessions, vocational rehabilitation
27. True, False, True, True, False, True, True, False
28. skeletal traction
29. The nurse will monitor for thrombophlebitis as evidenced by unilateral leg edema, erythema, and warmth. Entiembolism stockings, subcutaneous heparin.

30. The client will have reduced risk of constipation as evidenced by a bowel movement every 1–2 days. Bowel regimen to include digital stimulation to signal the body for reflex evacuation, 3000 ml fluid intake daily.
31. Seizures significantly increase metabolic requirements and cerebral blood flow and volume, increasing ICP.
32. muscle relaxants
33. False, False, True, True
34.

Medication	Indication for Use
Vasoactive agents	Support blood pressure
Steroids	Reduce inflammation/prevent damage
Thyrotropin-releasing hormone	Decrease post-traumatic ischemia
H₂ receptor blocking agents	Reduce risk of gastric/intestinal bleeding

35. Urecholine; Ditropan
36. Neurontin (Gabapentin)
37. etidronate disodium (Didronel)

CHAPTER 74

1. the nature of the presenting problem
2. a. very young, b. very old
3. 1, 2, 3
4. a. food, b. drug, c. blood, d. seasonal
5. because there is a consequent reduction in absorption of vitamin B_{12}
6. increased hemoglobin levels
7. 1, 2, 3
8. 1
9. a. loss of anatomic integrity from instrumentation (catheters), b. impaired dermatologic barrier function (burns), c. mucosal inflammation (cigarette smoke), d. mucociliary elevator dysfunction (cystic fibrosis)

10.

Anatomic area	Manifestation	Possible Cause
Eyes	Visual disturbances Blindness Scleral jaundice Conjunctivitis, tearing, eye rubbing, styes, and dark circles or "allergic shiners," or "raccoon eyes"	Anemia, polycythemia Retinal hemorrhage related to thrombocytopenia or bleeding disorder Hemolytic anemia Allergies
Ears	Vertigo or tinnitus Blood in the external auditory canal or bluish tympanic membrane, suggesting blood in the middle ear Chronic otitis media, mastoiditis Hearing impairment related to eardrum rupture, scarring, perforated tympanic membrane	Severe anemia Bleeding disorders Immunodeficiencies or chronic infections and treatment with ototoxic drugs
Nose	Epistaxis Crusting around nares, sinopulmonary drainage, and indications of chronic sinusitis sneezing, sniffling, rhinitis, nasal polyps, nasal voice quality	Thrombocytopenia and bleeding disorders Immunodeficiency Allergies
Mouth	Smooth, glossy, bright red, and sore tongue gingival bleeding Oral ulcers, candidiasis, gingivitis, periodontitis, dental caries, and tooth loss Tonsils may be enlarged, inflamed, or pustular; lip and tongue swelling; frequent throat clearing from postnasal drip; sore throat; itching of the palate, throat, or neck; and hoarseness can occur	Pernicious anemia, iron-deficiency anemia Thrombocytopenia, bleeding disorders Immunodeficiencies Allergies

11. True, False, True, True, True, True
12. 1
13. a. anemia, b. thrombocytopenia, c. bleeding disorders, d. congenital blood disorders, e. jaundice, f. frequent infections, g. delayed healing, h. cancer, i. autoimmune disease
14. a. superficial lymph nodes, b. liver, c. spleen
15. a. complete blood count, b. differential white blood count, c. coagulation studies, d. a peripheral blood smear for red blood cell morphology
16. dyspnea; orthopnea
17. a. platelet count, b. PT, c. PTT, d. bleeding time
18. a. low, b. normal, c. normal, d. low, e. high, f. low, g. high, h. normal, i. high, j. normal, k. high, l. normal, m. normal
19. True, True
20. Donating blood or blood products can affect laboratory values for days or weeks.
21. Toxic chemicals or ionizing radiation that occurs in the work environment such as plastics, ceramics, steel, or metal refinery can predispose an individual to blood disorders.
22. tachycardia
23. Coomb's test
24. bleeding tendencies
25. Some herbal preparations may have an anticoagulant effect such as ginkgo or garlic; Ephedra might reduce the effect of prednisone; St. John's wort can reduce warfarin levels.
26. cephalosporins; penicillin; sulfonamides
27. False, True

CHAPTER 75

1. 4
2. 2
3. a. severity of blood loss, b. speed of blood loss, c. chronicity of the anemia, d. other comorbid conditions
4. a. decreased hemoglobin, b. decreased RBCs, c. hypoxia
5. blood loss, most commonly from the GI tract
6. globin
7. RBCs; Vitamin B$_{12}$; folic acid
8. 3
9. hemolytic
10. oxygenation
11. pluripotent stem cells
12. joint pain
13. phlebotomy
14. neutrophils
15. bone pain
16. a. intact blood vessels, b. an adequate number of functioning platelets, c. sufficient amounts of 12

clotting factors, d. a well-controlled fibrinolytic system
17. idiopathic thrombocytopenic purpura
18. vitamin K
19. a. infection, b. introduction of tissue coagulation factors into the circulation, c. damage to vascular endothelium, d. stagnant blood flow
20. a. purpura, petechiae, and ecchymoses on the skin, mucous membranes, heart lining, and lungs, b. prolonged bleeding from venipuncture, c. severe, uncontrolled hemorrhage, d. excessive bleeding from gums and the nose, e. intracerebral and GI bleeding, f. renal hematuria, g. tachycardia and hypotension, h. dyspnea, hemoptysis, and respiratory congestion
21. males
22. False, True, False, True, True, False, True, True, True, True, False, True, True, True, True, True, True, True, True, False, False, True
23. 2
24. 2
25. 4
26. 1–6 decreased, 7 increased
27. 1
28. splenic rupture secondary to trauma; hypersplenism
29. False, True
30. a. iron therapy, b. nutritional therapy, c. surgery, d. splenectomy, e. removal of toxic agents, f. stem cell or bone marrow transplantation, g. corticosteroid therapy, h. immunosuppressive therapy
31. blood transfusion
32. Stop the transfusion and keep the IV open with normal saline, treat any respiratory or circulatory manifestations immediately, notify the physician and blood bank, recheck identifying tags and numbers on the blood and the client, monitor vital signs and urine output, treat symptoms per physician's orders, save blood bag and tubing and send it to the blood bank for examination with transfusion reaction report, complete transfusion reaction report in accordance with institutional policy, obtain blood and urine samples, document client's condition and all actions taken in the client's record and transfusion reaction forms per hospital policy
33. 170; trap fibrin clots; 4–6
34. Walking places stress on the long bones and thus increases calcium absorption.
35. emotional support due to the frightening nature of the symptoms
36. True, False, False, False, False, True, True, True, True
37. reticulocytes; 5–10 days

38. high doses of folate, cobalamin, and pyridoxine
39. an opioid
40. 2
41. allopurinol 100–300 mg/daily
42. True, False, True, True, False, False, False
43. 4
44. 3
45. 4

CHAPTER 76

1. 1
2. 1, 2, 4
3. a. inhalation, b. injection, c. ingestion, d. direct contact
4. 2, 3
5. 5, 1, 3, 2, 4
6. T cells
7. a. immediate/anaphylactic, b. cytolytic/cytotoxic, c. immune complex, d. cell-mediated or delayed
8. 4
9. 4, 1, 3, 2
10. 4
11. Arthus
12. 3
13. a. client history, b. clinical manifestations during or after an allergic exposure, c. results of commonly used allergy tests
14. a. food allergies, b. food intolerances
15. 4
16. a. 5, b. 3, c. 1, d. 2
17. 6, 4, 1, 3, 2, 5
18. True, True, False, False, True, True
19. 4
20. 1, 2, 3, 4
21. 3
22. a. stop the transfusion, b. maintain an open IV line, c. assess the client's vital signs, d. notify the physician
23. Obtain an allergy history and document findings in the medical record.
24. 3
25. a. apply a cool compress, a topical steroid or antihistamine, b. administer an oral antihistamine
26. Clients are asked to wait so that immediate reactions can be treated.
27. client education
28. double-blind, placebo-controlled food challenge
29. 1, 2, 3, 4
30. 3
31. The newer agents do not cross the blood-brain barrier and therefore do not cause significant drowsiness.
32. 4

33. a. antihistamines, b. topical corticosteroids, c. antibiotics
34. antihistamine
35. True, True

CHAPTER 77

1. Arthritis
2. 1, 2, 4, 5, 6, 7
3. 2, 3, 4
4. a. swan-neck deformity, b. boutonniere deformity, c. carpal tunnel syndrome
5. C: calcium deposits in the tissues
   R: Raynaud's phenomenon
   E: esophageal hardening
   S: scleroderma of the digits
   T: telangiectasis (capillary dilations on face, lips and fingers)
6. WHITE: Vasospasm causes constriction of blood vessels: pallor of fingers
   BLUE: Venous congestion and cyanosis: blue coloring
   RED: Vasospasm resolves with hyperemia due to vasodilation: red coloring
7. Lyme disease
8. ACR 20
9. 1, 2, 3, 4, 5
10. impingement syndrome
11. systemic lupus erythmatosus
12. Repetitive actions can produce trauma to the joint and result in bursitis. This information will also aid in measures to prevent further trauma.
13. 1, 2, 3
14. 3
15. a. Improve joint motion; passive ROM can assist in preventing contractures
    b. Preserve or improve the muscle's ability to do work
16. a. making the client comfortable according to what has worked in the past, b. listening to and learning from clients, c. reducing anxiety, d. enlisting family and community support
17. 1, 2, 3, 4
18. 1, 2, 4, 5
19. 1, 2, 3, 4, 5
20. steroids; immunosuppressive agents
21. impaired renal function
22. Nifedipine
23. Penicillamine
24. a. l-tryptophan for sleep, b. tricyclic antidepressants to inhibit serotonin uptake, c. benzodiazepines for anxiety and depression, d. glucocorticoids for pain, e. NSAIDs for pain
25. It decreases the production of rheumatoid factors which cause inflammation, edema, and

pain. It also decreases the number of immune complexes which are deposited in the synovium, causing inflammation and pain

26. The inflammation releases lysosomal enzymes which attack the synovial tissue resulting in swelling and eventual loss of joint space.
27. Glucocorticoids, ASA, and NSAIDs
28. Inflammation causes release of macrophages and leukocytes to the area, which normally attack "foreign" tissue. Rheumatoid arthritis is an autoimmune disease that causes immune cells to attack "self," causing destruction.
29. joint swelling, muscle spasms
30. Joint fusion, loss of joint space. Rheumatoid nodules are most often temporary.

CHAPTER 78

1. 65 million
2. 4.9 million
3. 4th
4. a. minority populations, b. men who have sex with other men, c. injecting drug users, d. women, e. older adults, f. adolescents
5. $28,000.00
6. Adequate economic resources
7. HIV-1
8. a. sexual practices, b. exposure to blood, c. perinatal (vertical) transmission
9. needle stick
10. 2, 1, 5, 4, 6, 8, 3, 7
11. $22/mm^3$
12. A long-term nonprogressor is a person who is HIV+, but who, after many years, shows no sign of disease progression. A long-term survivor is a client who has lived > 8 years after diagnosis.
13. 4–12
14. 4
15. a. bacterial, b. fungal, c. protozoal, d. viral
16. a. fulminant course, b. disseminated throughout the body, c. results in shorter survival
17. Local: radiation, localized chemotherapy, cryotherapy
    Systemic: doxorubicin, alpha interferon, bleomycin, paclitaxel, daunorubicin
18. postcoital bleeding, metrorrhagia, blood-tinged vaginal discharge
19. cough, other respiratory manifestations
20. True, True, False, True, False, True
21. a. CD4 count, b. clinical presentation
22. 3
23. existing level of knowledge
24. a. ability to safely maintain independent living, b. medication compliance
25. False, True, False

26. standard precautions, appropriate disposal of sharps
27. a. Initial HIV diagnosis
    b. Initial AIDS diagnosis
    c. Changes in treatment
    d. New manifestations
    e. Recurrence of problems or relapse
    f. Terminal illness
28. 1, 4, 5, 6
29. megestrol acetate, dronabinol, human growth hormone
30. a. keep the client in a warm room to prevent shivering, b. apply sheets loosely and use woven blankets/sheets, c. avoid fanning or exposing the skin
31. tepid baths cause vasoconstriction and shivering
32. 3
33. True, False, True, False, True
34. Absolutely safe: do not inject drugs
    Very safe: use only sterile injection paraphernalia, do not share any paraphernalia
    Probably safe: reuse paraphernalia after cleaning with a bleach solution
35. Completely safe: autosexual activities such as masturbation, mutually monogamous relationships between noninfected partners, and abstinence
    Very safe: noninsertive activity, insertive practices with a properly used condom as long as no exposure to body fluids occurs
36. 4
37. zidovudine (Retrovir, AZT)
38. 3, 4, 5, 2, 1
39. 95%
40. True, True, True, True, False, False
41. 1
42. a. education, b. simplify the regimen, c. use "adherence promoting" devices

CHAPTER 79

1. a. 2, b. 4, c. 1, d. 3
2. a. genetic factors, b. exposure to ionizing radiation and chemicals, c. congenital abnormalities, d. primary immunodeficiency and infection
3. acute lymphoblastic leukemia (ALL)
4. acute myeloid leukemia (AML)
5. a. anemia, b. thrombocytopenia, c. leukopenia
6. tumor lysis syndrome
7. 1, 2, 3
8. Allogeneic bone marrow is obtained from a relative or unrelated donor having a closely matched HLA type. Syngeneic bone marrow is donated by an identical twin. Autologous marrow is removed from the intended recipient during the remission

phase to allow another course of ablative therapy to be given if relapse occurs.
9. 7; 30
10. True, True, True
11. 3
12. bone marrow aspiration
13. 4
14. a. the blood should be human leukocyte antigen (HLA) matched, b. the blood should be cytomegalovirus (CMV) negative
15. 4
16. 3
17. 2
18. True
19. to prevent infection, detect and treat infection early in an effective manner as evidenced by absence of fever, no respiratory difficulty, and neutrophil count greater than 1000/mm³
20. (1% + 42%) × 1650 = 709.50
21. No; protective isolation is indicated when the ANC count falls below 500.
22. The nurse should explain that because of the risk of infection the client is on a low-bacteria diet that prohibits raw fresh fruits and vegetables.
23. d. The nurse should question the order for Tylenol because the client should not receive rectal suppositories and the Tylenol may mask the fever.
24. During the acute phase there is an increased risk of introducing blast cells into the CNS.
25. Teach the client that he or she needs a high-carbohydrate diet; cold foods are tolerated better than hot, spicy foods; small, frequent meals may be tolerated more easily; and to space activities with rest to avoid fatigue.
26. Explain to the client that the hair loss is temporary; however, the hair may have a different texture and color when it returns.
27. They assist the client and family in understanding the disease process and treatment, and in identifying strategies for successful transition from the hospital to home and outpatient care.
28. 1
29. Aspirin decreases platelet aggregation and further contributes to the risk for bleeding.
30. a. adriamycin, b. bleomycin, c. vinblastine, d. dacarbazine. This treatment regimen can be easily delivered with full doses, has fewer side effects, and carries less risk of developing subsequent leukemia.
31. apoptosis; Philadelphia test

CHAPTER 80

1. 2

2. Infection
3. the first 3 months after transplantation
4. after the first 3 months after transplantation
5. 1, 2, 3
6. 1, 2, 3, 4
7. 3
8. 1
9. 1, 2, 3, 4
10. 1, 2, 3, 4
11. Social Security Act
12. 1, 2
13. 4
14. Xenotransplantation
15. 1
16. 1, 2, 3
17. True, True
18. 1, 2, 3
19. 1, 2, 3
20. 1, 2, 3
21. 1, 2, 3
22. 1, 2, 3, 4, 5
23. 1, 2
24. 1, 2, 3, 4, 5
25. Answers will vary.

CHAPTER 81

1. 1
2. 1, 2, 3
3. 1
4. 1, 2
5. 2
6. 1, 2, 3
7. 1, 2
8. 1
9. 1, 2, 3
10. 1, 2, 3, 4
11. respiratory failure
12. 1
13. 2
14. 1, 2
15. 1
16. 1
17. 1
18. 1, 2
19. 1, 2
20. 1, 2, 3, 4
21. 1, 2, 3
22. 1, 2, 3
23. 1, 2, 3, 4
24. 1, 2
25. 1
26. 1, 2, 3, 4
27. 1
28. 2

29. There is a significant reduction in mortality and morbidity in ICU clients when intensive insulin therapy is provided and tight glycemic control is maintained

CHAPTER 82

1. mid-60s
2. 100 million
3. decreased; 12%
4. 50; 64
5. treatment of acute conditions that threaten loss of life, limb, or vision; management of nonurgent chronic conditions
6. Emergency nursing is defined by the ENA as "the assessment, diagnosis, and treatment of perceived, actual or potential, sudden or urgent, physical or psychosocial problems that are primarily episodic or acute. These may require minimal care or life-support measures, education of client and significant others, appropriate referral, and knowledge of legal implications."

7. Rh-O negative
8. 7, 4, 2, 5, 8, 6, 3, 1
9. 1, 2, 3, 4
10. 4, 7, 6, 1, 5, 3, 2, 8
11. Patient Self-Determination Act
12. 1, 2, 3
13. 5
14. 2, 3, 4
15. 1, 2, 3, 4
16. 1
17. 1, 2
18. 1, 2, 3
19. 2, 3
20. 2
21. 2
22. 1, 2, 3, 4
23. 1, 2, 3, 4
24. 2
25. 2, 3

Notes

Notes

Notes

Notes

Notes

Notes

Notes

Notes

Notes